A NIOSH Technical Guide . . .

NIOSH GUIDE TO INDUSTRIAL RESPIRATORY PROTECTION

Nancy J. Bollinger
Robert H. Schutz

U.S. DEPARTMENT OF HEALTH AND HUMAN SERVICES
Public Health Service
Centers for Disease Control
National Institute for Occupational Safety and Health
Division of Safety Research

September 1, 1987

DISCLAIMER

Mention of company name or product does not constitute endorsement by the National Institute for Occupational Safety and Health.

DHHS (NIOSH) Publication No. 87-116

Copies of this and other NIOSH documents are available from:

Publications Dissemination, DSDTT
National Institute for Occupational Safety and Health
4676 Columbia Parkway
Cincinnati, Ohio 45226
(513) 841-4287

For sale by the U.S. Government Printing Office
Superintendent of Documents, Mail Stop: SSOP, Washington, DC 20402-9328

TABLE OF CONTENTS

TABLE OF CONTENTS *(Continued)*

TABLE OF CONTENTS *(Continued)*

LIST OF FIGURES

LIST OF FIGURES *(Continued)*

Acknowledgements

The initial development of this document was performed under an interagency agreement between NIOSH and Los Alamos Scientific Laboratory (now Los Alamos National Laboratory) with John A. Pritchard as the author.

We would like to express our gratitude to Samuel L. Terry for information on atmosphere-supplying respirators, Christopher Coffey for information on air-purifying respirators, Nancy Morgan for her word processing support, and Howard Ludwig for his review.

In addition, we would like to thank the respirator manufacturers who provided National Institute for Occupational Safety and Health (NIOSH) with pictures of their products to be used as illustrations, and the American National Standards Institute Z88.2 Respirator Committee, and the American Industrial Hygiene Association Committee on Respirators for their technical review of the document.

A special thanks goes to Herb Linn for his editorial review, art work, document preparation, and cover design.

CHAPTER 1

NIOSH AND RESPIRATORY PROTECTION

This report is intended to provide respirator users with a single source of respirator information. It covers the selection, use, and maintenance of respiratory protective devices available in 1987, and therefore serves as an update to the 1976 ***Guide to Industrial Respiratory Protection.***

When the National Institute for Occupational Safety and Health (NIOSH) was established in 1971, the professional staff recognized the crucial need for establishing the correct role of respiratory protection in workplaces. While dedicating the majority of its resources to the fundamental concepts of industrial health and safety, NIOSH has devoted a significant part of those resources to three areas of respiratory protection--research, training, and certification.

NIOSH has had an ongoing respirator research program since the early 1970s. Most of the recent research has been dedicated toward improving the quality and reliability of respirators through development of new and revised performance requirements for respirator certification.

Respirator training has been a focal point of the NIOSH activities in respiratory protection. The basic respirator training courses which are available from several sources today are based on the respirator course developed by NIOSH personnel.

NIOSH and OSHA established a Joint Respirator Committee in 1973, for the purpose of developing standard respirator selection criteria and tables for the approximately 400 hazardous materials regulated by OSHA. This committee, assisted by contractors from Los Alamos Scientific Laboratory and Arthur D. Little, Inc., developed the respirator selection tables that appear in NIOSH criteria documents and in the initial ***NIOSH/OSHA Pocket Guide to Chemical Hazards.*** The committee also participated in development of the initial ***Respirator Decision Logic,*** which has been revised for this publication.

The respirator certification work of NIOSH is a direct offshoot of the approval of mine rescue breathing apparatus by the Bureau of Mines. Under authorization of the Coal Mine Health and Safety Act of 1969 and the Federal Mine Safety and Health Act of 1977, NIOSH has established an evaluation and certification program for respirators. All certifications are issued jointly with the Mine Safety and Health Administration (MSHA).

The goal of the certification program is to help increase worker protection from airborne contaminants by certifying respirators that meet the minimum

performance requirements which appear in Title 30, Code of Federal Regulations, Part 11 (30 CFR 11). NIOSH certification evaluations include a laboratory evaluation of the respirator, an evaluation of the manufacturer's quality control (QC) plan, audit testing of certified respirators, and investigations of problems with MSHA/NIOSH certified respirators.
In accordance with 30 CFR 11, MSHA/NIOSH certifications are issued for respirators specifically for use in mines and mining. However, the wide variety of respirators used in mines and mining ensures the availability of certified respirators for most other applications.

NIOSH has proposed significant revisions to 30 CFR 11. Once revised regulations are in effect, NIOSH expects to push vigorously for other improvements in respirator performance standards over the ensuing several years.

NIOSH also monitors respirators over the lifetime of their certification. Samples of "off the shelf" respirators are evaluated in NIOSH laboratories to see if they continue to meet applicable minimum performance requirements. In addition, NIOSH performs in-plant QC audits in order to determine if manufacturers are complying with the QC plans submitted in their approval applications. Reports of problems received from regulatory agencies, labor organizations, respirator users, and respirator manufacturers are investigated and resolved.

CHAPTER 2

TYPES OF RESPIRATORS

The basic purpose of any respirator is, simply, to protect the respiratory system from inhalation of hazardous atmospheres. Respirators provide protection either by removing contaminants from the air before it is inhaled or by supplying an independent source of respirable air. The principal classifications of respirator types are based on these categories.

A respirator that removes contaminants from the ambient air is called an **air-purifying respirator**. A respirator that provides air from a source other than the surrounding atmosphere is an **atmosphere-supplying respirator**. Both types can be further subclassified by the type of inlet covering and the mode of operation. Figures 2-1 through 2-6 detail the subclassifications of respirators that will be discussed in this chapter.

I. Respiratory Inlet Coverings

The respiratory inlet covering serves as a barrier against the contaminated atmosphere and as a framework to which air-purifying or atmosphere-supplying elements may be attached.

A. Tight-fitting coverings

Tight-fitting coverings, usually called "facepieces," are made of flexible molded rubber, silicone, neoprene, or other materials. Present designs incorporate rubber or woven elastic headstraps that are attached at two to six points. They buckle together at the back of the head, or may form a continuous loop of material.

Facepieces are available in three basic configurations. The first, called a "quarter-mask," covers the mouth and nose, and the lower sealing surface rests between chin and mouth (Fig. 2-7). Good protection may be obtained with a quarter-mask, but it is more easily dislodged than other types. Quarter-masks are most commonly found on dust and mist respirators.

A second type, the "half-mask," fits over the nose and under the chin (Fig. 2-8). Half-masks are designed to seal more reliably than quarter-masks, so they are preferred for use against more toxic materials.

A third type, the "full-facepiece," covers from roughly the hairline to below the chin (Fig. 2-9). On the average they provide the greatest protection, usually seal most reliably, and provide some eye protection

AIR-PURIFYING RESPIRATORS

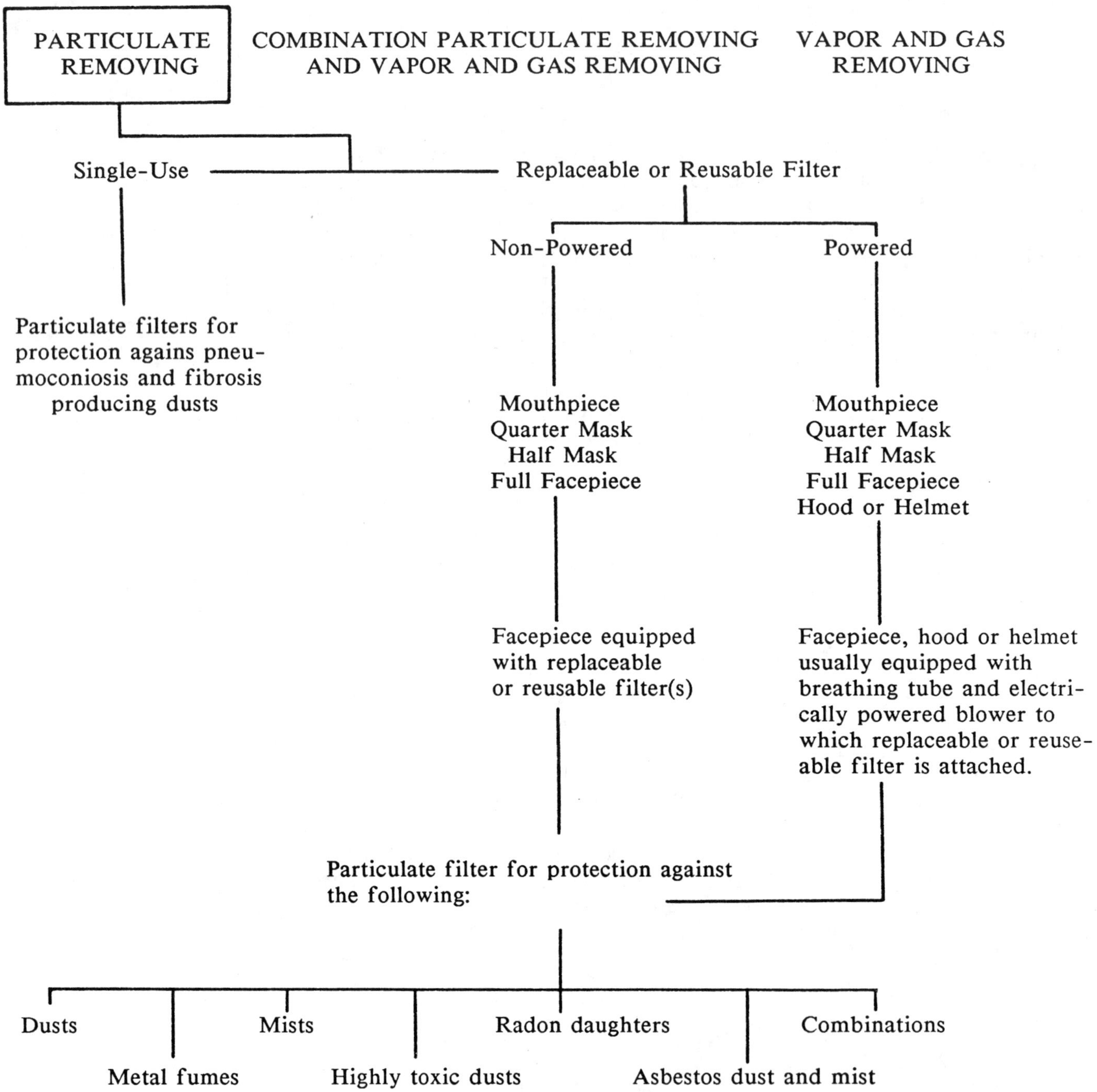

Figure 2-1. **Particulate removing respirators**

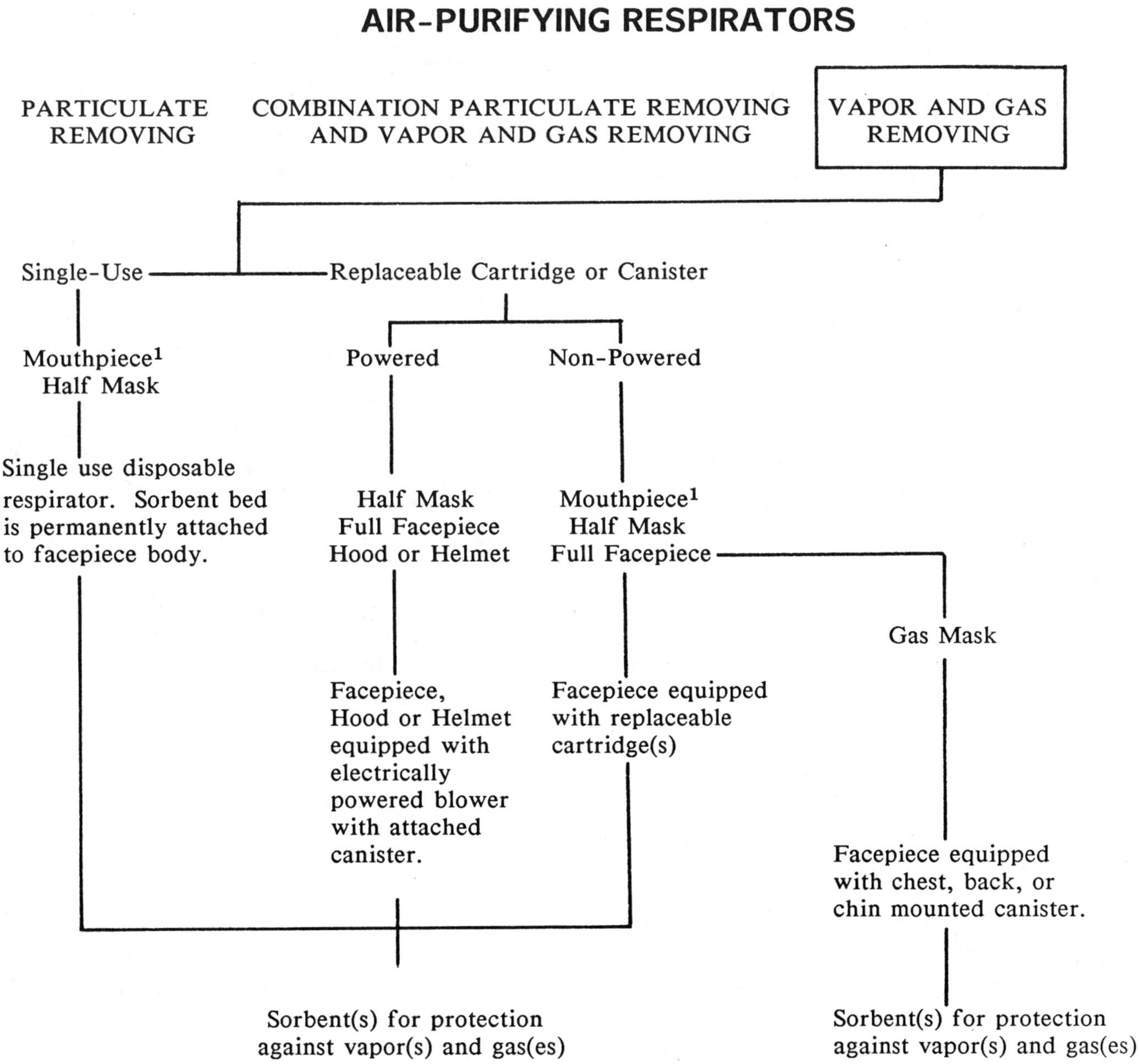

[1] Escape Only

Figure 2-2. **Vapor and gas removing respirators**

AIR-PURIFYING RESPIRATORS

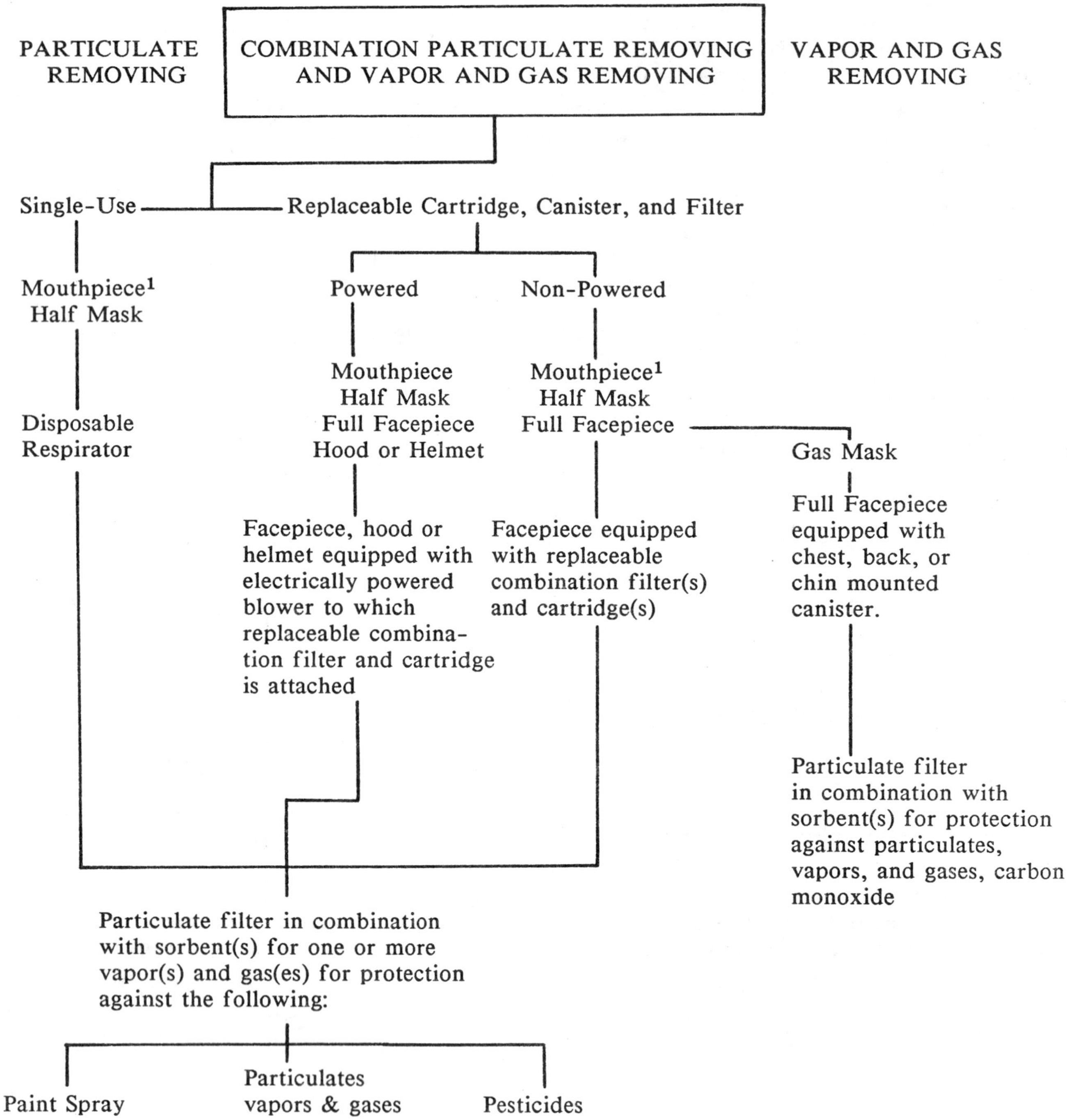

[1] Escape Only

Figure 2-3. **Combination particulate and vapor and gas removing respirators**

ATMOSPHERE-SUPPLYING RESPIRATORS

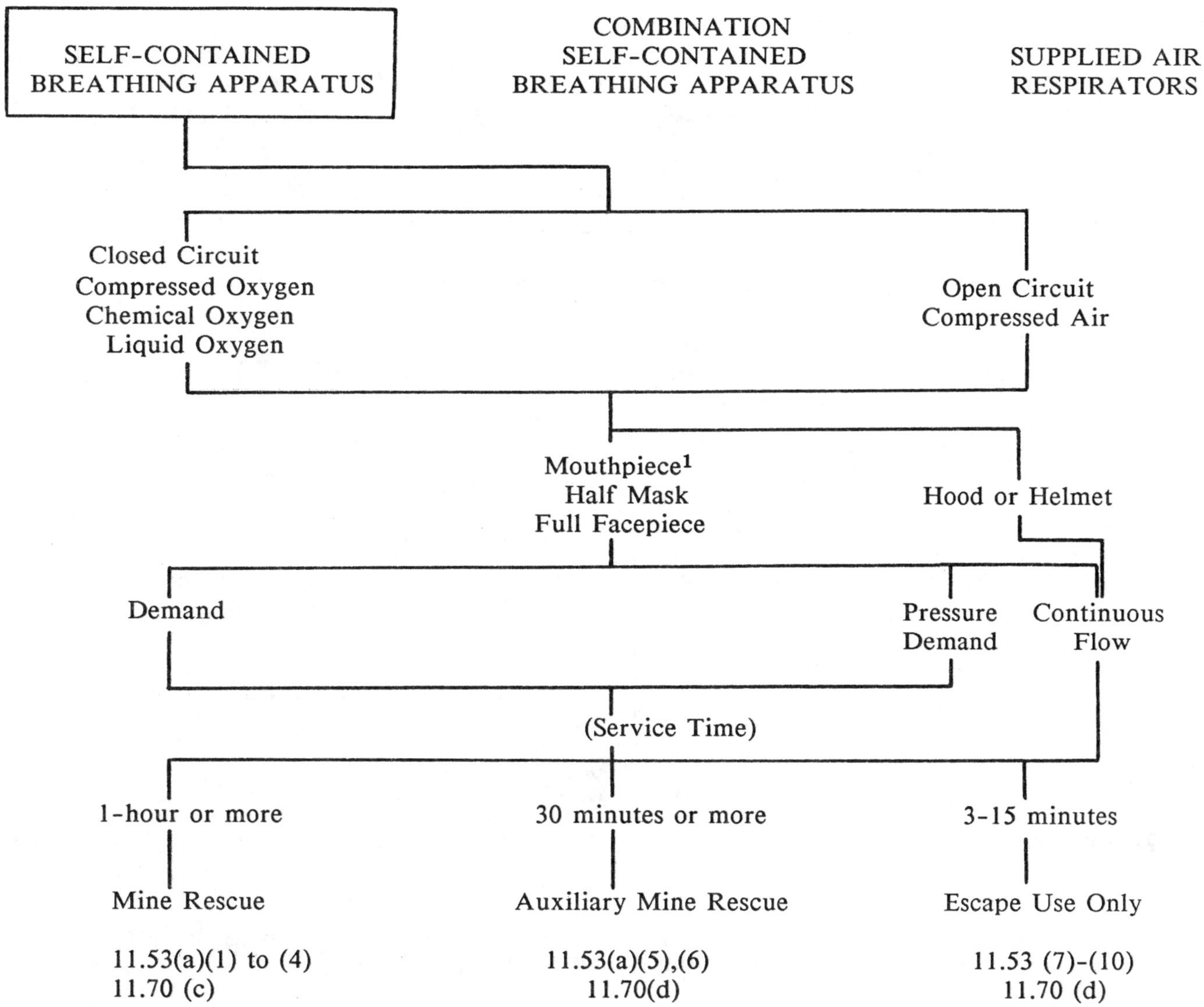

[1] Escape Only

Figure 2-4. **Self-contained breathing apparatus**

ATMOSPHERE-SUPPLYING RESPIRATORS

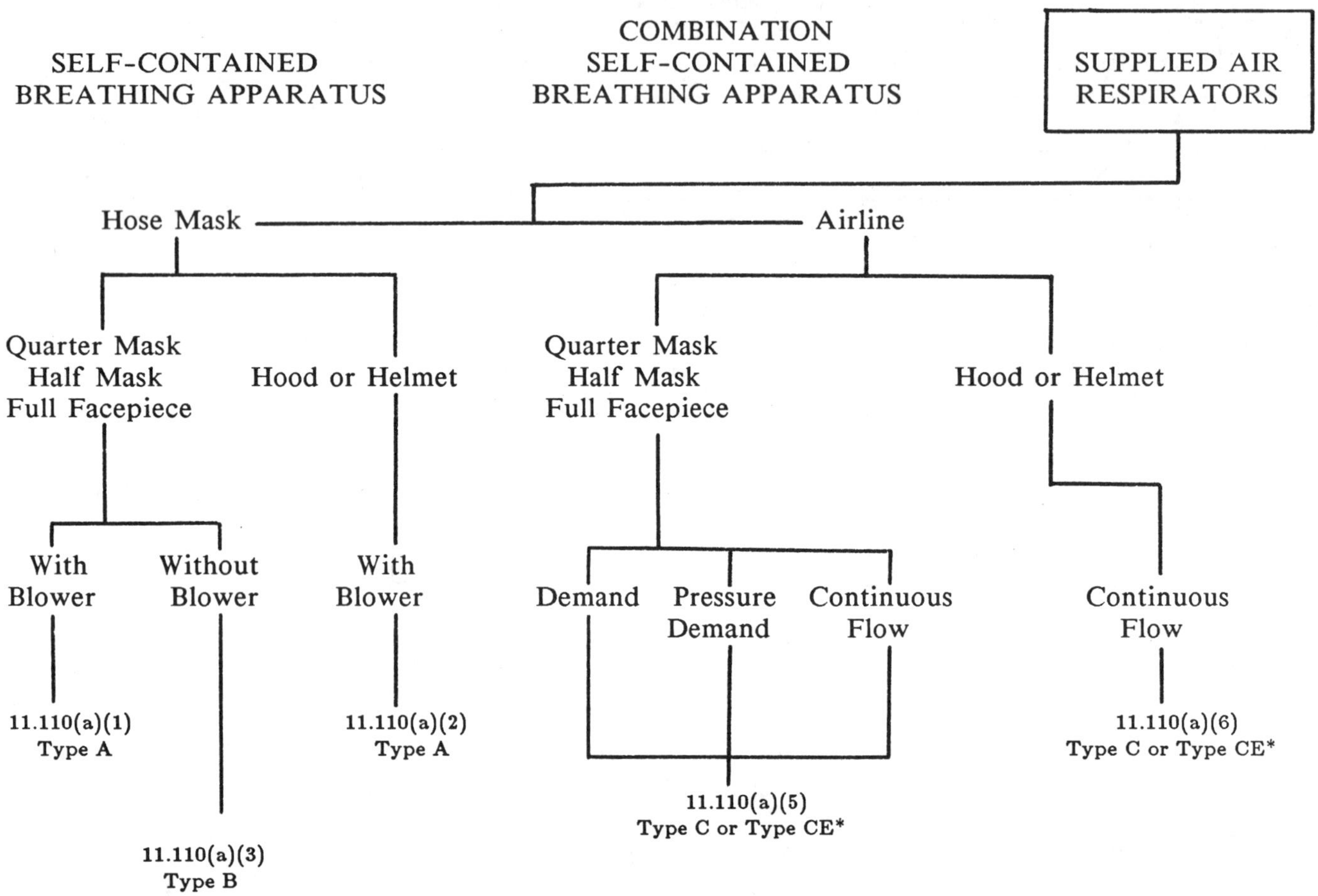

* Type CE respirators must have a means of protecting the wearer's head and neck against impact and abrasions from rebounding abrasive material and with shielding material such as plastic, glass, woven metal wire, etc.

Figure 2-5. **Supplied-air respirators**

ATMOSPHERE-SUPPLYING RESPIRATORS

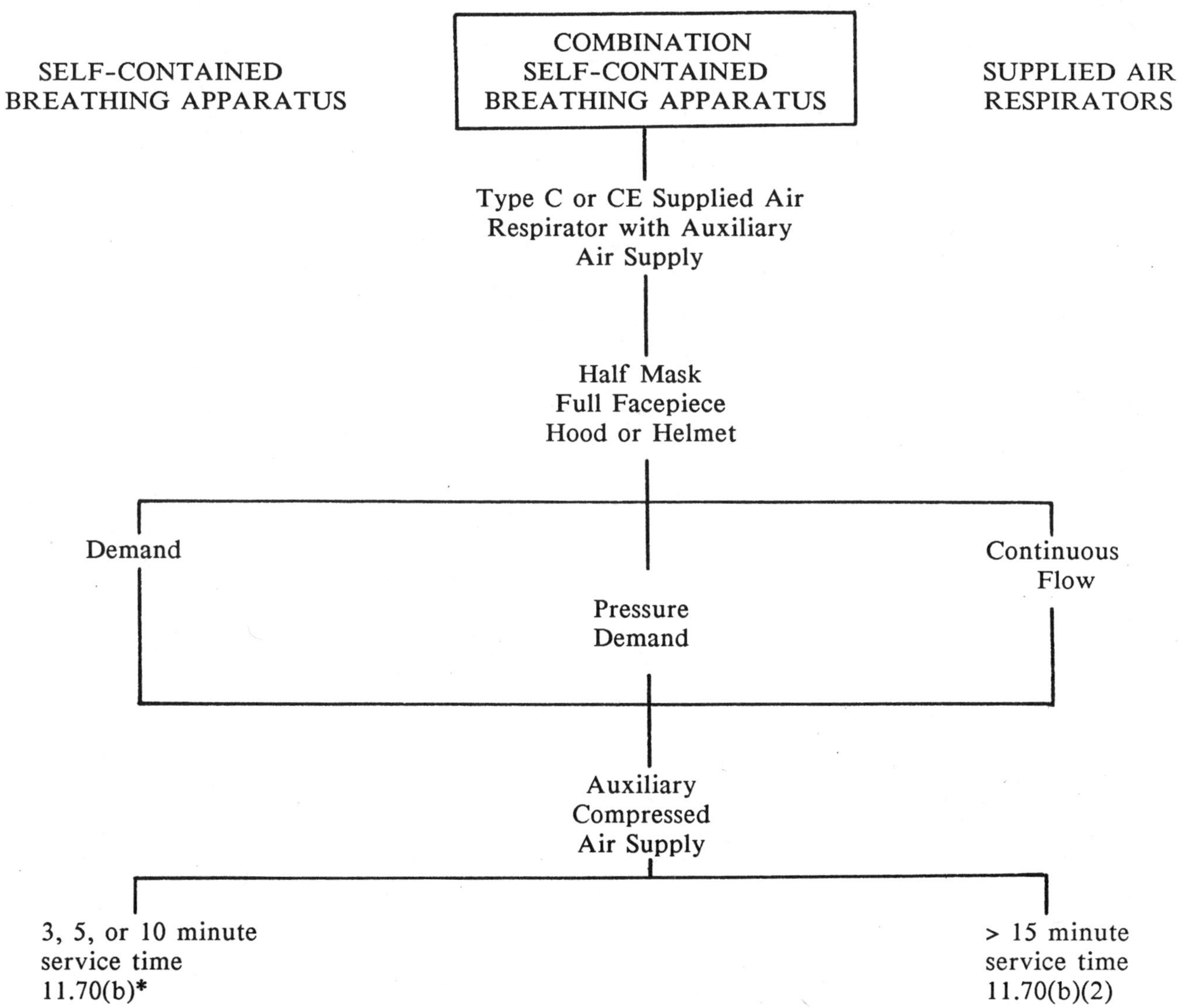

* SCBA can be used for egress only.

Figure 2-6. **Combination SCBA and supplied-air respirators**

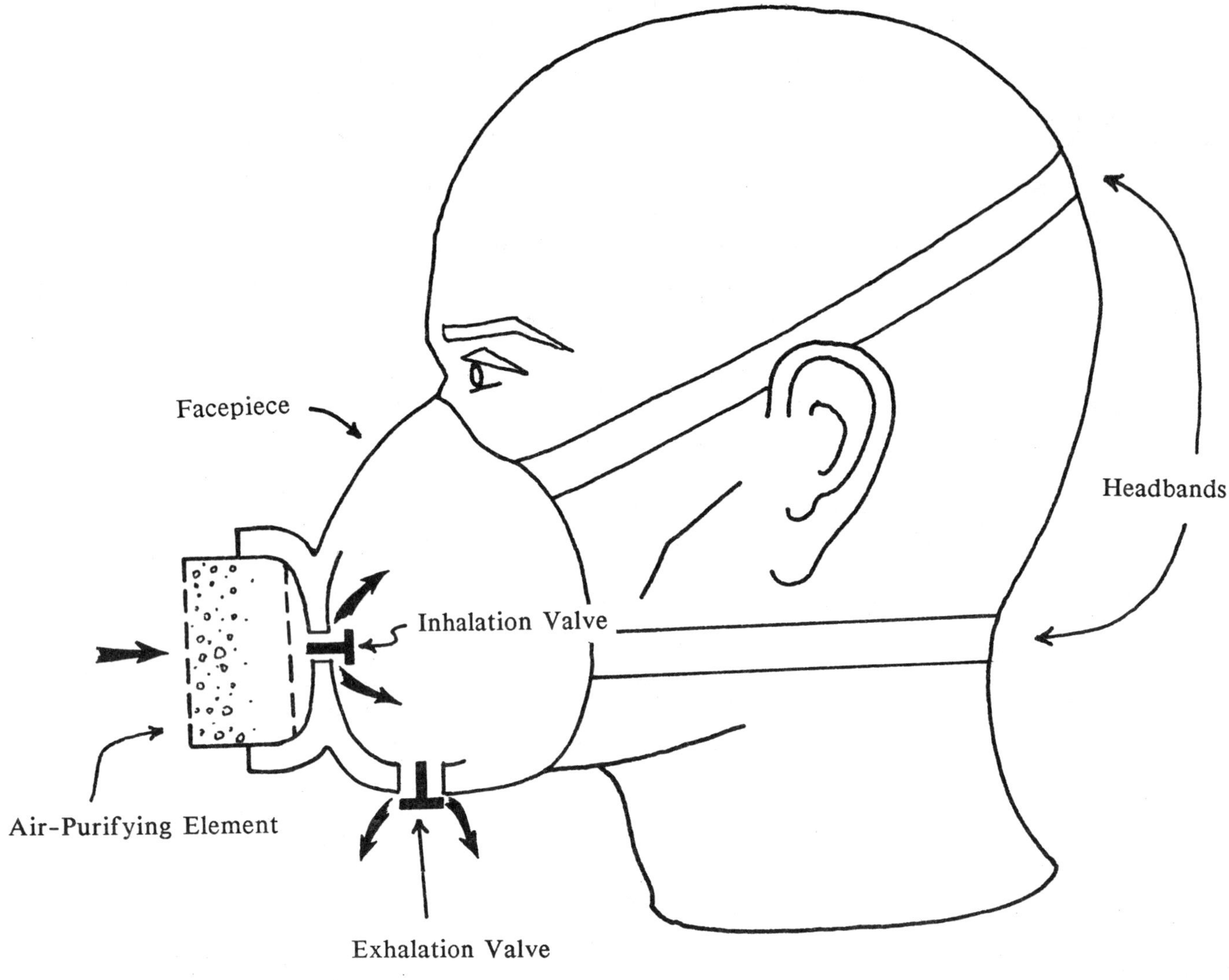

FIGURE 2-7. **Typical quarter-mask respirator**

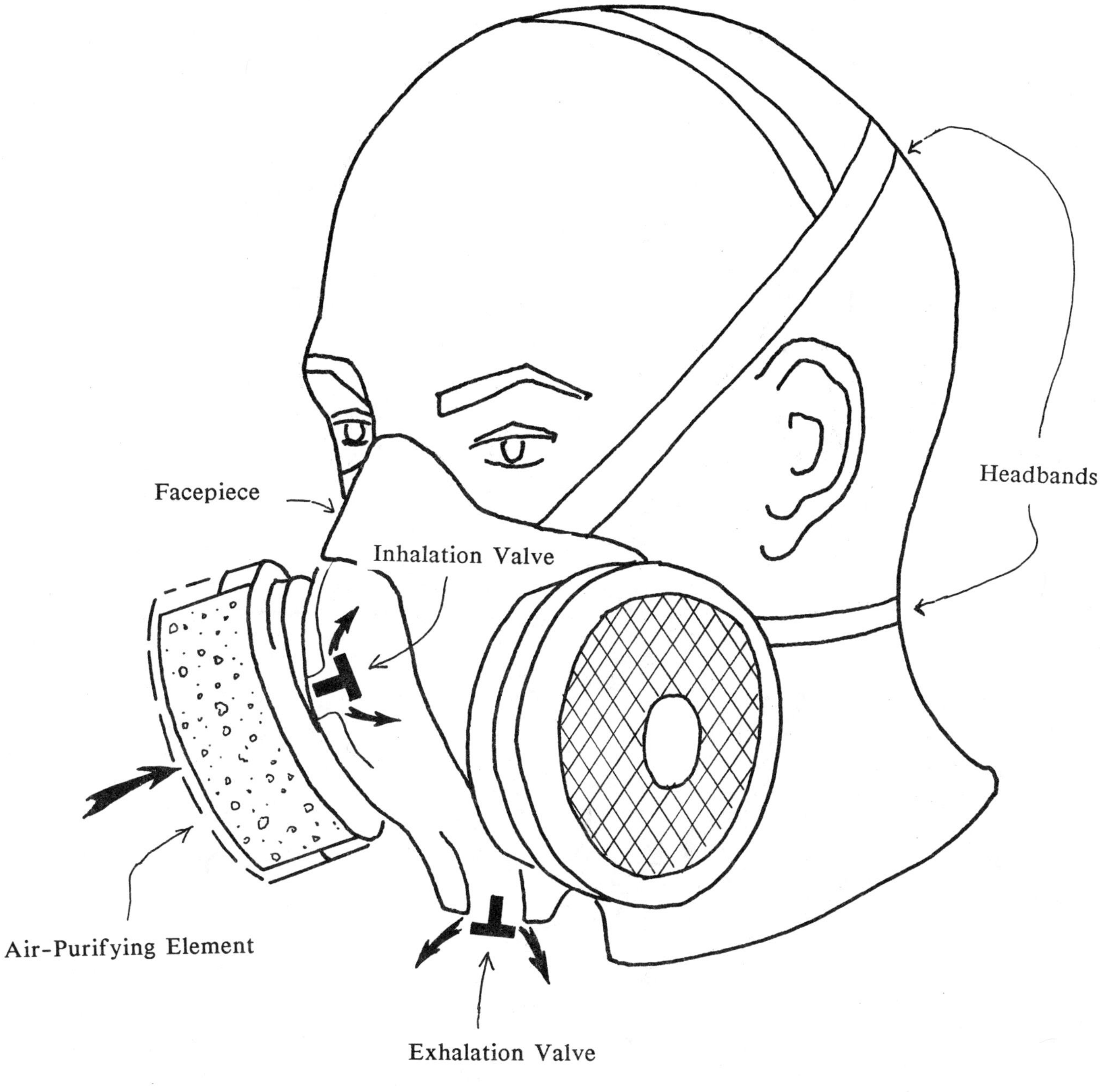

FIGURE 2-8. **Typical half-mask respirator**

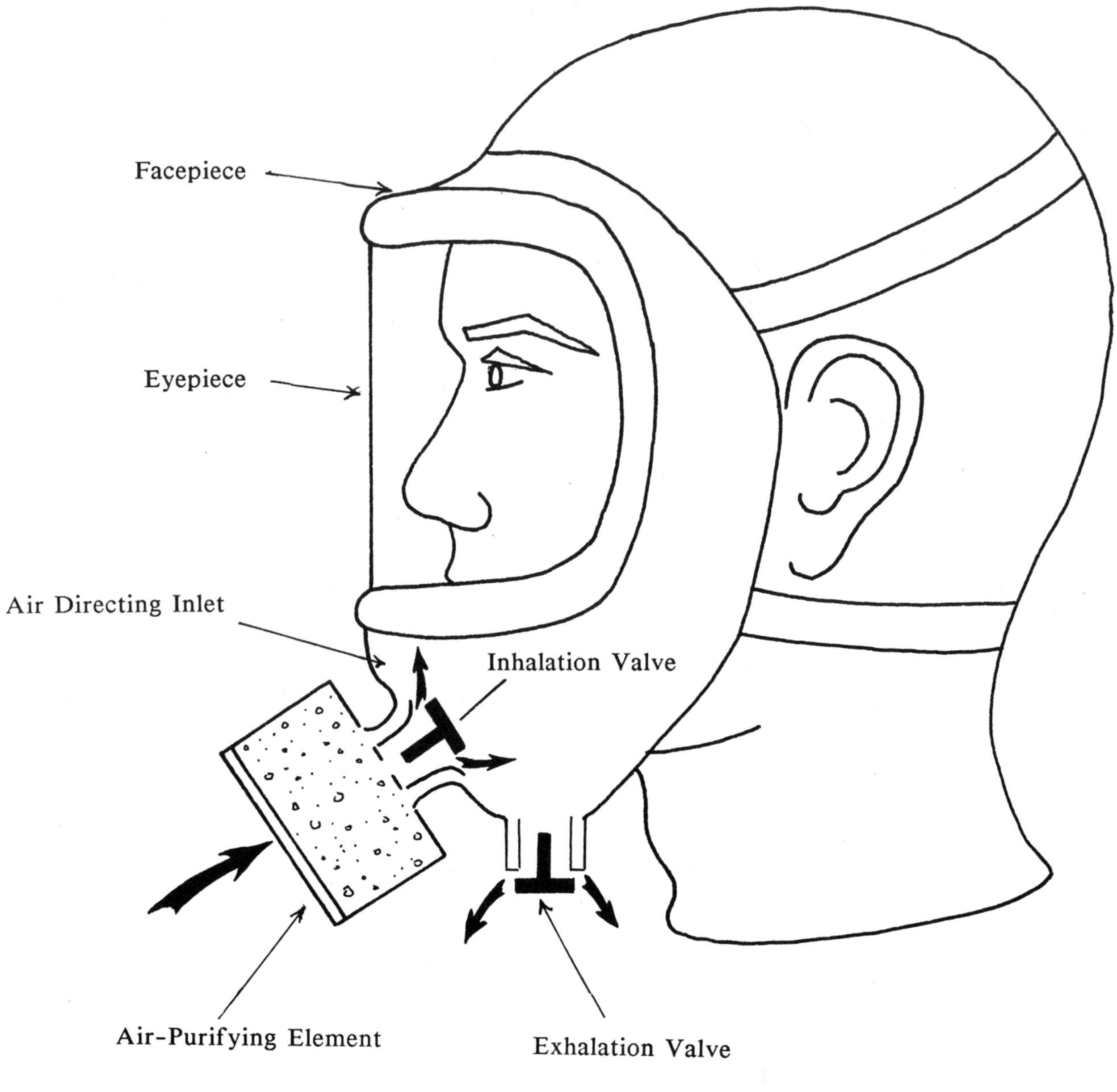

FIGURE 2-9. **Typical full-facepiece respirator**

as well. Full-facepiece respirators, both air-purifying and atmosphere-supplying, are designed for use in higher concentrations of toxic materials than are quarter- or half-mask respirators.

The mouthpiece consists of a mouthpiece held in the teeth (the lips seal around it) and a clamp that closes the nostrils (Fig. 2-10). Mouthpiece respirators should provide a good seal, but they eliminate communication, may cause fatigue, and provide no eye protection. Therefore, mouthpiece respirators are certified for use as escape-only respirators.

B. Loose-fitting coverings

Loose-fitting coverings include hoods, helmets, suits, and blouses. The wide variety of designs precludes any simple description, but Fig. 2-11 shows a blouse which typifies the basic principles of construction and operation of all such devices.

Generally, loose-fitting respirators enclose at least the head. A light flexible device covering only the head and neck, or head, neck, and shoulders is called a hood. If rigid protective headgear is incorporated into the design, it is called a helmet. Blouses extend down to the waist, and some have wrist-length sleeves. The enclosure includes a system through which clean compressed air is distributed around the breathing zone.

A special type of loose-fitting covering in common use is the abrasive-blasting hood (Fig. 2-12). The hood material is designed to withstand rebounding particles of abrasive material. Also, there is usually an impact-resistant glass or plastic viewing lens with additional plastic, glass, or woven wire shielding that deflects the rebounding particles.

II. Air-Purifying Respirators

A. Particulate Filtering Respirators

Particulate filtering respirators are used for protection against dusts, fumes, and/or mists. A dust is a solid, mechanically produced particle. A fume is a solid condensation particulate, usually of a vaporized metal. A mist is a liquid condensation particle.

Presently, all particulate filtering respirators use fibrous material (a filter) to remove the contaminant. As a particle is drawn onto or into the filter, it is trapped by the fibers. The probability that a single particle will be trapped depends on such factors as its size relative to the fiber size; its velocity; and, to some extent, the composition, shape, and electrical charge of both particle and fiber. With current filter media, any filter designed to be 100% efficient in removing particles would be unacceptably difficult to breathe through.

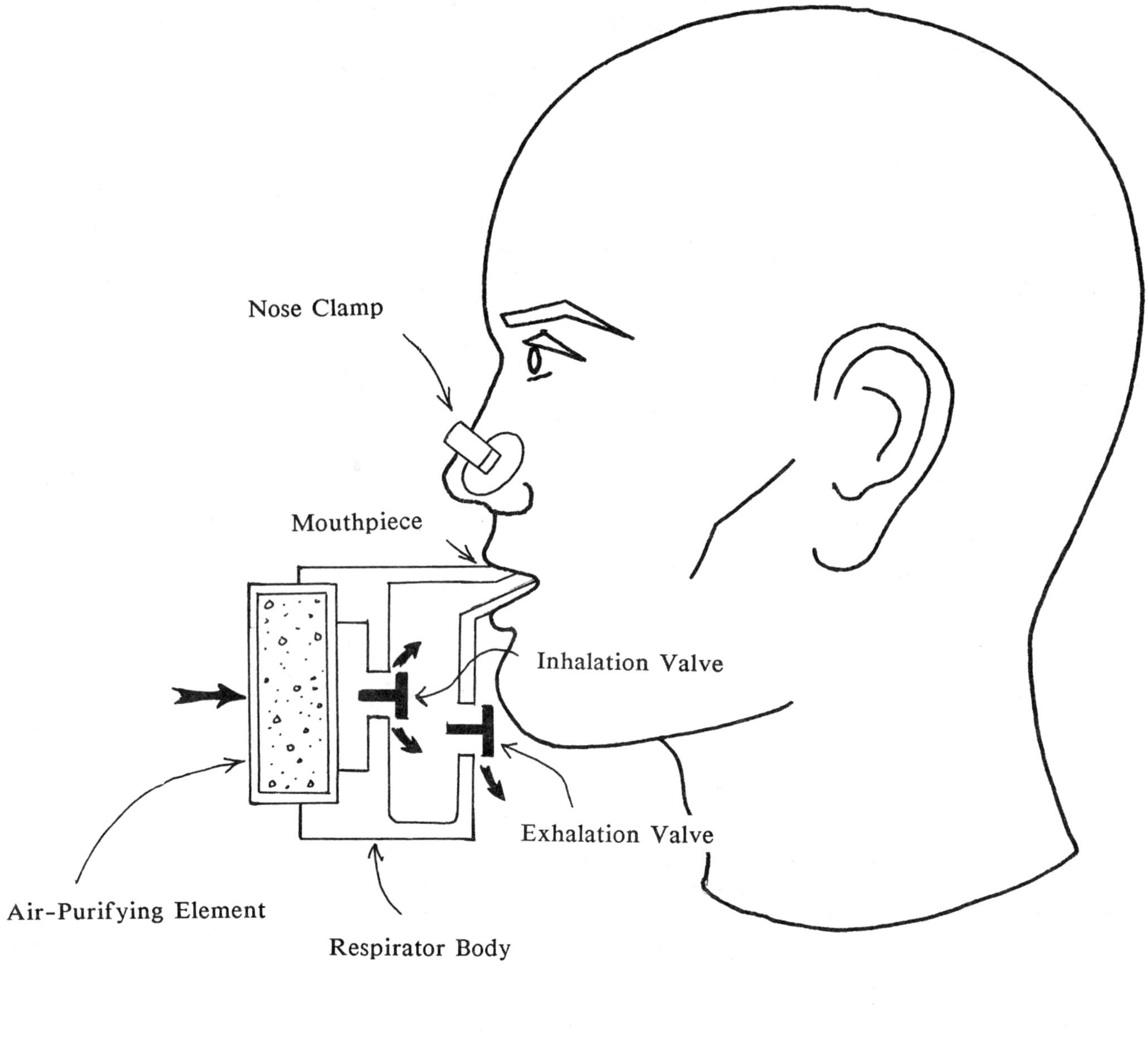

FIGURE 2-10. **Typical "mouthpiece" respirator**

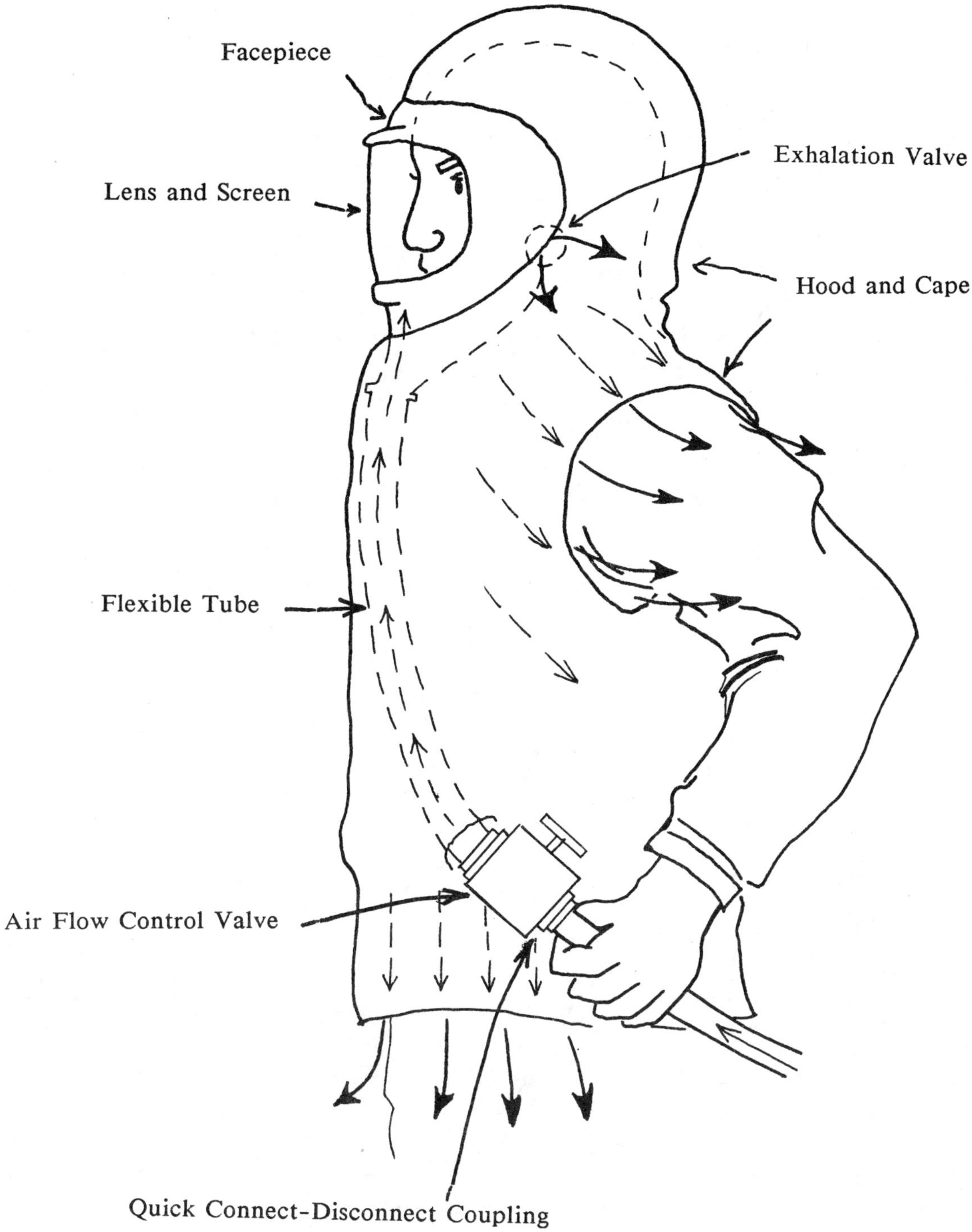

FIGURE 2-11. **Loose-fitting blouse**

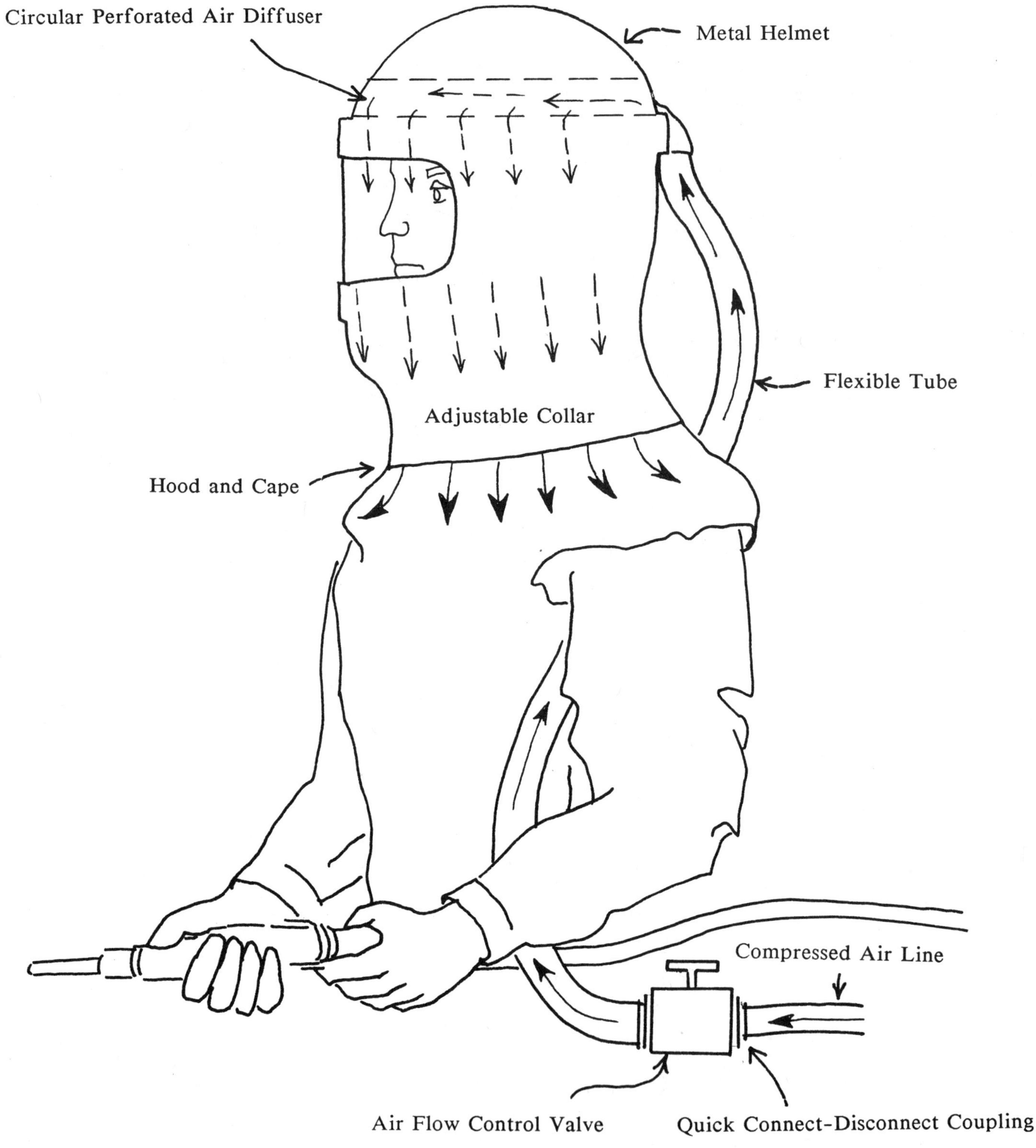

FIGURE 2-12. **Typical abrasive blasting hood**

Manufacturers try to produce the most efficient filter with the lowest breathing resistance. As the particulate respirator is used particulate material collects on the filter and the openings between fibers become smaller. This results in an increase in the breathing resistance. The filter may also become more efficient.

There are several designs of respirator filters. Each can be described by its filtration mechanism(s), production methods or type, the aerosol against which it is designed to provide protection, and the filtering efficiency.

1. Filtration Mechanisms

Particulate filters are of two types: absolute and non-absolute. Absolute filters use screening to remove particles from the air; that is, they exclude the particles which are larger than the pores. However, most respirator filters are non-absolute filters, which means they contain pores which are larger than the particles to be removed. They use combinations of interception capture, sedimentation capture, inertial impaction capture, diffusion capture, and electrostatic capture to remove the particles. The exact combination of filtration mechanisms which come into play depends upon the flowrate through the filter and the size of particle. Brief descriptions of these filtration mechanisms follow.

a. Interception Capture

As the air streams approach a fiber lying perpendicular to their path, they split and compress in order to flow around the fiber and rejoin on the other side (Figure 2-13). If the center of a particle in these airstreams comes within one particle radius of the fiber, it encounters the fiber surface and it is captured. As particle size increases, the probability of interception capture increases. The particles do not deviate from their original streamline in this mechanism.

b. Sedimentation Capture

Only large particles (2 μ and larger) are captured by sedimentation. Since this type of capture relies on gravity to pull particles from the airstream, flowrate through the filter must be low (Figure 2-14).

c. Inertial Impaction Capture

As the airstreams split and change direction suddenly to go around the fiber, particles with sufficient inertia cannot change direction sufficiently to avoid the fiber. Thus they impact on the surface of the fiber (Figure 2-15). A particle's size, density, speed and shape determine its inertia.

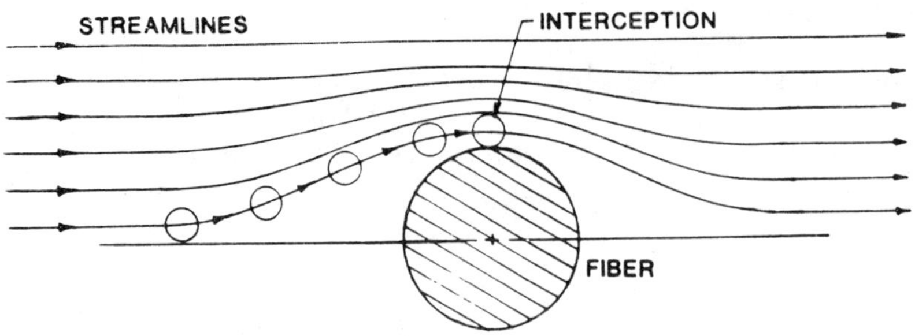

FIGURE 2-13. **Interception capture mechanism**[1]

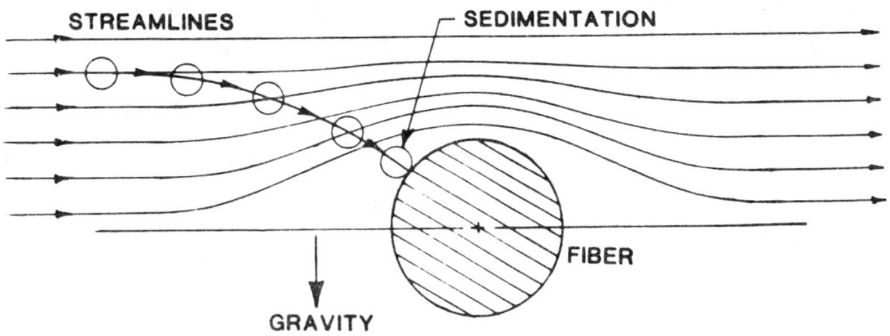

FIGURE 2-14. **Sedimentation capture mechanism**[1]

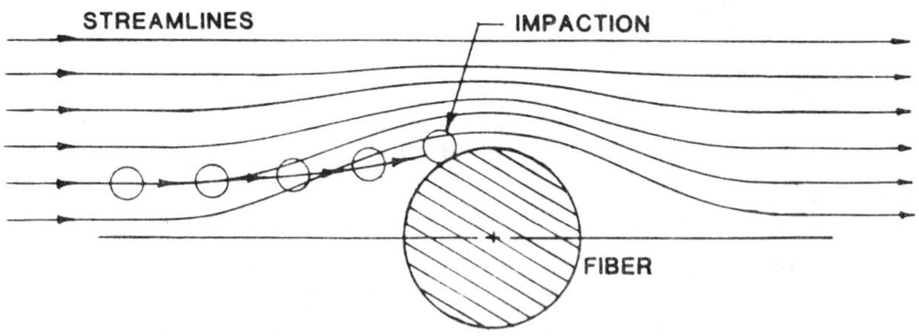

FIGURE 2-15. **Impaction capture mechanism**[1]

---

1 Japuntich, Daniel A. Respiratory Particulate Filtration. **J. Ind. Soc. Respir. Prot.** 1984; 2(1):137-169.

d. Diffusion Capture

The motion of smaller particles is affected by air molecules colliding with them. The particles then can randomly cross the airstream and encounter the fiber as they pass (Figure 2-16). This random motion is dependent on particle size and the air temperature. As the particle size decreases and air temperature increases the diffusive activity of the particle increases. This increases the probability of capture. Lower flowrate through the filter also increases the probability of capture because the particle spends more time in the area of the fiber.

e. Electrostatic Capture

In electrostatic capture, the particle is charged and the filter fibers have the opposite charge. Therefore, the particles are attracted to the fibers (Figure 2-17). The electrostatic capture mechanism aids the other capture mechanisms, especially interception and diffusion.

As was mentioned previously, the exact combination of capture mechanisms taking place depends upon several factors. However, some generalizations can be made. Large heavy particles are usually removed by inertial impaction and interception. Large light particles are removed by diffusion and interception. Diffusion removes very small particles.

2. Types of Filters

Three types of particulate filter predominate. The most common type presently available is a machine made flat disk of random laid non-woven fiber material which is carefully controlled to produce maximum filter efficiency and minimum resistance.

Another type (Figure 2-18) is a flat disk of compressed natural wool or synthetic fiber felt, or a blend, to which an electrostatic charge is imparted during manufacture by impregnating the material with a resin and mechanically beating or "needling" it. This charge increases the filter efficiency by electrostatically attracting the particles to the fibers. These filters protect adequately against most industrial dusts, but one precaution should be observed in their use. Certain agents, such as oil mists, and storage in very humid air remove the electrostatic charge. Therefore this type of filter should be stored in its original package, kept out of oil mists and high (>80%) humidity, and used as soon as possible after purchase.

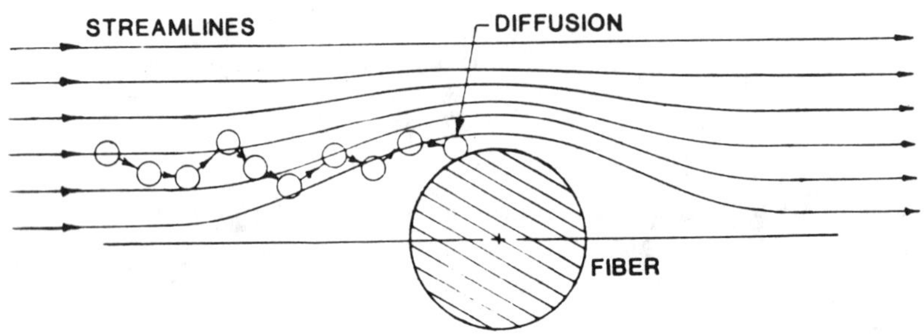

FIGURE 2-16. **Diffusion capture mechanism[1]**

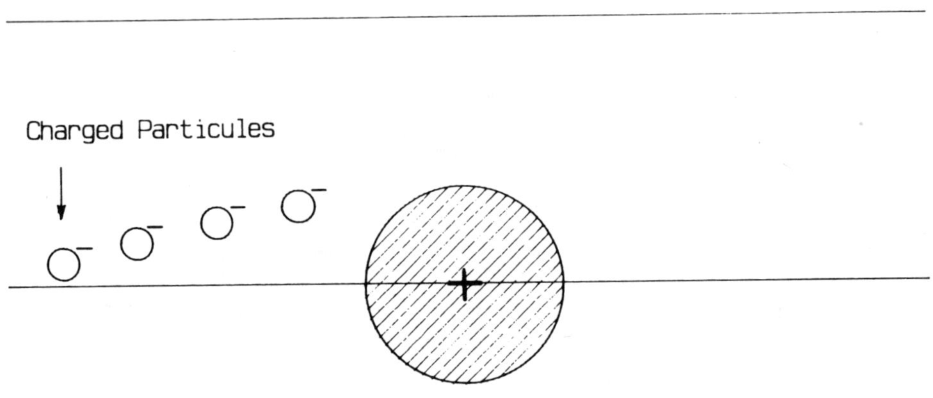

FIGURE 2-17. **Electrostatic capture**

---

1 Japuntich, Daniel A. Respiratory Particulate Filtration. **J. Ind. Soc. Respir. Prot.** 1984; 2(1):137-169.

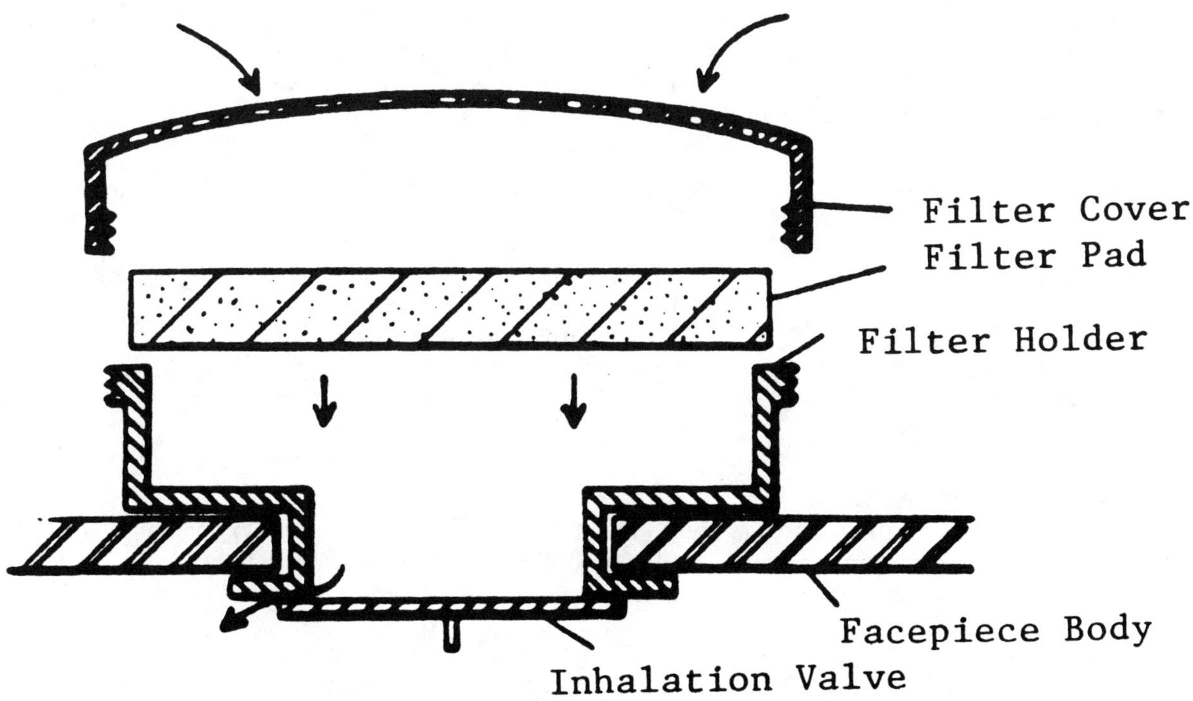

FIGURE 2-18. **Typical resin-impregnated felt dust filter**

The resin impregnated felt filter is readily identified by rubbing it between the fingers and then rubbing the fingers together. The fingers will feel slightly sticky.

Another type of dust filter is shown in Figure 2-19. The filtering medium is only loosely packed in the filter container so it is much thicker than the compressed type. Such filters are generally made of fibrous glass, although nonfelted, resin impregnated natural wool fibers have been used. They are not as common as the felted type. Typical dust respirators are shown in Figure 2-20.

Figure 2-21 shows a typical high efficiency dust, fume, and mist filter and Figure 2-22 shows high efficiency respirators. The filter is a flat sheet of material that is pleated and placed in the filter container. The pleating provides a large filtering area to improve the particle loading capacity and lower the breathing resistance. When viewed from the top, this type of filter shows a series of concentric rings or rows of pleats. This configuration is common, but other methods of construction are also used.

3. Particulate Respirator Classifications

For the 30 CFR 11 Subpart K certification tests particulate respirators are classified as designed for protection against a variety of dusts, fumes, mists. The following types are presently certified by MSHA/NIOSH:

a. Replaceable or Reusable Dust and Mist

Respirators, either with replaceable or reusable filters, designed as respiratory protection against (1) dusts and mists having an exposure limit not less than 0.05 milligram per cubic meter of air, or (2) dusts and mists having an exposure limit not less than 2 million particles per cubic foot of air.

b. Replaceable Fume

Respirators, with replaceable filters, designed as respiratory protection against fumes of various metals having an exposure limit not less than 0.05 milligram per cubic meter.

c. Replaceable Dust, Fume, and Mist

Respirators, with replaceable filters, designed as respiratory protection against dusts, fumes, and mists of materials having an exposure limit less than 0.05 milligram per cubic meter or 2 million particles per cubic foot of air.

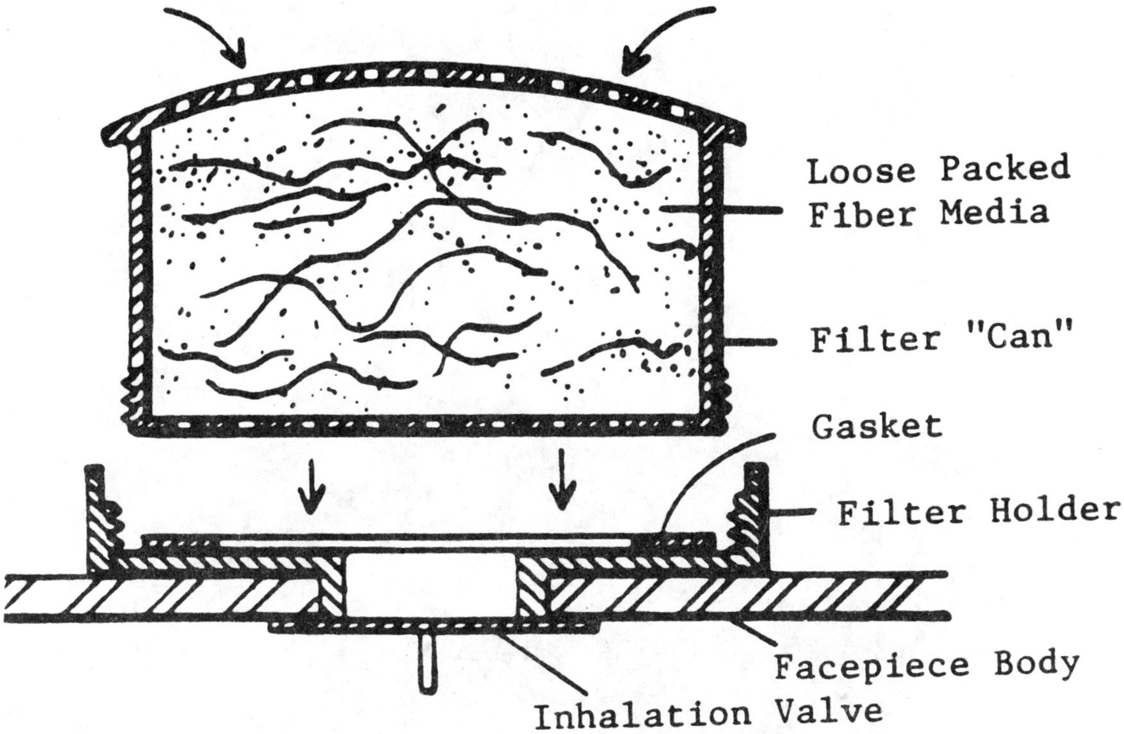

FIGURE 2-19. **Typical dust filter with loose packed medium**

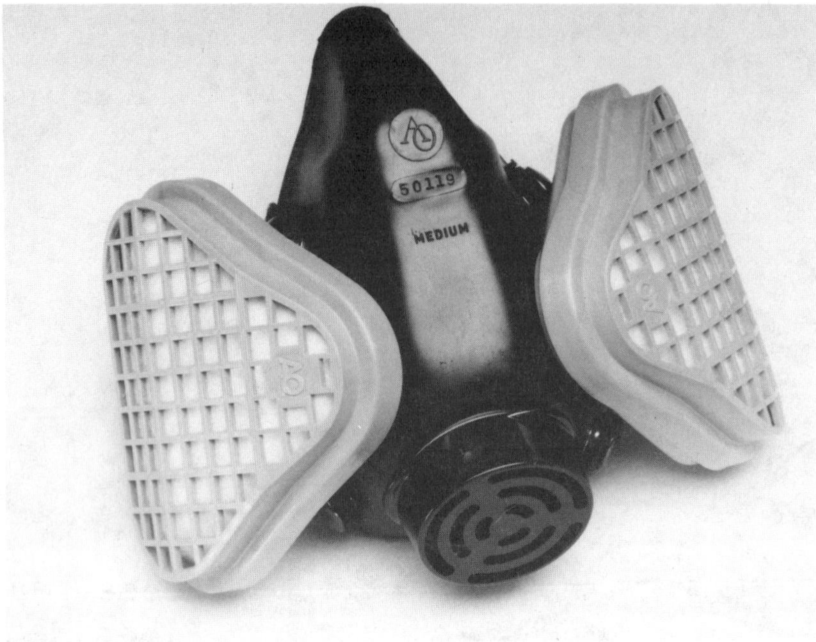

Photograph courtesy of American Optical Corporation

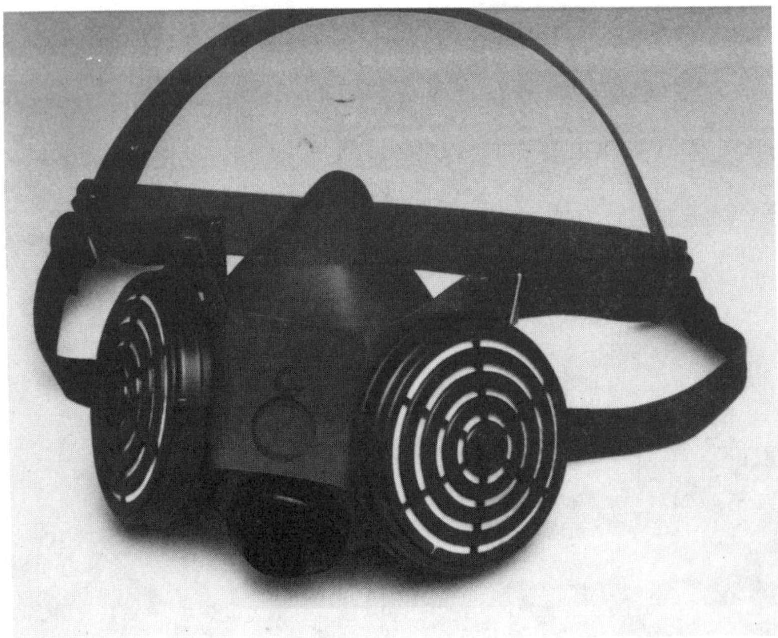

Photograph courtesy of U.S. Safety Service

FIGURE 2-20. **Typical dust respirators**

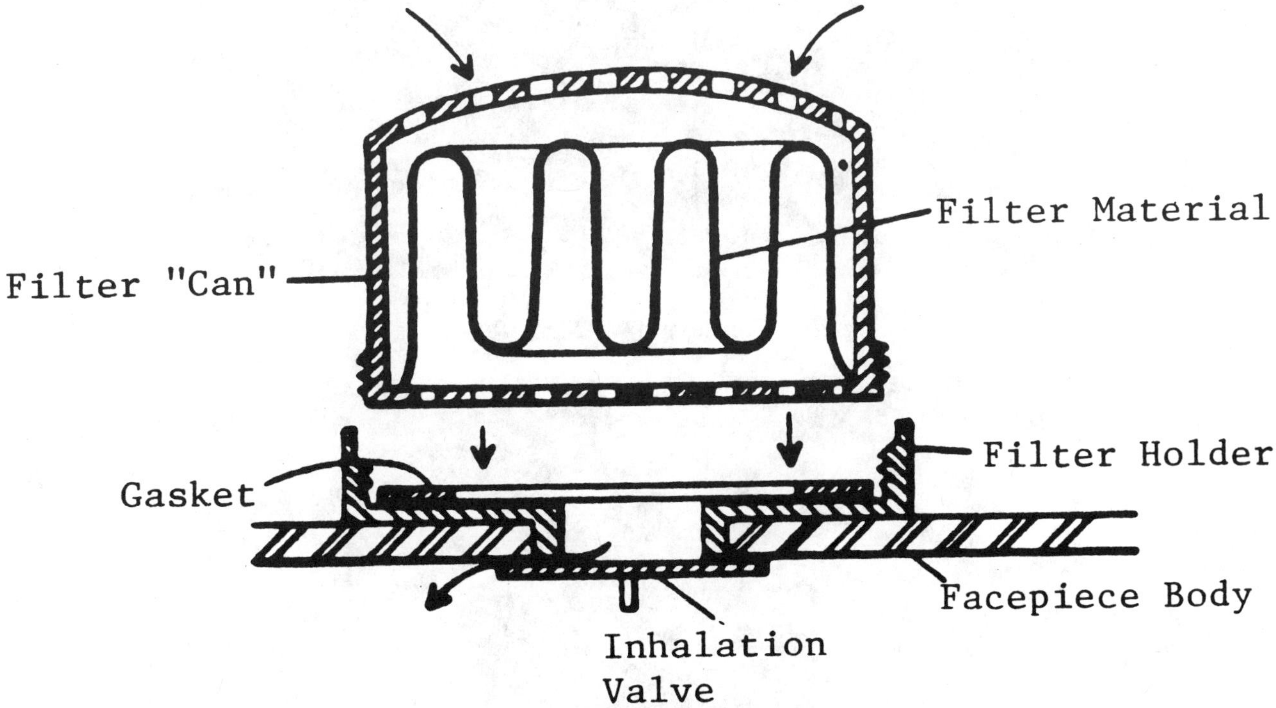

FIGURE 2-21. **Typical high efficiency filter**

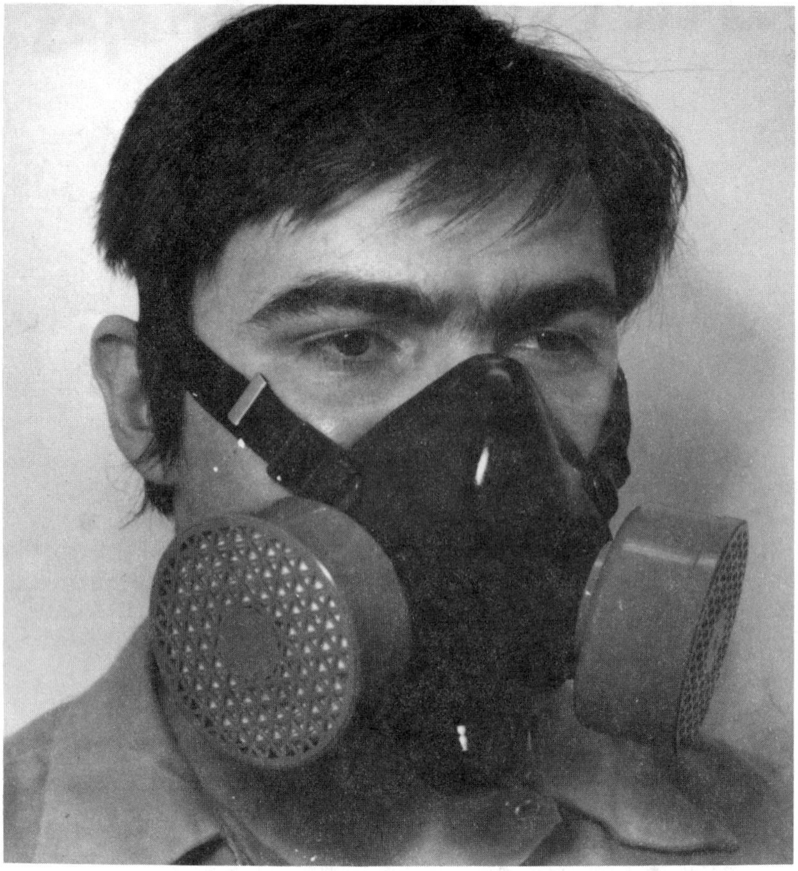

Photograph Courtesy of U.S. Safety Service

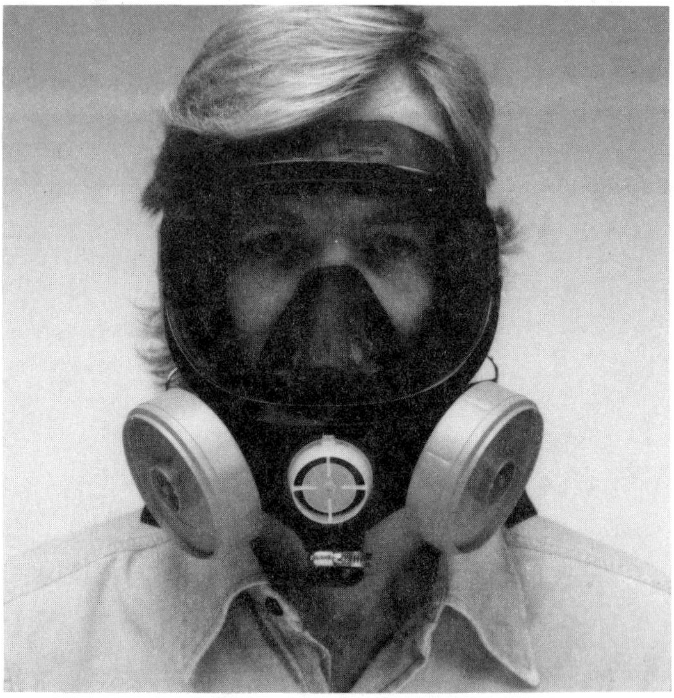

Photograph Courtesy of Willson Safety Products

FIGURE 2-22. **Typical half- and full-facepiece high efficiency respirators**

d. Single-use

Respirators designed as respiratory protection against pneumoconiosis- and fibrosis-producing dusts, or dusts and mist. In the single-use respirator, the filter is either an integral part of the facepiece or it is the entire facepiece itself (see Figure 2-23).

4. Filter Efficiency

Filter efficiency may be classified as follows:

a. High Efficiency

The highest efficiency filters (99.97 percent against 0.3μ dioctyl phthlate particle) are used on high efficiency respirators certified for protection against dusts, fumes, and mists having an exposure limit less than 0.05 milligram per cubic meter or 2 million particles per cubic foot of air.

b. Lower Efficiency

Respirators for dusts, fumes, and mists having an exposure limit not less than 0.05 milligram per cubic meter, have lower efficiency filters as classified in 30 CFR 11 (approximately 99 percent against a lead fume aerosol).

Dust, mist, single-use dust and mist respirators also have lower efficiency filters as classified in 30 CFR 11 (approximately 99 percent against a silica dust particle with a geometric mean diameter of 0.4 to 0.6μ and a standard geometric mean deviation not greater than 2).

B. Vapor and Gas Removing Respirators

The other major class of airborne contaminants consists of gases and vapors. Air-purifying respirators are available for protection against both specific gases and vapors, such as ammonia gas and mercury vapor, and classes of gases and vapors, such as acid gases and organic vapors. In contrast to filters, which are effective to some degree no matter what the particulate, the cartridges and canisters used for vapor and gas removal are designed for protection against specific contaminants.

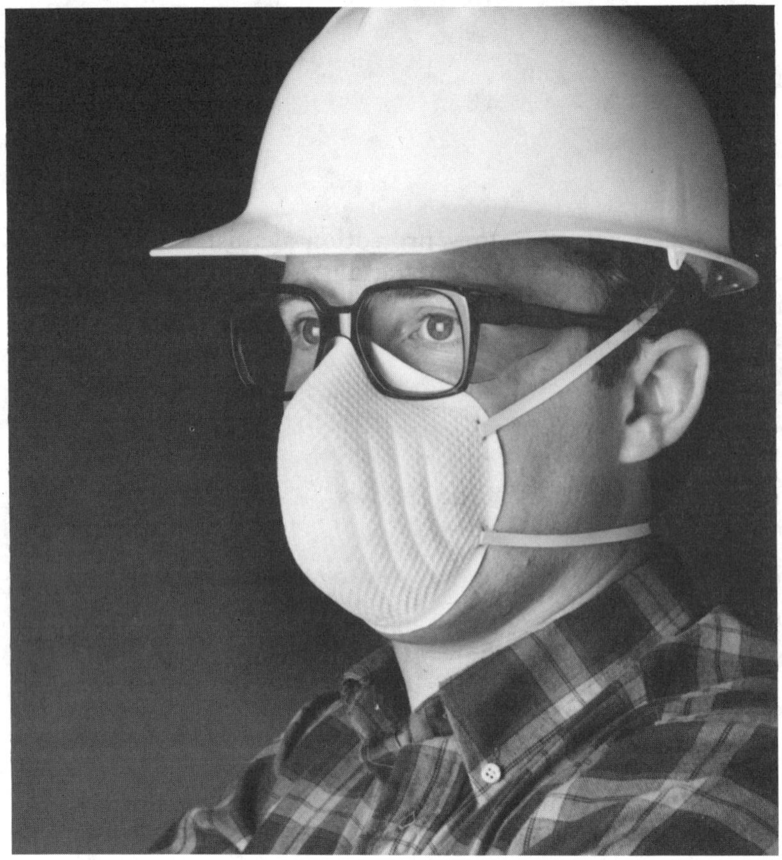

Photograph Courtesy of Moldex-Metric Inc.

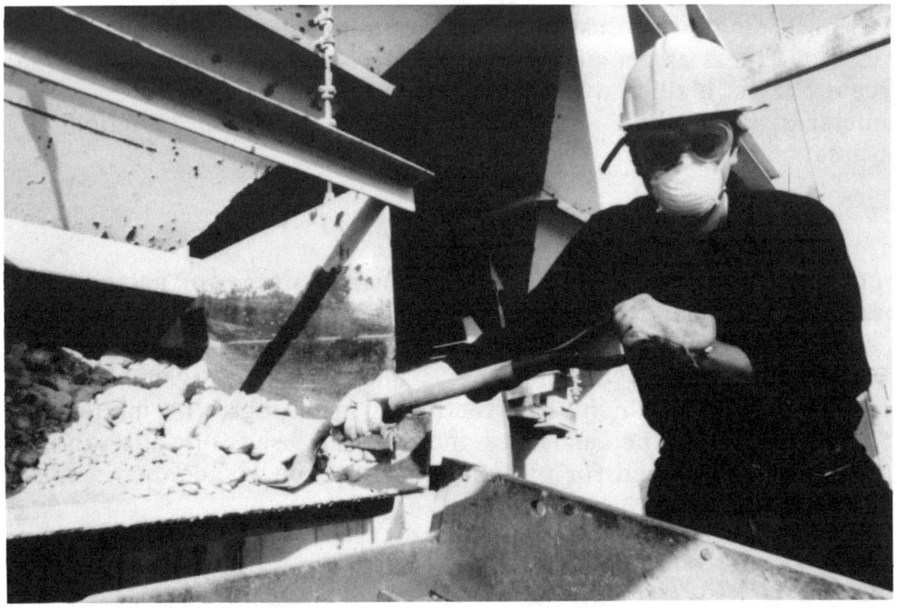

Photograph Courtesy of Louis M. Gerson Co., Inc.

FIGURE 2-23. **Typical single use respirators**

1. Removal Mechanisms

Vapor and gas removing respirators normally remove the contaminant by interaction of its molecules with a granular, porous material, commonly called the sorbent. The general method by which the molecules are removed is called sorption. In addition to sorption, some respirators use catalysts which react with the contaminant to produce a less toxic gas or vapor.

Three removal mechanisms are used in vapor and gas removing respirators.

a. Adsorption

Adsorption retains the contaminant molecule on the surface of the sorbent granule by physical attraction. The intensity of the attraction varies with the type of sorbent and contaminant. Adsorption by physical attraction holds the adsorbed molecules weakly. If chemical forces are involved, however, in the process called chemisorption, the bonds holding the molecules to the sorbent granules are much stronger and can be broken only with great difficulty.

A characteristic common to all adsorbents is a large specific surface area, up to 1500 m^2/g of sorbent. Activated charcoal is the most common adsorbent. It is used primarily to remove organic vapors, although it does have some capacity for adsorbing acid gases. Activated charcoal also can be impregnated with other substances to make it more selective against specific gases and vapors. Examples are activated charcoal impregnated with iodine to remove mercury vapor, with metallic oxides to remove acid gases, and with salts of metals to remove ammonia gas. Other sorbents which could be used in vapor and gas removing respirators include molecular sieves, activated alumina, and silica gel.

b. Absorption

Absorbents may also be used to remove gases and vapors. Absorbents differ from adsorbents in that, although they are porous, they do not have as large a specific surface area. Absorption is also different because the gas or vapor molecules usually penetrate deeply into the molecular spaces throughout the sorbent and are held there chemically. Probably, absorption cannot occur without prior adsorption on the surface of the particles. Furthermore, adsorption occurs instantaneously, whereas absorption is slower. Most absorbents are used for protection against acid gases. They include mixtures of sodium or potassium hydroxide with lime and/or caustic silicates.

c. Catalysis

A catalyst is a substance that influences the rate of chemical reaction between other substances. A catalyst used in respirator cartridges and canisters is hopcalite, a mixture of porous granules of manganese and copper oxides which speeds the reaction between toxic carbon monoxide and oxygen to form carbon dioxide.

As applied to respirators, the foregoing processes are essentially 100% efficient until the sorbent's capacity to adsorb gas and vapor or catalyze their reaction is exhausted. Then the contaminant will pass completely through the sorbent and into the facepiece. This is in contrast to mechanical particulate removing filters which become more efficient as matter collects on them and plugs the spaces between the fibers. This difference is important to remember. Water vapor reduces the effectiveness of some sorbents and increases that of others. For example, increasing moisture content of a sorbent designed to sorb acid gases may increase sorbent efficiency since most acid gases normally dissolve in water. Vapor and gas removing cartridges should be protected from the atmosphere while in storage.

2. ***Cartridges vs. Canisters.***

a. Sorbent Volume

The basic difference between cartridges and canisters is the volume of sorbent contained, not its function. Cartridges are vapor and gas removing elements that may be used singly or in pairs on quarter- and half-masks and on full-facepieces. The sorbent volume of a cartridge is small, about 50-200 cm^3, so the useful lifetime is usually short, particularly in high gas or vapor concentrations. Therefore, use of respirators with cartridges generally is restricted to low concentrations of vapors and gases. The user should refer to NIOSH recommendations, certification labels, or specific standards set forth by regulatory agencies for specific maximum use concentrations.

Canisters have a larger sorbent volume and may be chin-, front- or back-mounted. Respirators with canisters can be used in higher vapor and gas concentrations (up to the immediately dangerous to life or health level) than those with cartridges. Chin-style canisters have a volume of about 250-500 cm^3 and are used on full-facepiece respirators. Front- or back-mounted canisters are held in place by a harness and connected to the facepiece by a corrugated, flexible breathing tube. They have a sorbent volume of 1000-2000 cm^3. Front- or back-mounted and chin-style canisters are used with full-facepieces as part of "gas masks." The "gas mask" is certified for single or specific classes of gases and vapors. It differs from the chemical cartridge respirator only in its larger sorbent volume and the higher concentrations of vapors and gases against which it provides protection.

b. Labeling

As vapor and gas removing cartridges and canisters are designed for protection against specific contaminants, or classes thereof, how does the user know he has the proper device? The printed certification label clearly lists these contaminants. An American National Standard, ANSI K13.1-1973, established a color code for the various types of sorbent cartridges and canisters which identifies the contaminants they are designed to protect against. Users should not rely on memorizing the color code, but should always **READ THE LABEL!** This is the only foolproof way of ensuring use of the correct cartridge or canister. The color code of the ANSI K13.1 standard has been included verbatim in the OSHA regulations, 29 CFR 1910.134(g).

c. Construction

The type of sorbent found in vapor and gas removing cartridges and canisters for use against a particular substance may vary from manufacturer to manufacturer. However, cartridge and canister construction varies little. The basic construction problems are the same: to provide enough sorbent bed depth and volume to ensure that 1) the contaminant is totally removed in the times specified in 30 CFR 11 bench tests, and 2) the sorbent remains mechanically stable in the container.

Figure 2-24 shows a typical chemical cartridge certified for use with a half-mask. The bed of sorbent granules is retained in the cylindrical "can" by a screen and coarse filter pad at the top and by a coarse particulate filter pad and a screen at the bottom (Figure 2-25). The pads only keep the fine granules in the sorbent from escaping from the cartridge; they are not designed for protection against particulate contaminants. Various precautions for use of these cartridges are discussed in Chapter 5, **Respirator Use Under Special Conditions.**

One problem in design and manufacture of sorbent canisters is to prevent passage of large quantities of air through small areas of the bed of packed sorbent granules. Such air channeling through the canister reduces its useful service life. Selection of the proper sorbent granule size and careful packing in the canister minimize air channeling. There is a tendency toward channeling where the irregular sorbent granules touch the smooth canister wall. Sometimes channeling is prevented by forming ridges in the canister shell like those in Figure 2-26. The retaining screens and pads hold the granular sorbent bed in place. The spring ensures that the sorbent remains tightly packed.

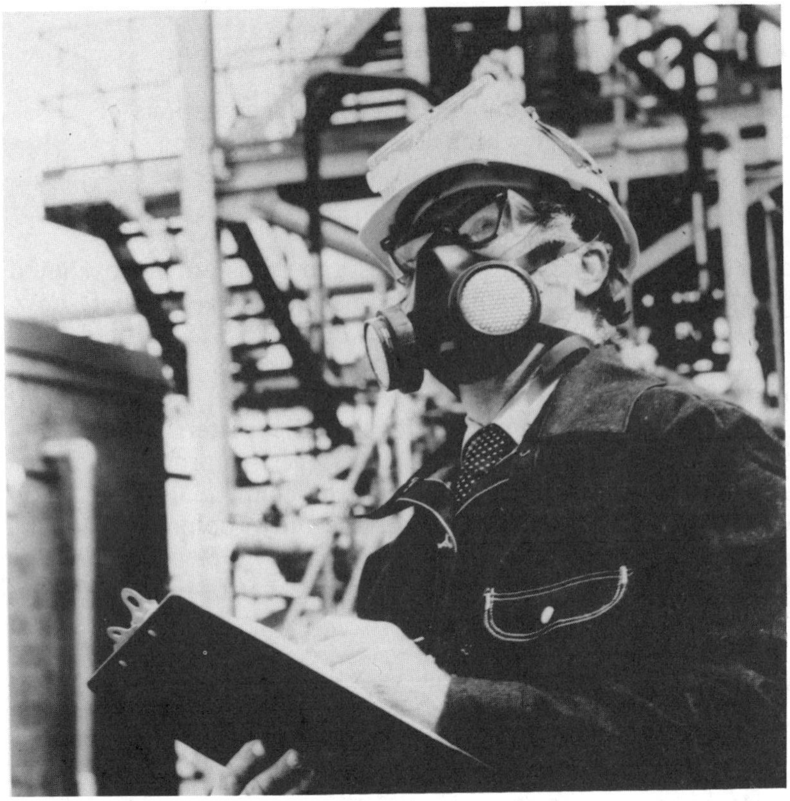

Photograph Courtesy of Glendale Protective Technology

FIGURE 2-24. **Typical half-mask chemical cartridge**

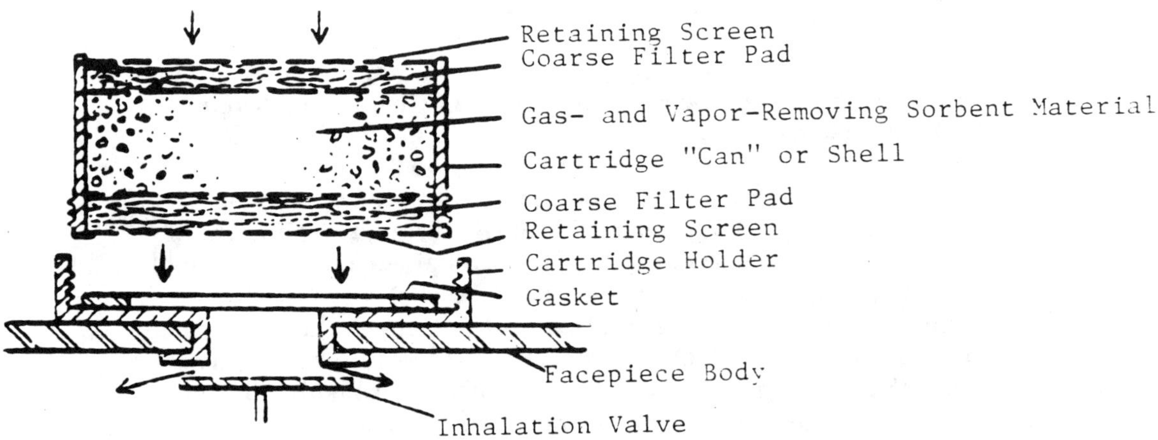

FIGURE 2-25. **Typical chemical cartridge**

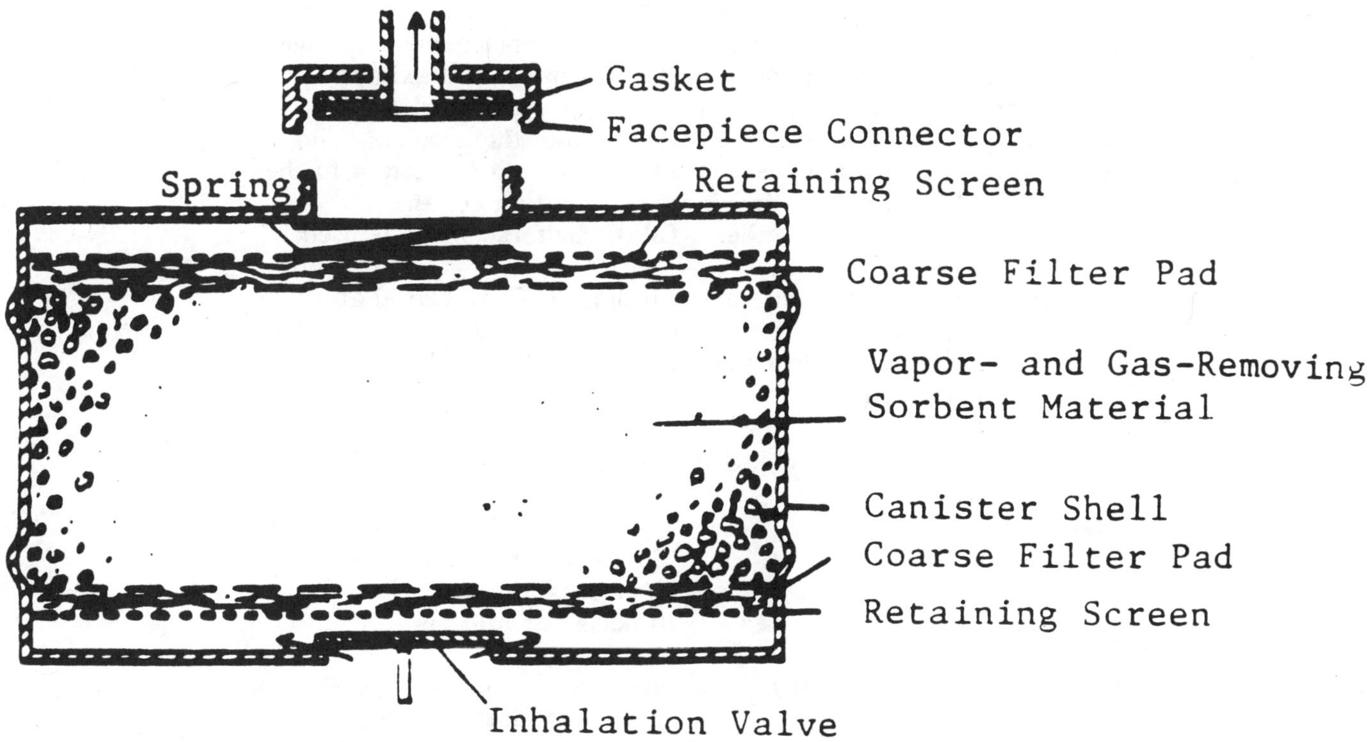

FIGURE 2-26. **Typical chin style canister**

Even with these precautions, sorbent canisters may be damaged by dropping. This can crush the granules, disturb the retaining screens or pads, or create channels between the sorbent granules and the canister wall. Cartridges and canisters should also be stored upright. In short, treat sorbent canisters with care.

3. *Vapor and Gas Respirator Classifications*

a. Chemical Cartridge Respirators

Figure 2-27 shows a typical chemical cartridge air-purifying respirator with an array of various cartridges that can be used with it. Chemical cartridge respirators can be either powered or non-powered, and either disposable or with replaceable cartridges or canisters. A listing of the vapors and gases and maximum concentrations for which chemical cartridge respirators are certified is included in 30 CFR 11.150. Note the accompanying restrictions on maximum use. These concentrations pertain to the cartridge and thus are the limiting concentration for the respirator regardless of whether a full or half facepiece is used.

In addition to the gases and vapors listed, 30 CFR 11.150 also allows MSHA/NIOSH to certify chemical cartridge respirators for gases and vapors other than those listed. Fox example, MSHA/NIOSH have certified respirators for use against:

Gas/Vapor	*Maximum Use Concentration*
Mercury*	0.5 mg/m^3
Hydrogen sulfide*	100 parts per million
Chlorine dioxide	1 part per million
Formaldehyde	30 parts per million

*Respirators may be certified for gases and vapors with poor warning properties if there is a regulatory agency standard which permits their use and an effective end-of-service-life indicator is provided (Reference: FR 49 No. 140 pages 29270-29272, July 19, 1984).

b. Gas Masks

The following types of gas masks have been certified by MSHA/NIOSH:

Front- or back-mounted canisters
Chin-style canisters
Escape

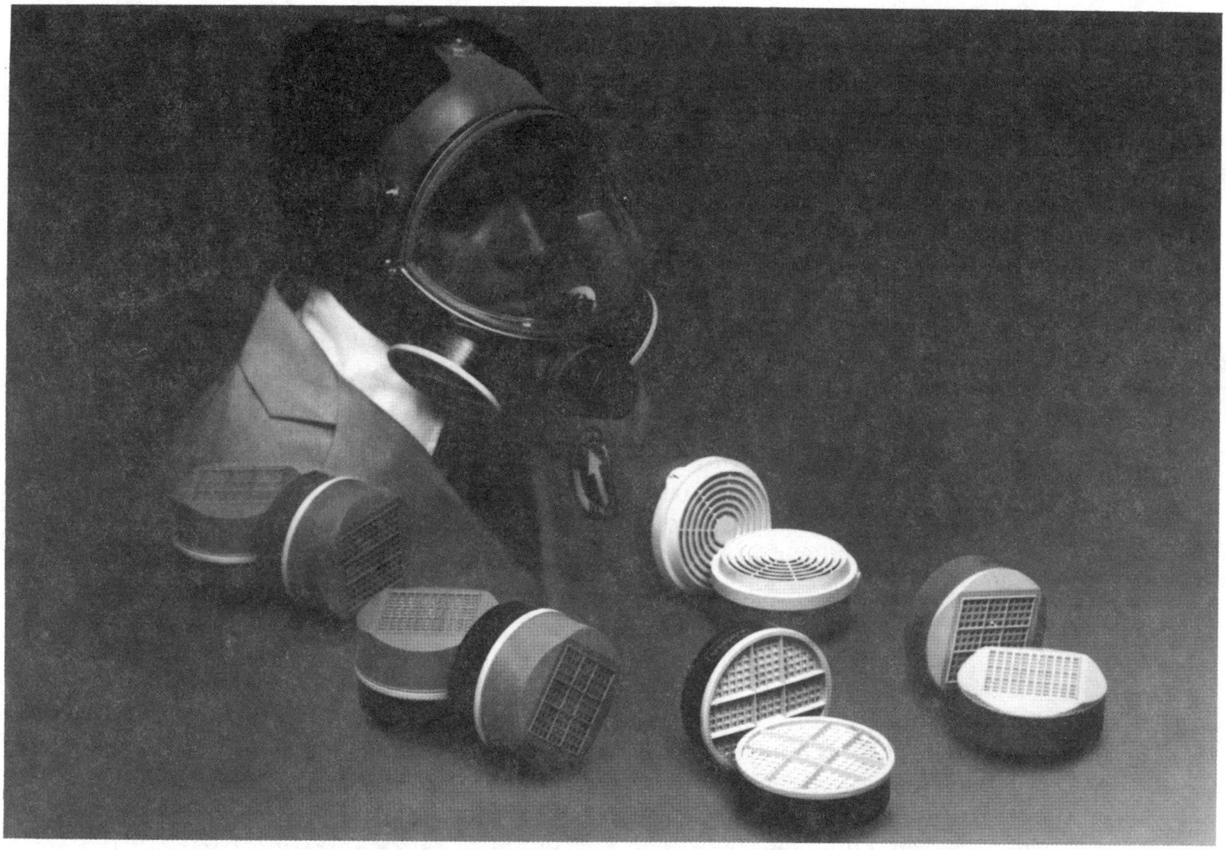

Photograph Courtesy of SurvivAir

FIGURE 2-27. **Full-facepiece chemical cartridge respirator with alternate cartridges**

Front- or back-mounted. Front- or back-mounted canisters are usually certified for use with a full-facepiece. However, some half-mask or mouthpiece gas masks are certified. A "super size" or "industrial" size canister is fastened to the user's body, and a breathing tube connects the canister to the facepiece inlet. A typical front-or back-mounted canister is shown in Figure 2-28. Note that the construction does not differ markedly from that of the chemical cartridge shown in Figure 2-24. Other than the volume of sorbent contained (1000-2000 cm^3), the greatest difference is that the canister, rather than the facepiece, usually contains the inhalation valve. Figures 2-29 and 2-30 show typical front- and back-mounted canister gas masks.

Canisters can be designed for one or more type(s) of gas(es) or vapor(s). Several specific gases and vapors for which MSHA/NIOSH can issue certifications are listed in 30 CFR 11.90. In addition, MSHA/NIOSH have certified gas masks for gases and vapors not listed but which have adequate warning properties (e.g., hydrogen fluoride, formaldehyde and phosphine). MSHA/NIOSH have also certified gas masks for ethylene oxide. However, since ethylene oxide has poor warning properties, these canisters are required to have an end-of-service-life indicator.

Canisters designed for protection against more than one vapor or gas have their sorbents either arranged in layers or intermixed. Figure 2-31 shows these two arrangements as either might appear in a chin-style canister. In certain instances, one type of construction has an advantage over the other, but mostly it is a matter of manufacturing convenience.

Chin-style. Chin-style gas masks typically have a medium-sized (250-500 cm^3) canister rigidly attached to a full-facepiece (Figure 2-32). The useful lifetime is less than that of a front- or back-mounted canister (owing to the smaller sorbent volume), but greater than that of chemical cartridges. Gas masks can either be powered or non-powered. The maximum use concentration for both the front- or back-mounted and chin style gas masks is the immediately dangerous to life or health (IDLH) level of the substance.

Escape masks. Gas masks for use during escape from (not entry or reentry into) atmospheres immediately hazardous to life and health are certified under 30 CFR 11, Subpart I. They consist of a facepiece or mouthpiece, a canister, and associated connections. Where eye irritation is a consideration, a full-facepiece gas mask is necessary. An example of an escape gas mask is the "filter" self-rescuer for carbon monoxide used in escaping from mines (Figure 2-33).

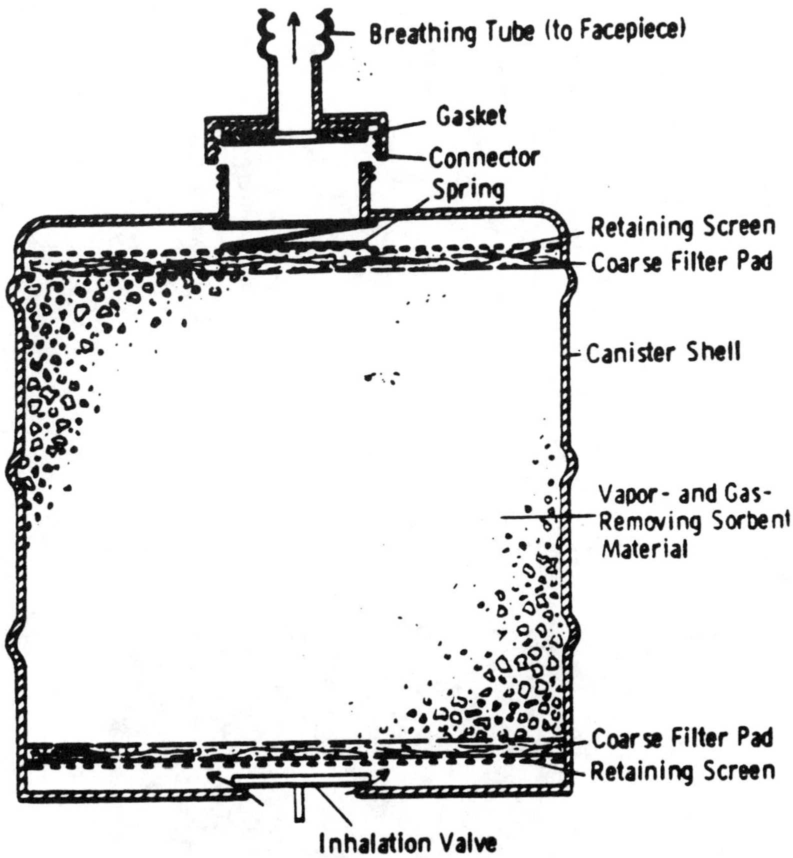

FIGURE 2-28. **Typical front- or back-mounted canister**

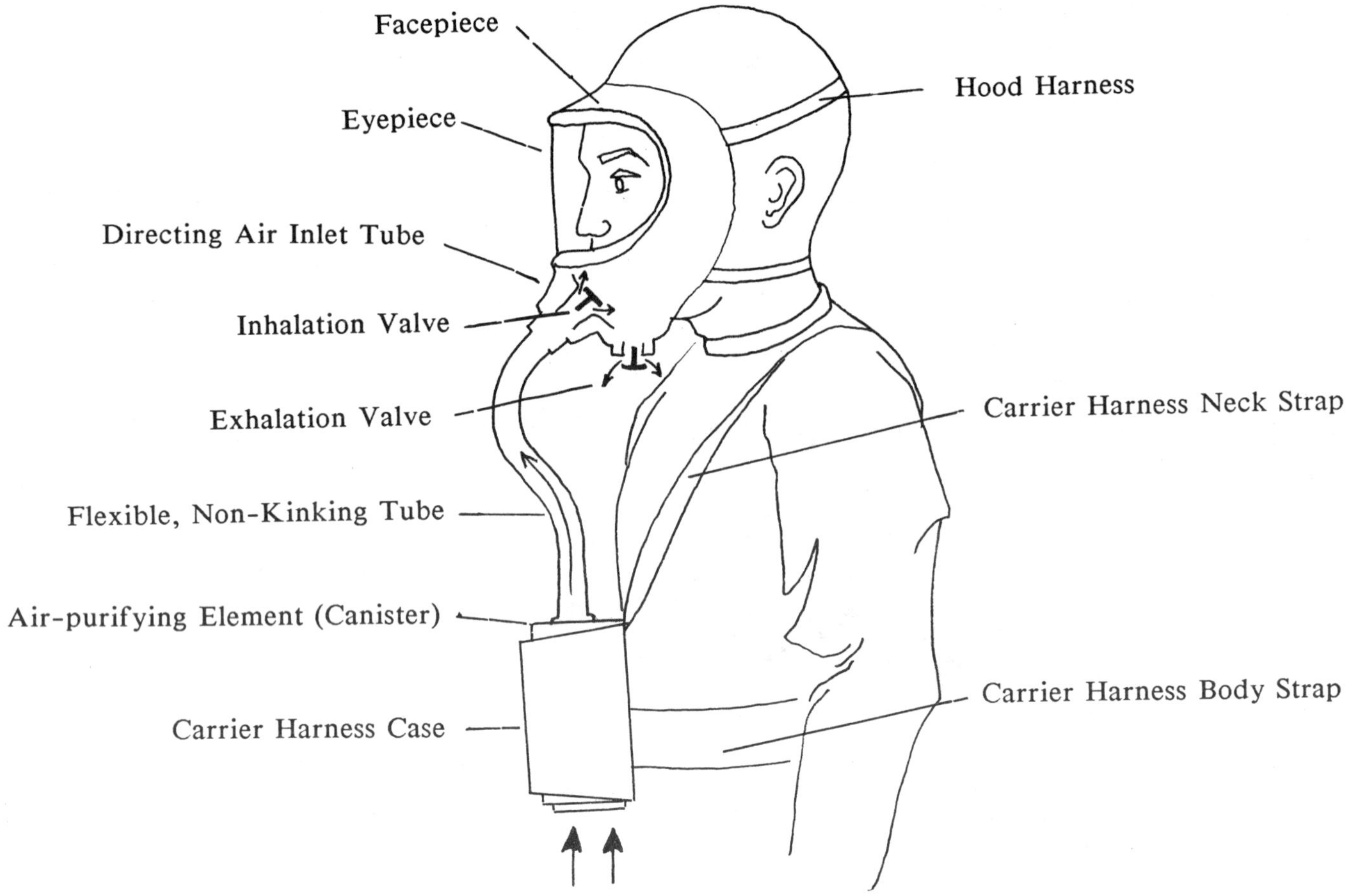

FIGURE 2-29. **Typical front- and back-mounted canister gas mask**

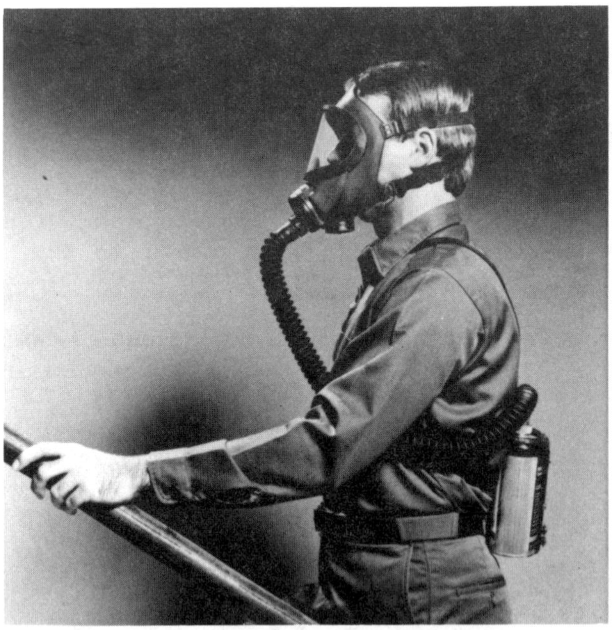

Photograph Courtesy of Mine Safety Appliances

FIGURE 2-30. **Typical back-mounted canister gas mask**

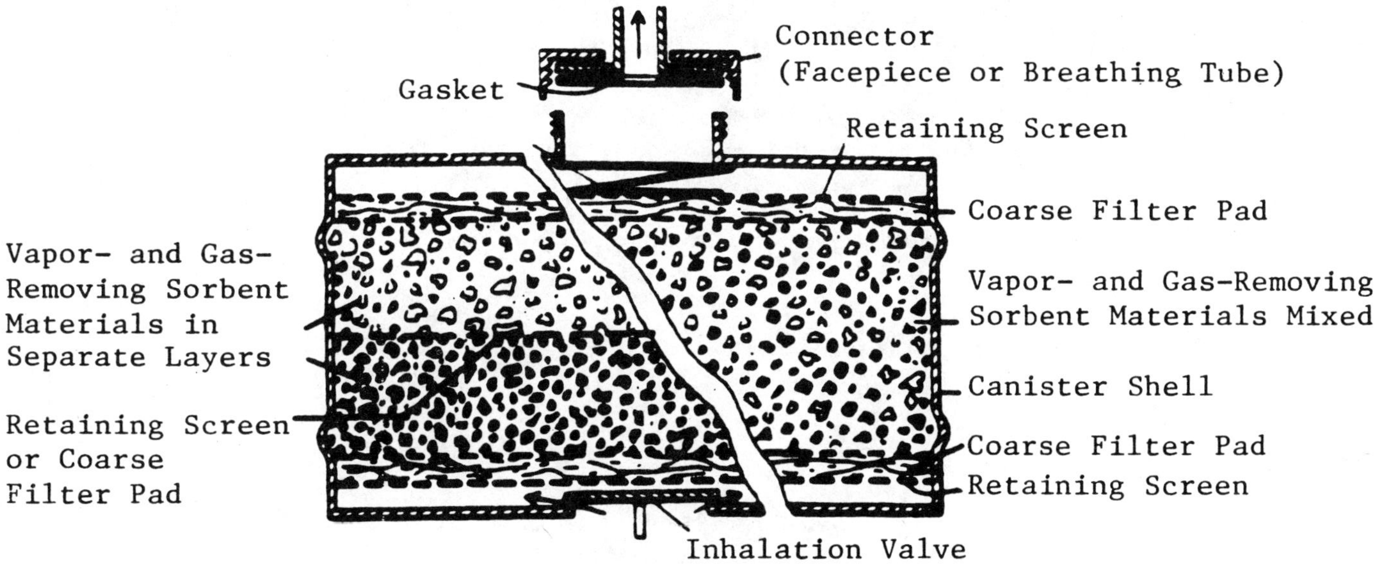

FIGURE 2-31. **Typical chin-style canister for more than one vapor**

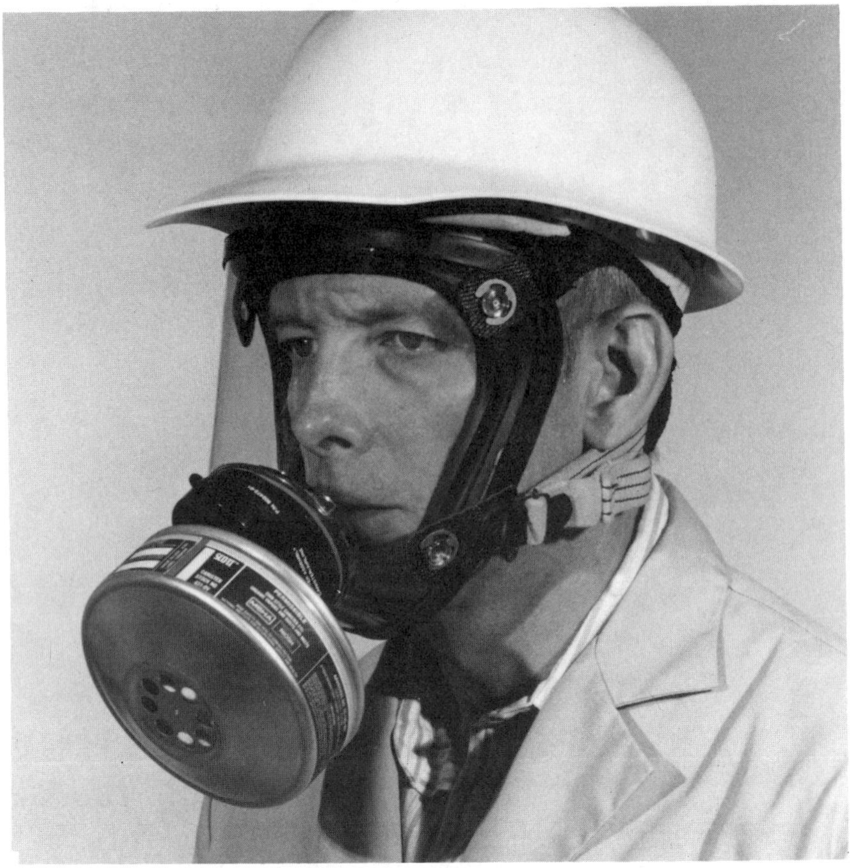

Photograph Courtesy of Scott Aviation

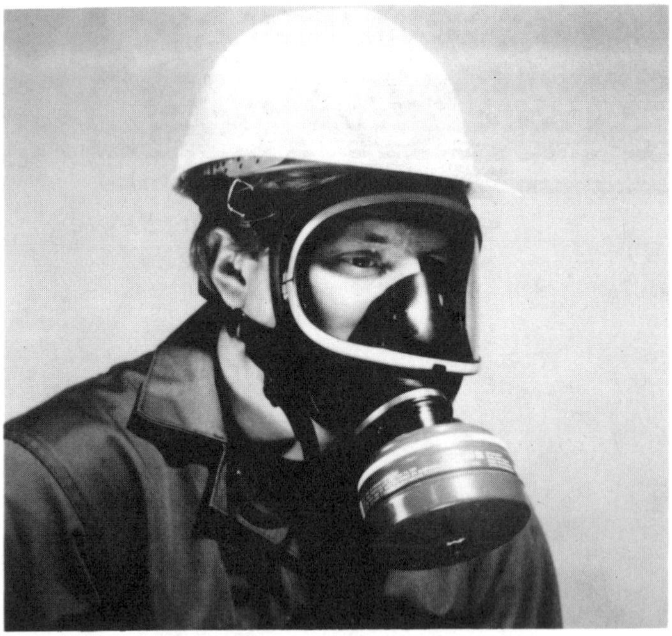

Photograph Courtesy of Draeger

FIGURE 2-32. **Chin-style canister gas masks**

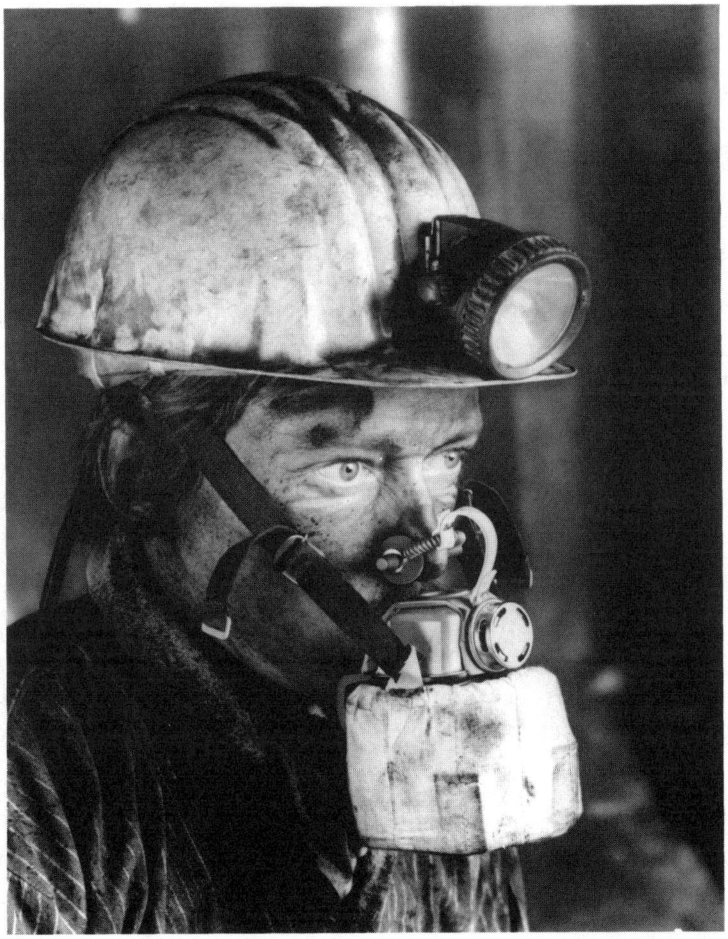

Photograph Courtesy of Draeger

FIGURE 2-33. **Filter self-rescuer**

c. Particulate Vapor and Gas Removing Air-Purifying Respirators

Cartridges and canisters are available to protect against both particulates and vapors and gases. These devices look much like the sorbent cartridge or sorbent canister alone. Figure 2-34 shows the two methods of attaching a particulate filter to a typical cartridge. In A, the particulate filter is inside the cartridge container, in B it is outside the can and held in place by a snap-on cover. Other variations may be found, but the principle is the same. Where filters are used in combination with cartridges, the filter must always be located on the inlet side of the cartridge. Pesticide and paint spray respirators use combination respirator cartridges, although paint spray respirators are certified under Subpart L of 30 CFR 11 (Chemical Cartridge Respirators), and pesticide respirators under Subpart M. Typical combination particulate, vapor, and gas removing respirators are shown, in Figure 2-35, being used in paint spraying.

High efficiency particulate filters are included on some types of combination canisters like the front-mounted canisters shown in Figure 2-30.

A very specialized type of combination particulate and vapor and gas removing canister is the so called "Type N," or "Universal" canister (Figure 2-36). It looks much like a front- or back-mounted canister, being about the same size and held on the body in the same way. Internally, however, there is a great deal of difference. The Type N canister may contain several different sorbents for ammonia, acid gases, and organic vapors; a catalyst, hopcalite, to convert carbon monoxide to carbon dioxide; layers of drying agent to protect the catalyst from water vapor; and a high efficiency filter for particulates.

All of these layers are packed into a space equivalent in size to the conventional canister; therefore, the sorptive capacity of any single layer of sorbent in the Type N canister is less than that of the large sorbent bed in the industrial size canister for use against a single contaminant. Consequently, the useful service life of the Type N canister is relatively short.

All canisters approved for entry into carbon monoxide atmospheres must have an indicator, usually behind a small window, that shows when the canister will no longer remove the carbon monoxide. Actually, it indicates the condition of the drying agent upstream of the catalyst. The CO catalyst, hopcalite, is rendered useless by moisture, and this indicator tells only the condition of the hopcalite, not that of the acid gas, ammonia gas, or organic vapor sorbent. Therefore, it cannot be used as an indication of the overall canister condition.

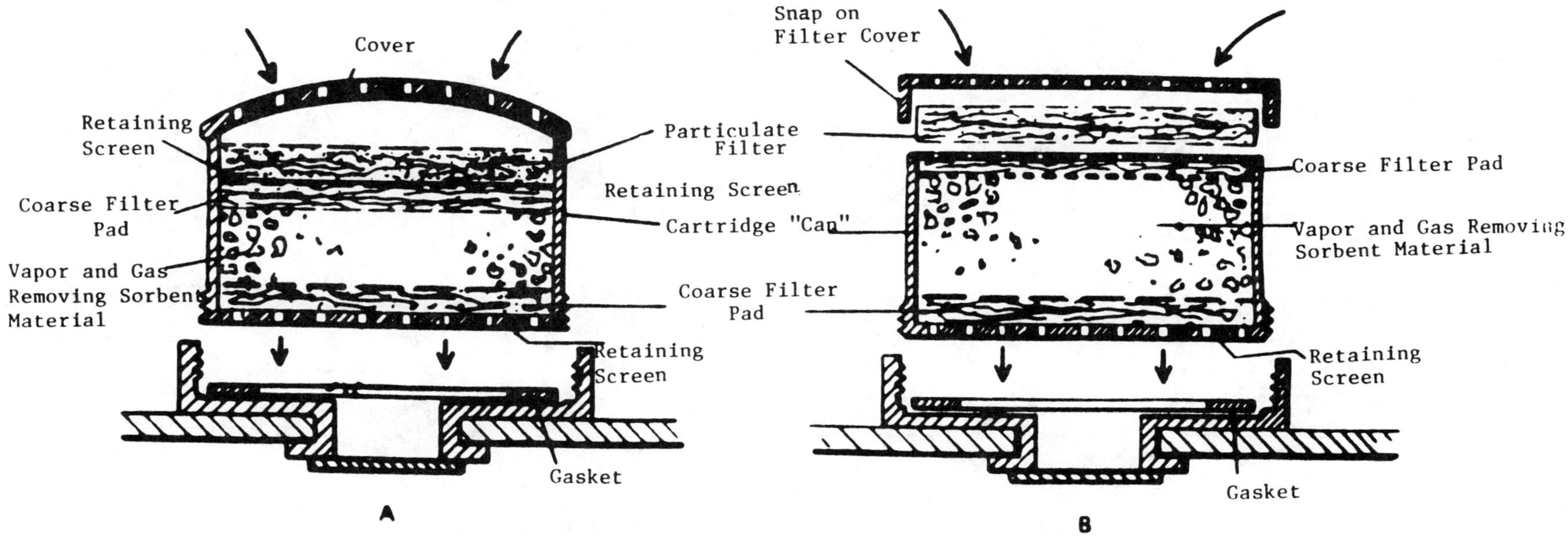

FIGURE 2-34. **Typical combination particulate- and gas- and vapor-removing cartridges**

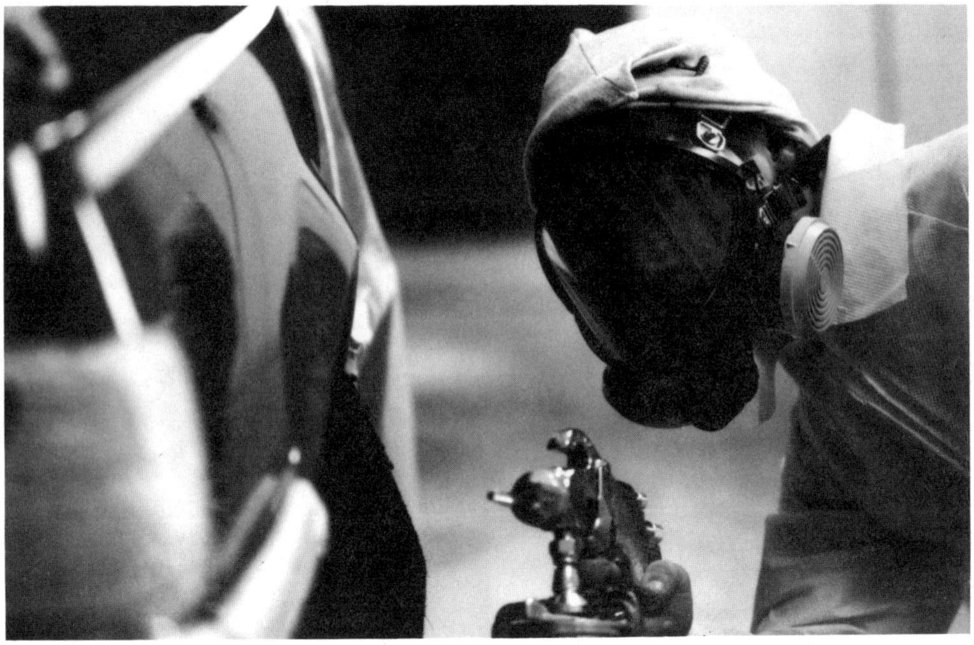

Photograph Courtesy of SurvivAir

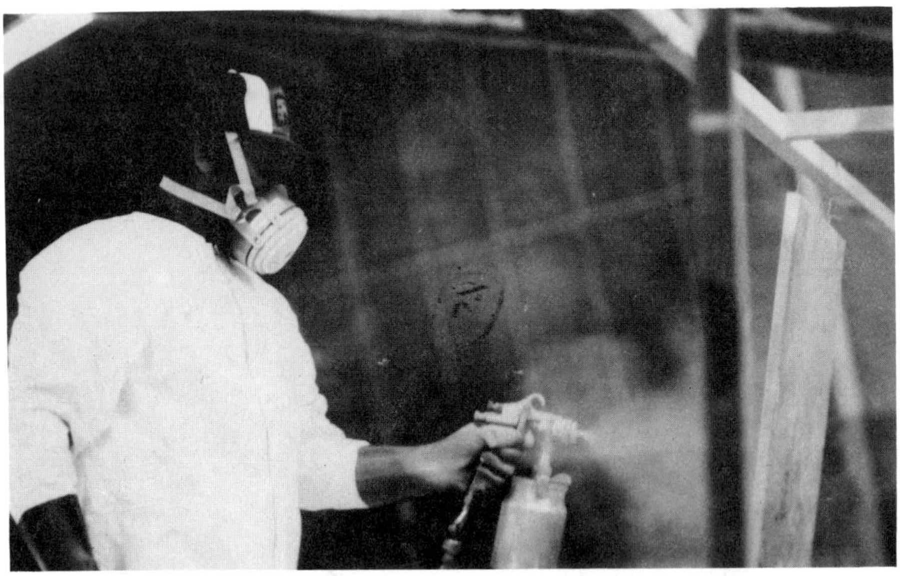

Photograph Courtesy of North

FIGURE 2-35. **Combination particulate-, gas- and vapor-removing respirator**

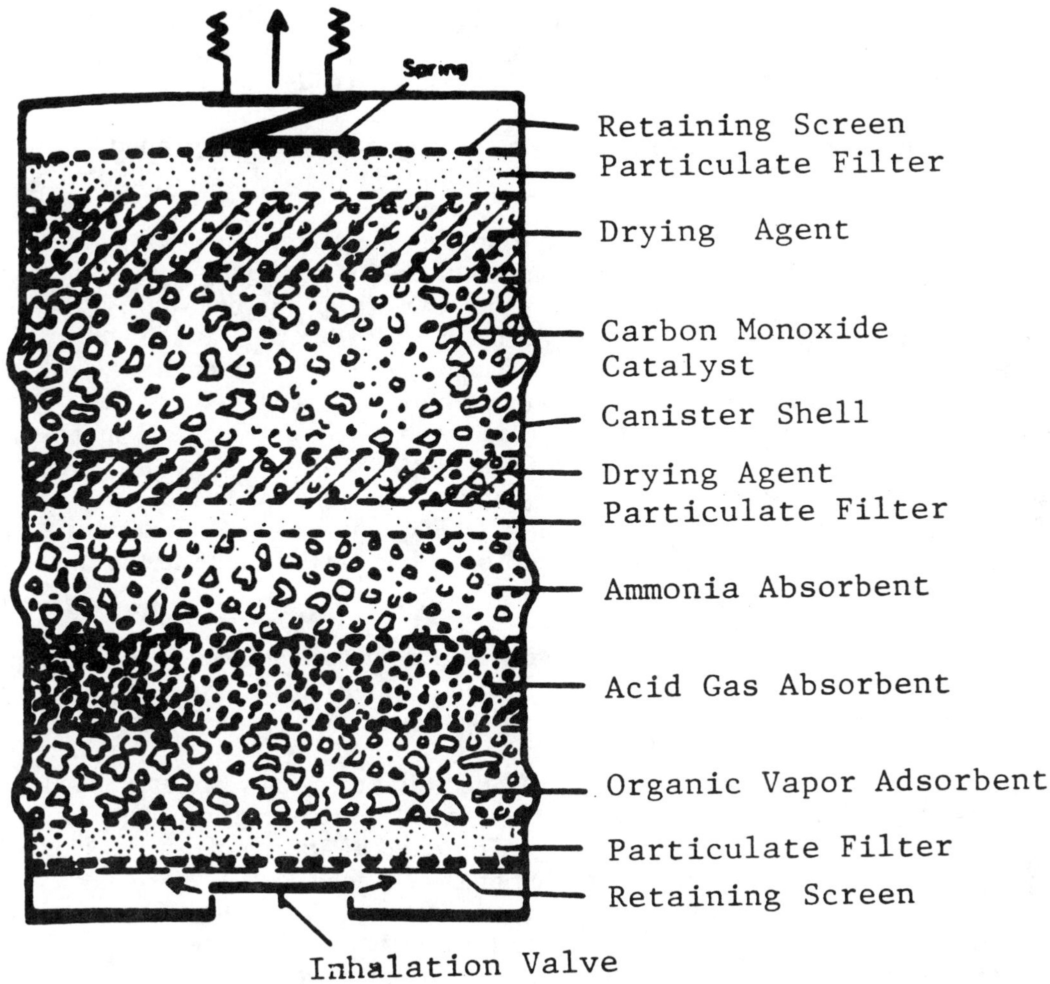

FIGURE 2-36. **Typical Type N canister**

Figure 2-37 shows a typical front-mounted Type N canister attached to a full-facepiece.

C. Powered Air-Purifying Respirators

The powered air-purifying respirator (PAPR) uses a blower to pass contaminated air through an element that removes the contaminants and supplies the purified air to a respiratory inlet covering. The purifying element may be a filter to remove particulates, a cartridge to remove vapors and gases or a combination filter and cartridge, canister or canister and filter. The covering may be a facepiece, helmet, or hood. These respirators are certified under 30 CFR 11, Subparts I, K, L, and M.

Powered air-purifying respirators come in several different configurations. One configuration consists of the air-purifying element(s) attached to a small blower which is worn on the belt and is connected to the respiratory inlet covering by a flexible tube as shown in Figure 2-38. This type of device is usually powered by a small battery (either mounted on the belt separately or as part of the blower), although some units are powered by an external DC or AC source.

Another type consists of the air-purifying element attached to a stationary blower, usually mounted on a vehicle, powered by a battery or an external power source and connected by a long flexible tube to the respiratory inlet covering.

The third type of powered air-purifying respirator consists of a helmet or facepiece to which the air-purifying element and blower are attached. Only the battery is carried on the belt.

The respiratory inlet covering for a powered air-purifying respirator may be a tight fitting half-mask (Figure 2-39) or full-facepiece, or a loose fitting hood or helmet (Figure 2-40). A powered air-purifying respirator with a tight fitting facepiece must deliver at least four cubic feet of air per minute (115 liters per minute). A powered air-purifying respirator with a loose fitting hood or helmet must deliver at least six cubic feet of air (170 liters per minute) at all times.

One potential disadvantage of powered air-purifying respirators is that since there is a constant flow through the air-purifying element instead of flow only during inhalation; the useful service lifetimes of the air-purifying elements on powered air-purifying respirators could be shorter than the service lifetimes of comparable elements attached to a negative pressure respirator. In order to overcome this problem, some powered air-purifying respirators have a spring loaded exhalation valve assembly. This causes the blower assembly to slow down when the wearer exhales. This helps to extend the service lifetime of the air-purifying elements.

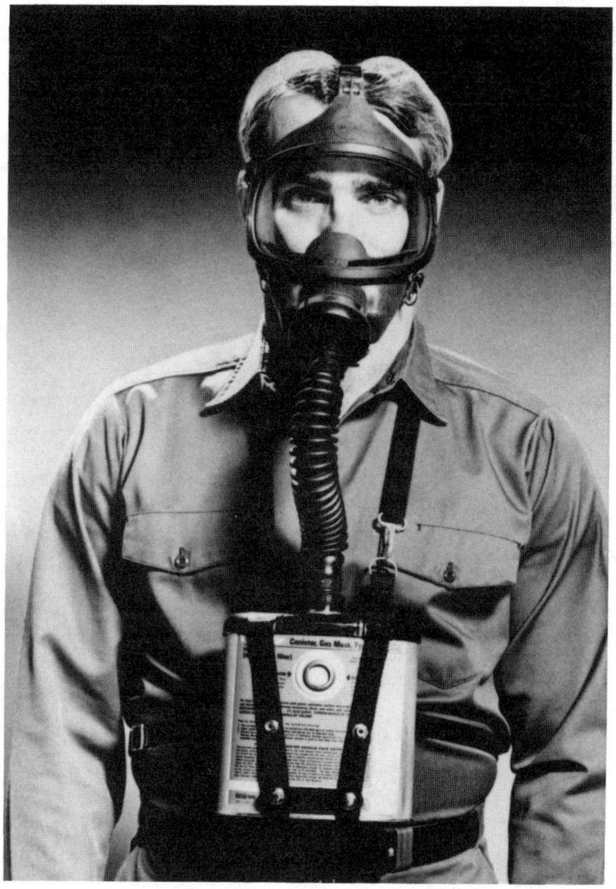

Photograph Couresy of Mine Safety Appliances

FIGURE 2-37. **Typical front-mount Type N canister gas mask**

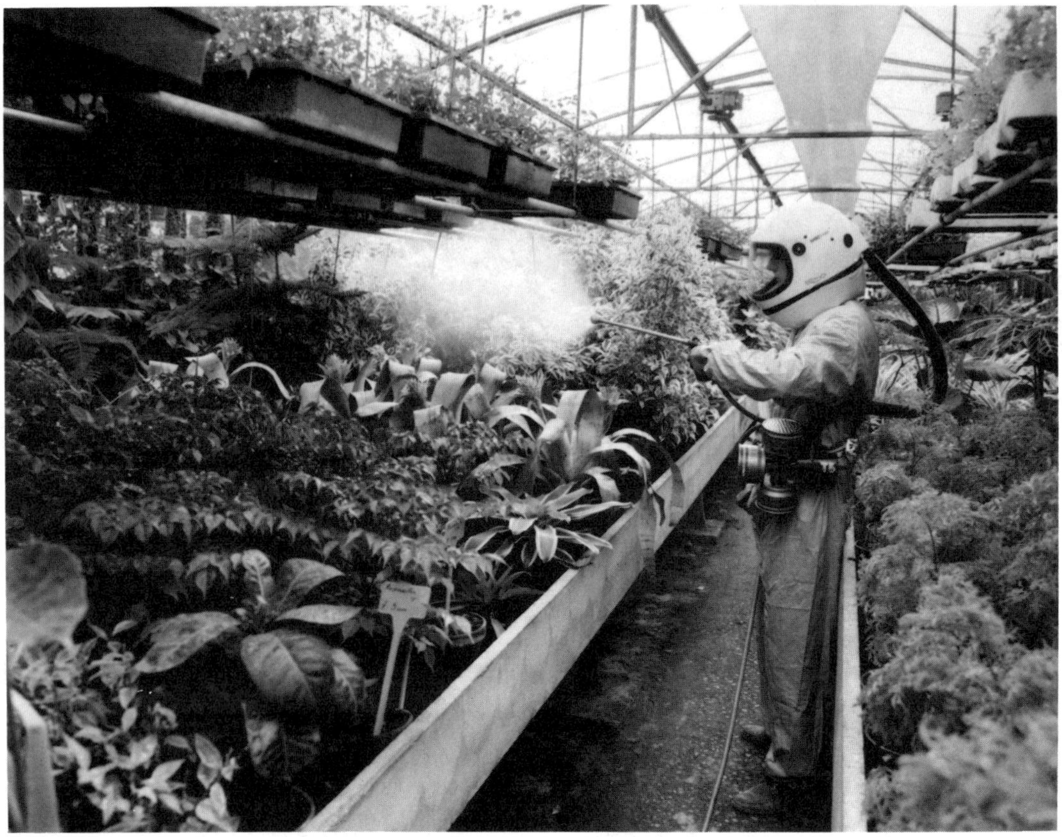

Photograph Courtesy of Kasco Inc.

FIGURE 2-38. **Powered air-purifying respirator with chemical cartridges and breathing tube**

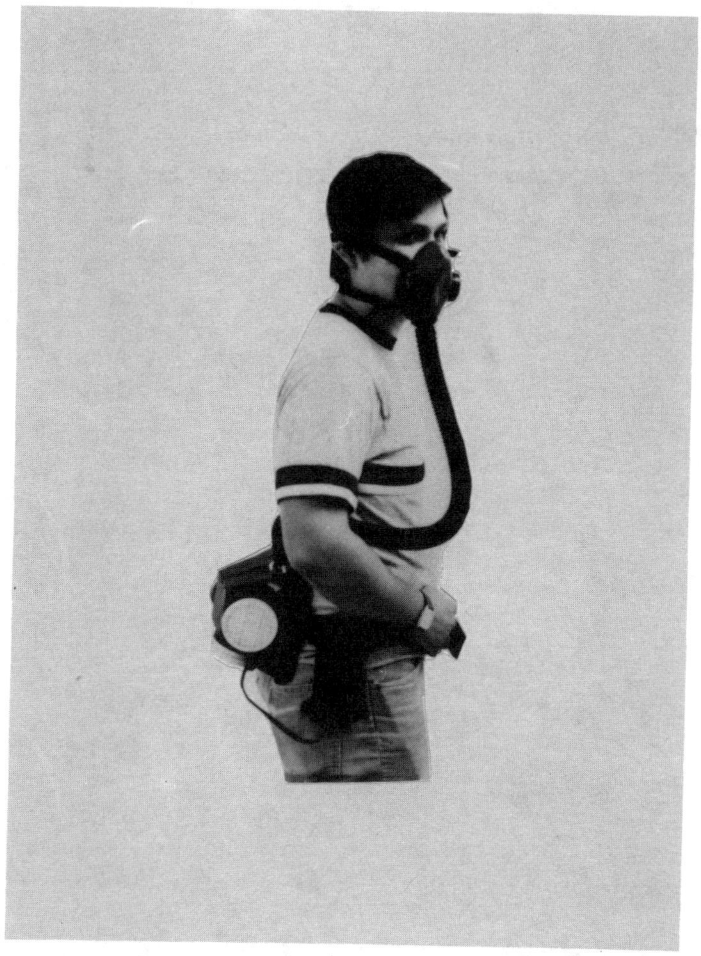

Photograph Courtesy of Neoterik

FIGURE 2-39. **Tight fitting half-mask powered air-purifying respirator**

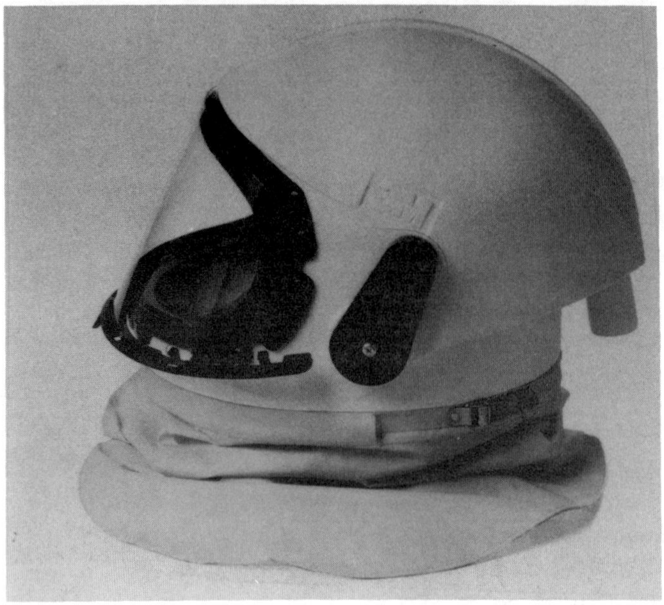

Photograph courtesy of 3M Company

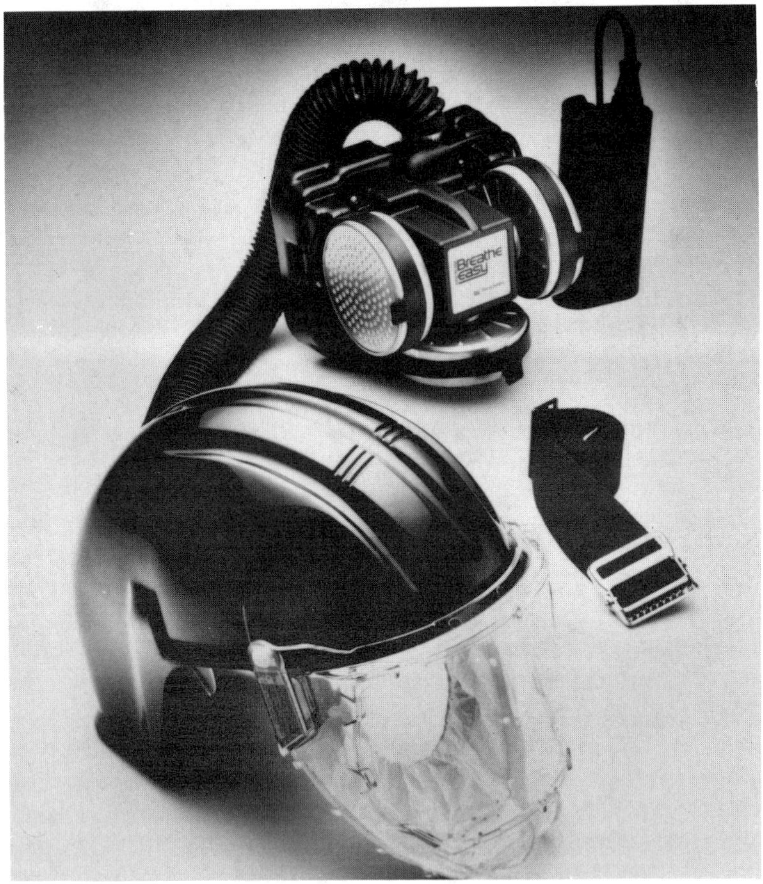

Photograph Courtesy of Racal Airstream

FIGURE 2-40. **Helmeted powered air-purifying respirator**

Powered air-purifying respirators using chemical cartridges and canisters have the same limitations, insofar as the air-purifying elements are concerned, as the negative pressure respirators approved for the same gases or vapors.

In the past, powered air-purifying respirators were considered positive pressure respirators, since they normally supplied air at positive pressure. It was assumed that any leakage was outward from the facepiece. They were given correspondingly high protection factors. However, recent field studies by NIOSH and others have indicated that the level of protection provided by these respirators may not be as high as previously reported. Because of the potential for overbreathing at the minimum airflow rates, NIOSH now recommends much lower protection factors.

D. Advantages and Disadvantages of Air-Purifying Respirators

Air-purifying respirators are generally small and are easily maintained. (The exceptions to this are the combination Type C supplied-air and air-purifying respirator and powered air-purifying respirator.) They restrict the wearer's movements the least. The many combinations of facepieces, mouthpieces, filters, cartridges and canisters allow the user to match the respirator to the particular situation.

Air-purifying respirators should not be used in atmospheres containing less than 19.5 percent oxygen nor in atmospheres immediately dangerous to life or health (except escape gas masks). They should not be used for protection against gases or vapors with poor warning properties except for escape only or where permitted by a regulatory agency and the respirator is equipped with an end of service life indicator for that particular substance. The cost of replacement elements for air-purifying respirators can be high. Chemical cartridge respirators have fairly low maximum use concentrations, even when used with a full-facepiece.

1. Particulate Respirators

The advantages of particulate filter respirators include their light weight, small size and ease of maintenance. In general, these respirators will not affect the mobility of the worker and may present little physiological strain to the wearer. The air flow resistance of a particulate-removing respirator filter element increases as the quantity of particles it retains increases. This resistance increases the breathing resistance offered by a nonpowered respirator and may reduce the rate of air flow in a powered respirator. Filter element plugging by retained particles may also limit the continuous use time of a particulate filter type respirator. Rapid plugging means that the element has to be replaced frequently. Elements should be replaced at least daily or more often if breathing resistance becomes excessive or if the filter suffers physical damage (tears, holes, etc.). Filter elements designed to be cleaned and reused also should be cleaned at least daily in accordance with the manufacturer's instructions. Between uses, reusable respirators should be packaged to reduce exposure to conditions which cause filter degradation, such as high humidity.

Performance of some fibrous filter materials (electrostatic felts) is hurt by storage in very humid atmospheres, so care should be taken in storing filter elements. Performance also may deteriorate during use because of water vapor or oil mists in the workplace atmosphere. Airborne liquid particles (aqueous and nonaqueous) and extremely small solid particles may deteriorate the functioning of these materials. Solid particles plug fibrous filter materials (including electrostatic felts), and, although this plugging increases the resistance to air flow and hence may exacerbate respirator faceseal leakage, significant plugging increases the materials' efficiency in removing particles from air.

2. *Vapor and Gas Removing Cartridges and Canisters*

Gas and vapor removing cartridges and canisters have the same advantages as particulate filter respirators. Certain cartridges and canisters have higher breathing resistance than particulate filter respirators and thus will present a slightly higher physiological burden to the wearer. If a vapor or gas lacks adequate warning properties (odor, taste, irritation) in a concentration above the established breathing time-weighted average concentration (TWA), a vapor and gas removing air-purifying respirator should not be used unless the respirator incorporates an adequate end of service life indicator .

Another disadvantage is the limited capacity of the cartridges and canisters in these respirators to remove vapors and gases from air, or to catalyze a reaction converting toxic vapors or gases to nontoxic products or products that can be removed from air. Theoretically, cartridges and canisters containing sorbents are totally efficient against vapors and gases until their capacity for adsorption or catalysis is exhausted. Then, the vapor or gas passes through the sorbent bed of the cartridge or canister and into the facepiece. If the wearer detects an odor or taste of gas in the inspired air, or feels eye or throat irritation, he/she should leave the hazardous area immediately and go to a safe area that contains respirable air. Then the wearer should replace the cartridge or canister. Because of the limited useful service time of canisters and cartridges, they should be replaced daily or after each use, or even more often if the wearer detects odor, taste, or irritation. Discarding the cartridge/canister is recommended at the end of the day, even if the wearer does not detect odor, taste or irritation. This is due to the possibility of desorption of the gas or vapor occurring during overnight storage.

If a respirator wearer detects an odor, taste, or irritation for a very short time and then the sensation disappears, penetration of an air contaminant into the respiratory inlet covering has not necessarily ceased. The nerve endings that cause a sensation of odor, taste, or irritation often are fatigued or their response is dulled by low concentrations of substances. Thus, one may fail to detect low concentrations of some substances in air. This often happens when the concentration increases very slowly.

In addition to odor thresholds, users can institute change-out schedules based on reliable service-life data. Users should be warned to replace cartridges whenever they detect the odor of the substance and at the end of the service time indicated by the change-out schedule.

Some sorbents used in cartridges and canisters are harmed by high humidity, whereas others are harmed by very dry atmospheres. Therefore, when replacing these elements, unsealed cartridges and canisters should not be used. Also, remember that if the hazardous atmosphere is very moist or dry, the useful service time may be markedly reduced.

3. *Nonpowered Air-Purifying Respirators*

In addition to those limitations imposed by respiratory inlet coverings (see Chapter 2), particulate filter elements, and sorbent cartridges and canisters, further limitations of nonpowered air-purifying respirators should be considered.

An important disadvantage is the negative air pressure created inside the respiratory inlet covering during inhalation which can cause air contaminants to penetrate the covering if it fits poorly. Care should be taken to provide each wearer with a respirator that fits properly. This can best be accomplished by individual fittings and fit tests.

Other disadvantages of nonpowered air-purifying respirators include resistance to breathing and need for frequent replacement of air-purifying elements (except for disposable respirators).

4. Powered Air-Purifying Respirators

One advantage of powered air-purifying respirators is that they provide an airstream to the wearer. This airstream has the advantage of providing a cooling effect in warm temperatures, but can present a problem in cold temperatures. The decreased inhalation resistance makes the respirator possibly more comfortable to wear. Powered air-purifying respirators with loose fitting hoods or helmets have the advantage that since there are no large sealing surfaces on the face, some people who cannot wear a tight-fitting facepiece for such a reason as facial scars or facial hair can wear them.

Powered air-purifying respirators normally do not restrict mobility. In addition, these respirators offer minimal breathing resistance since the blower supplies the filtered air to the breathing zone of the wearer. Powered air-purifying respirators have limitations in addition to those imposed by respiratory inlet coverings, particulate filter elements and cartridges containing sorbents. A powered respirator's battery should be recharged periodically to ensure that the blower will deliver enough respirable air to the respiratory inlet covering. A battery has a limited useful life and cannot be recharged indefinitely. Battery replacement can be expensive.

The blower in most powered respirators has a high speed motor which will eventually wear out. Therefore, the blower will have to be replaced periodically. If the blower fails, the wearer of a powered respirator should go to the nearest safe area.

Other disadvantages include weight, bulk, complex design, the need for continual maintenance, at least daily replacement of air-purifying elements, and periodic replacement of batteries and blowers. Out-of-doors use presents special problems if hot or very cold air is supplied to the respiratory inlet covering.

Until recently, powered air-purifying respirators were considered positive pressure devices. Field studies by NIOSH as well as others, have indicated that these devices are not positive pressure, and that their assigned protection factors are inappropriately high.

III. Atmosphere-Supplying Respirators

Examples of respirators that provide breathing gas from a source independent of the surrounding atmosphere instead of purifying the atmosphere are shown in Figures 2-4 thru 2-6. The different types are classified according to the method by which the breathing gas is supplied and used and the method used to regulate the gas supply.

A. Self-Contained Breathing Apparatus

The distinguishing feature of all self-contained breathing apparatus (SCBA) is that the wearer need not be connected to a stationary breathing gas source, such as an air compressor. Instead, enough air or oxygen for up to 4 hours, depending on the design, is carried by the wearer. As Fig. 2-4 shows, SCBAs are classified as "closed circuit" or "open circuit."

1. Closed Circuit

Another name for closed-circuit SCBAs is "rebreather" device, indicative of the mode of operation. The breathing gas is rebreathed after the exhaled carbon dioxide has been removed and the oxygen content restored by a compressed or liquid oxygen source or an oxygen generating solid. Descriptions and certification tests for the closed-circuit apparatus are given in Subpart H of 30 CFR 11.

These devices are designed primarily for 1 to 4 hour use in oxygen deficient and/or IDLH atmospheres such as might be encountered during mine rescues or in confined spaces. They have been used since the early 1900's when the Gibbs and McCaa devices were developed. Few major design changes have been made since then, a significant commentary on their acceptance and good performance. [NOTE: 30 CFR 11 prescribes certification for mine rescue only devices that give 1-hour or more performance. Devices that give 30-minute or longer performance may be certified for auxiliary mine rescue service.]

Because negative pressure is created in the facepiece of non-positive pressure apparatus during inhalation, there is increased leakage potential. Therefore, negative pressure closed-circuit SCBA should be used in atmospheres immediately dangerous to life or health (IDLH) only where their long term use capability is necessary, as in mine rescue. For use in oxygen deficient atmospheres over long periods, closed-circuit SCBA are satisfactory. Positive pressure closed-circuit SCBA are a significant new respirator development and are described in Chapter 6, **New Developments at NIOSH.**

Two basic types of closed-circuit SCBA are presently available. One uses a cylinder of compressed oxygen and the other a solid oxygen generating substance. Figure 2-41 shows a typical closed-circuit SCBA with a small cylinder of compressed oxygen. Breathable air is supplied from an inflatable bag. The exhaled air passes through a granular solid adsorbent that removes the carbon dioxide, thereby reducing the flow back into the breathing bag. The bag collapses so that a pressure plate bears against the admission valve, which opens and admits more pure oxygen that reinflates the bag. Thus, the consumed oxygen is replaced. The advantage of the rebreathing process is that only the oxygen supply need be provided, as all the other air constituents except the waste carbon dioxide are recirculated. The advantage of this type of device is its long term (1- to 4-hour) protection. Disadvantages include the bulk of the SCBA and the negative pressure created in the facepiece during inhalation from some closed-circuit SCBA. As previously discussed, it is now possible for certification of positive pressure devices which offer a higher level of protection. Figure 2-42 shows a closed-circuit SCBA in use.

The second type of closed-circuit SCBA (Fig. 2-43) uses an oxygen-generating solid, usually potassium superoxide (KO_2). The H_2O and CO_2 in the exhaled breath react with the KO_2 to release O_2.

$$2\ KO_2 + CO_2 + H_2O \dashrightarrow K_2CO_3 + 1.5\ O_2 + H_2O,$$
$$2\ KO_2 + 2CO_2 + H_2O \dashrightarrow 2KH\ CO_3 + 1.5\ O_2.$$

The O_2 is not released until the wearer's exhaled breath reaches the canister. Thus, there is a short time lag between when the canister is initiated and O_2 flow begins. This has been overcome in some devices by providing a "quick start" feature known as a chlorate candle, a canister section filled with mixed sodium chlorate and iron. Oxygen flow is started by striking the device, somewhat like lighting a match. This is designed to provide enough oxygen until the potassium superoxide in the canister begins to function.

Oxygen is continually released at a high flow rate into the breathing bag(s) which acts as a reservoir to accommodate breathing fluctuations. A pressure relief valve and saliva trap release the excess pressure created in the facepiece by oxygen flow and nitrogen buildup.

This closed-circuit apparatus is lighter and simpler than the cylinder type. However, it is useful for only about one hour and, once initiated, cannot be turned off. The precautions are the same as for the compressed oxygen unit.

Recently, as a result of regulations promulgated by MSHA under the Coal Mine Health and Safety Act, a new device of closed-circuit SCBA, known as a self-contained self-rescuer (SCSR) was certified for use in underground mines in emergency situations. These devices are similar in design and operation as those already described. They include both compressed-oxygen and oxygen-generating types and offer a duration of one hour.

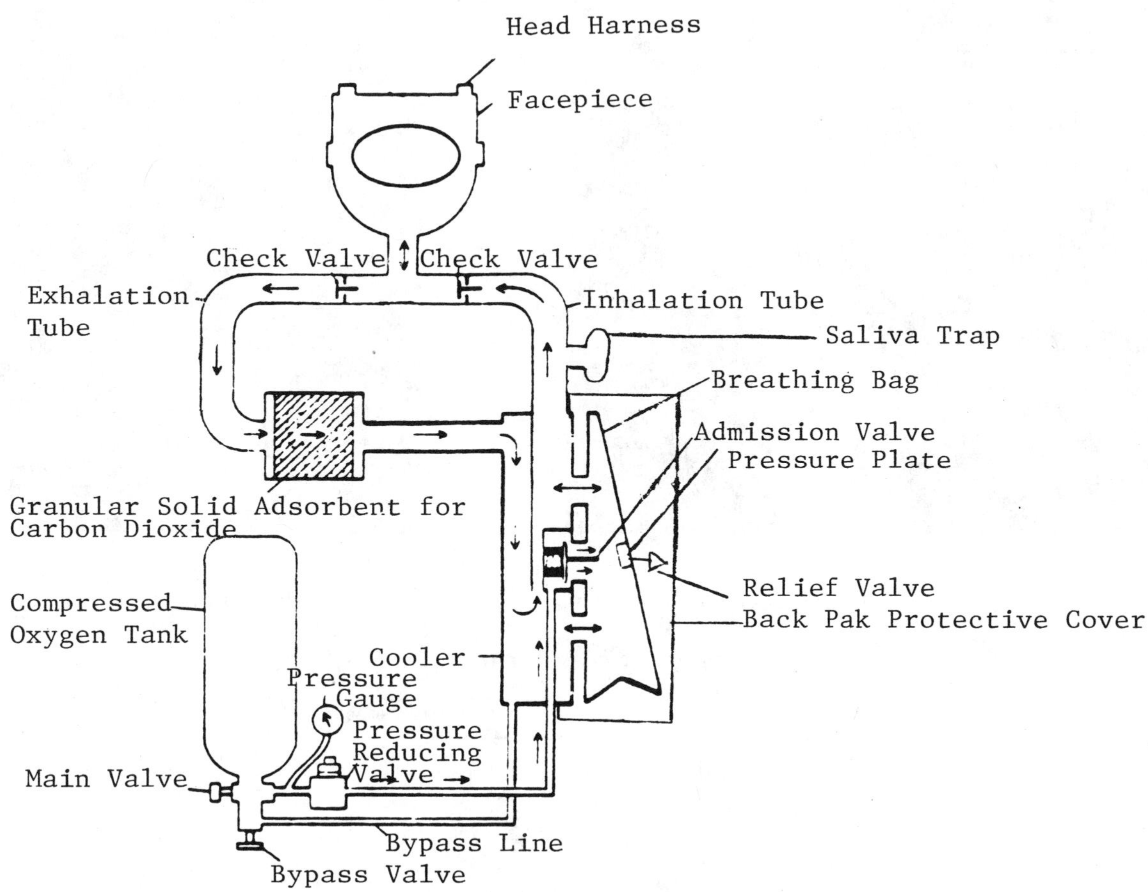

FIGURE 2-41. **Closed-circuit SCBA**

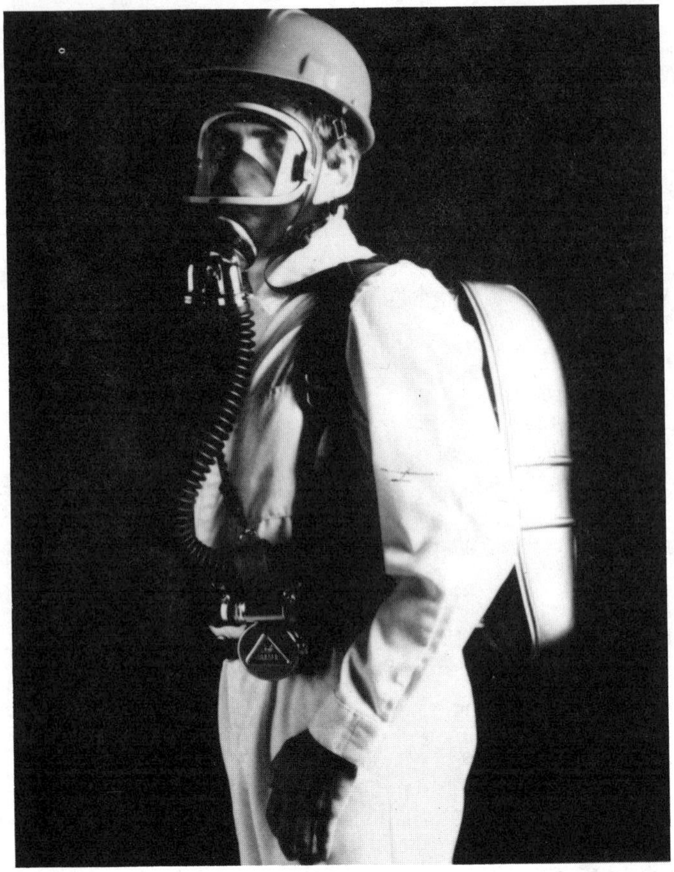

Photograph Courtesy of Draegerwerk

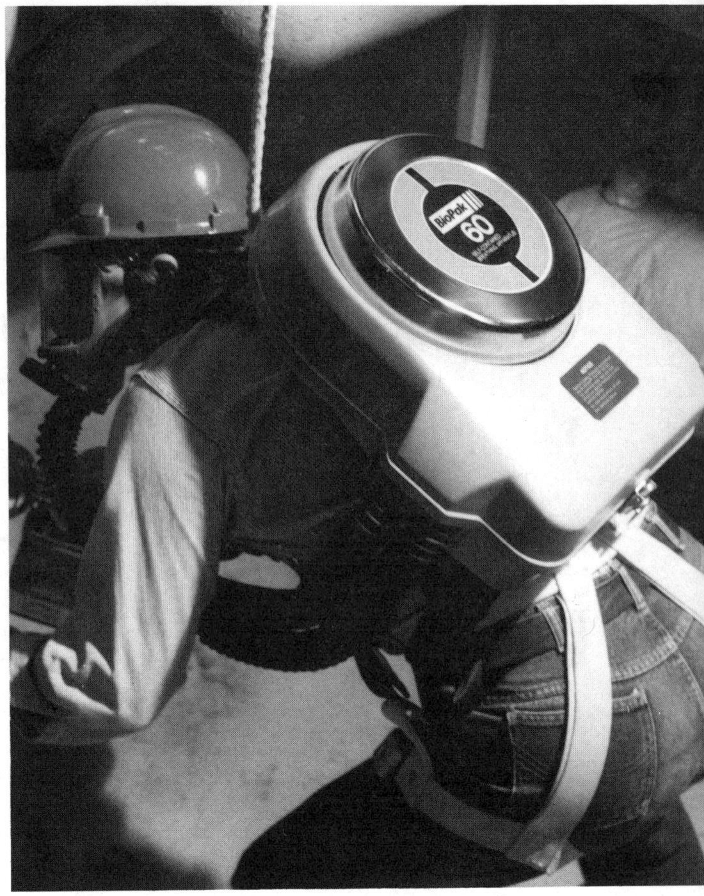

Photograph Courtesy of Rexnord

FIGURE 2-42. **Closed-circuit SCBA**

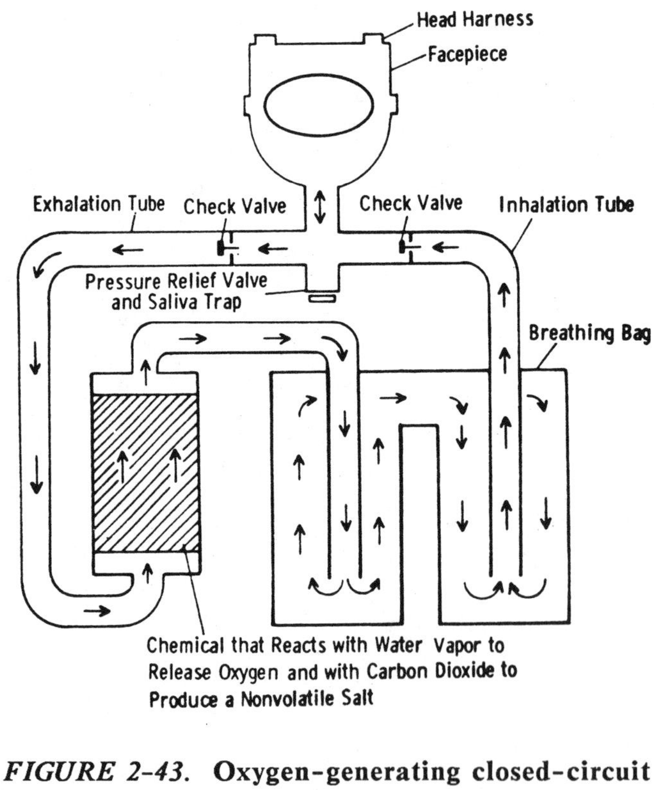

FIGURE 2-43. **Oxygen-generating closed-circuit SCBA**

SCSR are much smaller and weigh considerably less than closed-circuit SCBA for entry. Their weights range between 7 and 16 pounds. The SCSR are escape only apparatus and need not meet all the entry unit requirements of 30 CFR 11. Factors contributing to size and weight reduction include: a mouthpiece in place of a facepiece; the elimination of structural breathing bag protection; filament wound pressure gas vessels; smaller candles; lighter breathing bag material; single pendulum flow breathing tube; the elimination of bypass valve and warning whistle requirements; a more efficient utilization of carbon dioxide sorbent and/or oxygen-generating chemicals; lighter weight packaging material; and others. Figure 2-44 shows an oxygen-generating SCSR. These devices are not usually worn by the miner during mining operations as were the former filter self-rescuers (CO scrubbing only or air-purifying respirators), because they are larger and heavier than the filter self-rescuer. MSHA has strict enforceable storage and location requirements for SCSR. Since they are sealed and may not be opened except for emergency use, there are specific daily and 90 day required SCSR inspection periods and inspection procedures. SCSR with pressure vessels use active pressure gauge indicators. The chemical SCSR use passive storage life color indicators and inspection criteria.

2. Open Circuit

An open-circuit SCBA exhausts the exhaled air to the atmosphere instead of recirculating it. 30 CFR 11 does not specify which breathing gas must be used for these devices, but it is almost always compressed air. Compressed oxygen cannot be used in a device designed for compressed air because minute amounts of oil or other foreign matter in the device components can cause an explosion. In fact, 30 CFR 11 prohibits certification of any device designed to permit interchangeable use of oxygen and air. It is an accepted safety rule that :

OXYGEN NEVER BE USED IN A DEVICE UNLESS IT IS SPECIFICALLY DESIGNED FOR THAT PURPOSE.

Figure 2-45 shows typical open-circuit SCBA. A cylinder of high pressure (2000-4500 psi) compressed air supplies air to a regulator that reduces the pressure for delivery to the facepiece. This regulator also serves as a flow regulator by passing air to the facepiece on demand. The regulator is either mounted directly to the facepiece or a flexible corrugated hose connects the regulator to the respiratory inlet covering, usually a full-facepiece.

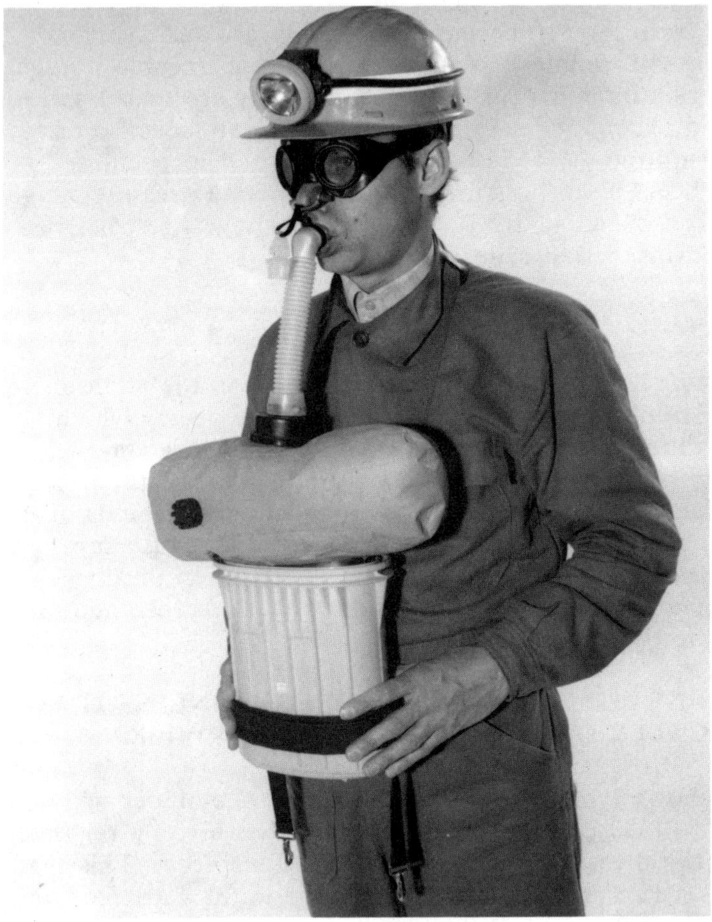

Photograph Courtesy of Draegerwerk

FIGURE 2-44. **Oxygen-generating self-contained self-rescuer**

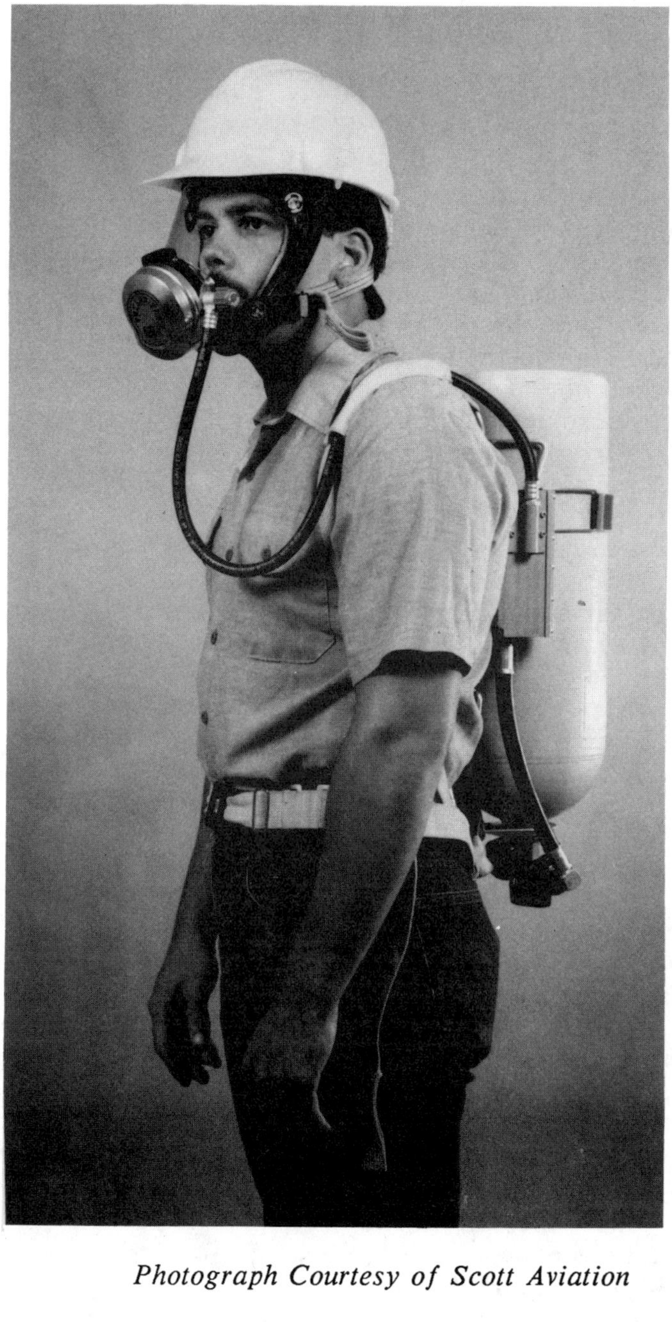

Photograph Courtesy of Scott Aviation

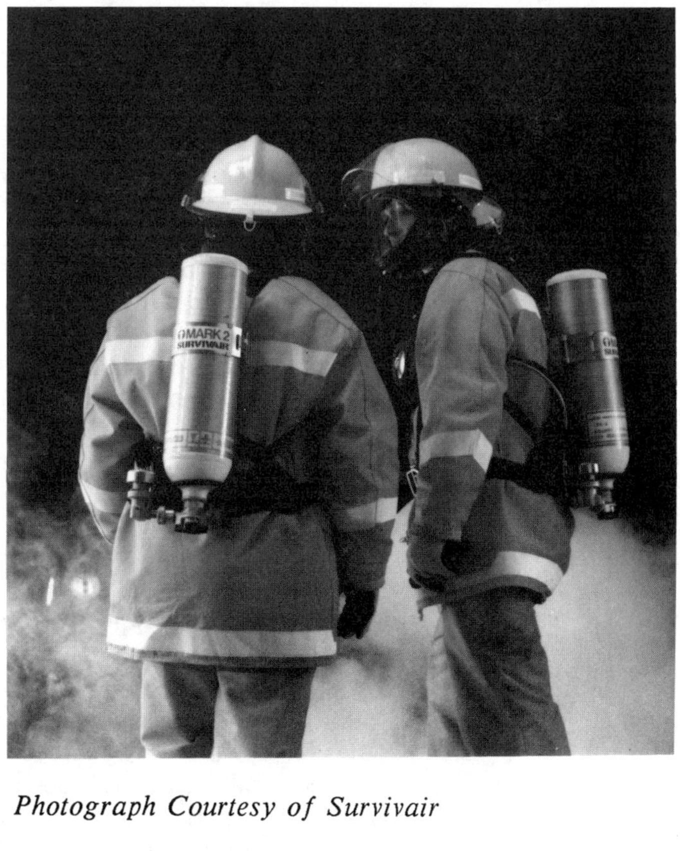

Photograph Courtesy of Survivair

FIGURE 2-45. **Open-circuit SCBA**

Because it has to provide the total breathing volume requirements, since there is no recirculation, the service life of the open-circuit SCBA is usually shorter than the closed-circuit SCBA. Most open-circuit SCBA have a service life of 30 minutes to 60 minutes based on NIOSH breathing machine tests as prescribed in 30 CFR 11 (11.85-10). NIOSH certifies units with less than 1 hour, but not less than 30 minutes service for auxiliary mine rescue. Open-circuit SCBA are widely used in fire fighting and for industrial emergencies. SCBA with less than 30 minutes service time are certified, generally for escape use only. Escape SCBAs are also certified in combination with supplied-air, airline respirators.

Two types of open-circuit SCBA are available, "demand" or "pressure demand." The difference is very important and best explained by describing the operation of a typical open-circuit SCBA regulator. In a "demand" or negative pressure type regulator, air at approximately 2000 psi is supplied to the regulator through the main valve (Fig. 2-46). A bypass valve passes air to the facepiece in case of regulator failure. Downstream from the main valve, a two-stage regulator reduces the pressure to approximately 50-100 psi at the admission valve, which is actuated by movement of a diaphragm and its associated levers. The admission valve stays closed as long as positive pressure in the facepiece (during exhalation) forces the diaphragm away from the valve assembly. Inhalation creates negative pressure in the facepiece, and the diaphragm contracts, opening the admission valve and allowing air into the facepiece. In other words, air flows into the facepiece only on "demand" by the wearer, hence the name.

Recent studies indicate that a demand-type SCBA is no more protective than an air-purifying respirator with the same facepiece. Therefore, a demand-type open-circuit SCBA should not be used in IDLH atmospheres. Like closed-circuit SCBA, however, they may be adequate against oxygen-deficient atmospheres.

A pressure-demand or positive pressure regulator is very similar to a demand type except that there is usually a spring between the diaphragm and the outside case of the regulator. This spring tends to hold the admission valve slightly open, theoretically allowing continual air flow into the facepiece. This would be true except that all pressure-demand devices have a special exhalation valve that maintains about 1.5-3 inches H_2O positive back pressure in the facepiece, and opens only when the pressure exceeds that value. This combination of modified regulator and special exhalation valve is designed to maintain positive pressure in the facepiece at all times. Under certain conditions of work a momentary negative pressure may occur in the wearer's breathing zone, although the regulator still supplies additional air on

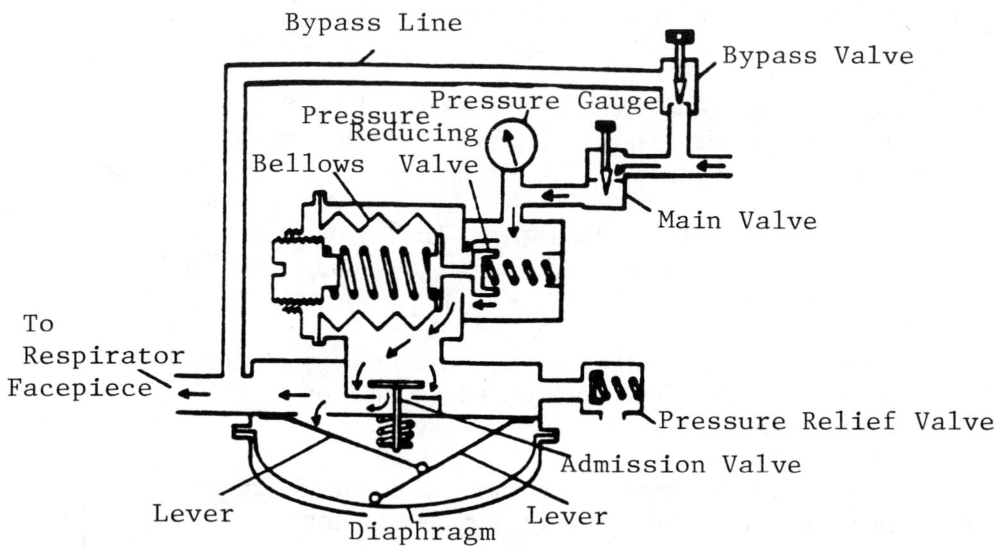

FIGURE 2-46. **Open-circuit demand SCBA regulator**

"demand." Because of the positive pressure, any leakage should be outward; therefore, a pressure-demand SCBA provides very good protection. Contrary to common belief, the pressure-demand SCBA has the same service time as a demand version of the same device, if it seals well on the wearer's face. Any leakage increases air consumption and decreases service time.

A FACEPIECE WHOSE EXHALATION VALVE IS DESIGNED FOR DEMAND OPERATION CANNOT BE USED WITH A PRESSURE-DEMAND REGULATOR, AS AIR WILL FLOW CONTINUALLY AND QUICKLY EXHAUST THE AIR SUPPLY.

Some open-circuit SCBA can be switched from demand to pressure-demand operation. The demand mode should be used **only** for donning and adjusting the apparatus in order to conserve air and should be switched to "pressure demand" for actual use.

Several required safety features on all certified entry (both closed and open circuit) SCBA provide additional protection. Among these are:

- o pressure gauges or liquid level gauges visible to the wearer which indicate the quantity of gas or liquid (air or oxygen) remaining in the cylinder

- o remaining service life indicators or warning devices that signal alarm when only 20-25% of service time or service volume remains

- o bypass valves, in case the first and second stage reducer or regulator fails and it is necessary to conserve or provide respirable air

- o fittings on devices that use compressed or liquid oxygen which are incompatible with compressed or liquid air fittings.

The choice of demand or pressure-demand open-circuit SCBA should be based on thorough evaluation of the respiratory hazards. MSHA and NIOSH continue to issue certifications for both types since the demand type is still used in many industrial applications. In a potentially IDLH atmosphere, a pressure-demand SCBA should most certainly be used.

In addition to entry, SCBA are also certified for escape from IDLH. These escape-only SCBA are generally of short duration, that is, 3, 5 or 10 minutes, and are small in both size and weight. The compressed-air container is usually hip- or back-mounted with the air valve in a readily accessible position for immediate activation. The facepiece may be donned quickly by simply tightening the headband straps or a hood may be furnished for quick donning of the escape SCBA. Figure 2-47 shows two hood-type, escape-only SCBA.

B. Supplied-Air Respirators

1. *Airline respirators (Types C and CE)*

Airline respirators as described in 30 CFR 11, Subpart J use compressed air from a stationary source delivered through a hose under pressure. 30 CFR 11 specifies that the pressure shall not exceed 125 psi at the point where the hose attaches to the air supply. A manufacturer submitting an airline respirator for certification must specify the operating pressure and the hose length, from 25 to 300 feet. At the lowest pressure and longest hose length, the device must deliver at least 170 Lpm to a helmet or hood. At the highest pressure and shortest hose length the flowrate must not exceed 425 Lpm to a helmet or hood. The equivalent airflows to a tight-fitting facepiece are 115 Lpm and 425 Lpm, respectively.

Airline respirators are available in demand, pressure-demand, and continuous-flow configurations (see Figure 2-5). The respiratory inlet covering may be a facepiece, helmet, hood, or complete suit, although there are presently no approval tests for suits.

A demand or pressure-demand airline respirator is very similar in basic operation to a demand or pressure-demand open circuit SCBA, except that the air is supplied through a small diameter hose from a stationary source of compressed air rather than from a portable air source. Because the air pressure is limited to 125 psi, regulators for demand and pressure-demand airline respirators need only single stage reduction. Otherwise, the demand and pressure-demand airline regulators are similar in operation to the demand and pressure-demand SCBA regulators respectively. Figure 2-48 shows a typical demand type regulator. Figure 2-49 shows a typical pressure-demand airline respirator with a tight-fitting facepiece. Note that the regulator sometimes is mounted on the facepiece or worn on the wearer's chest.

Continuous-flow airline respirators maintain air flow at all times, rather than only on demand. In place of a demand or pressure-demand regulator, an air flow control valve or orifice partially controls the air flow. According to 30 CFR 11, a flow of at least 115 Lpm to a tight fitting facepiece and 170 Lpm to

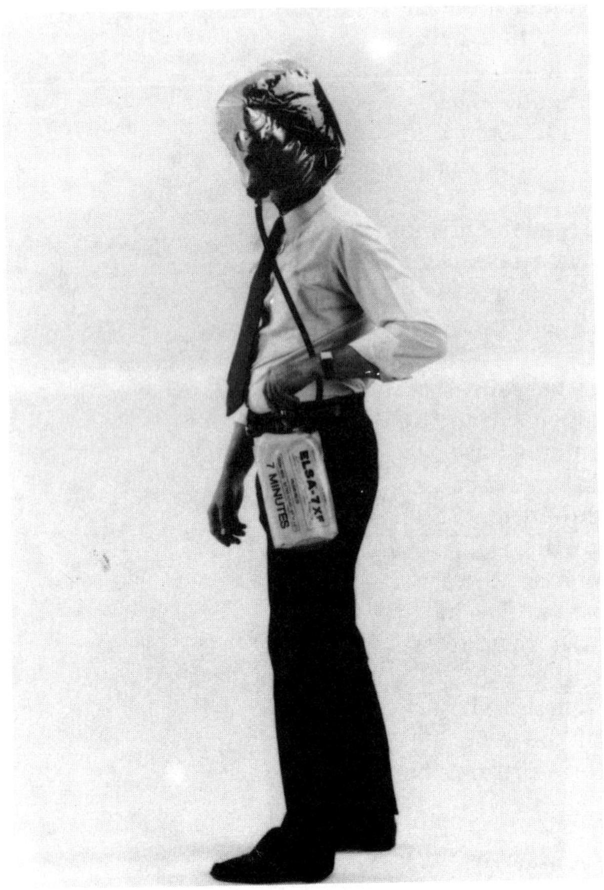

Photograph Courtesy of ISI

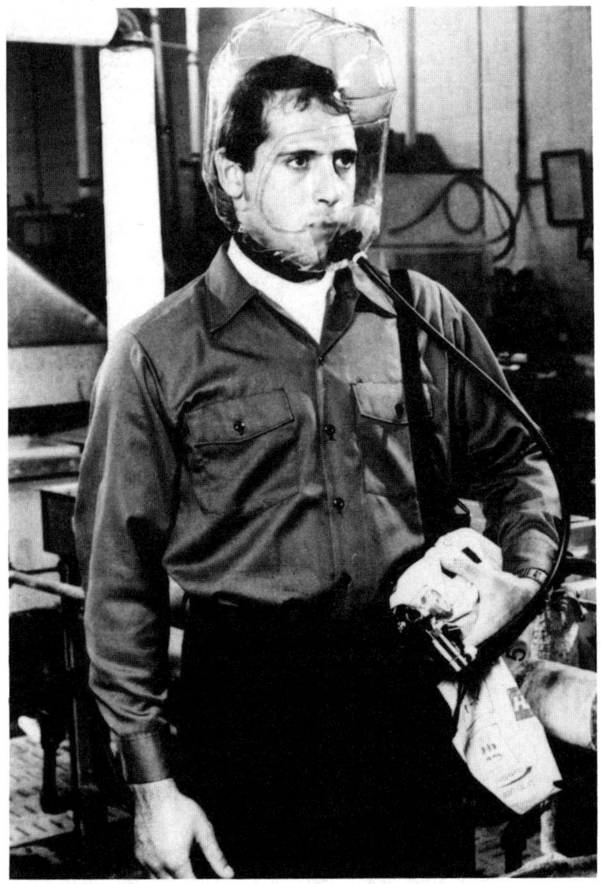

Photograph Courtesy of North

FIGURE 2-47. **Typical escape-only ESCBA**

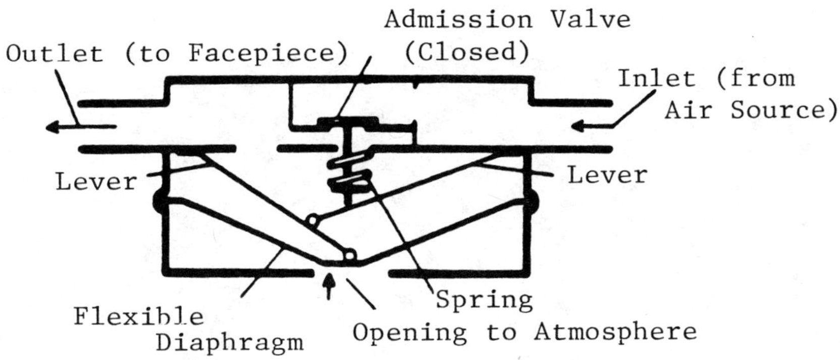

EXHALATION. High pressure of exhaled air stretches diaphragm. Resulting lever movement and spring action close admission valve, and air flow ceases.

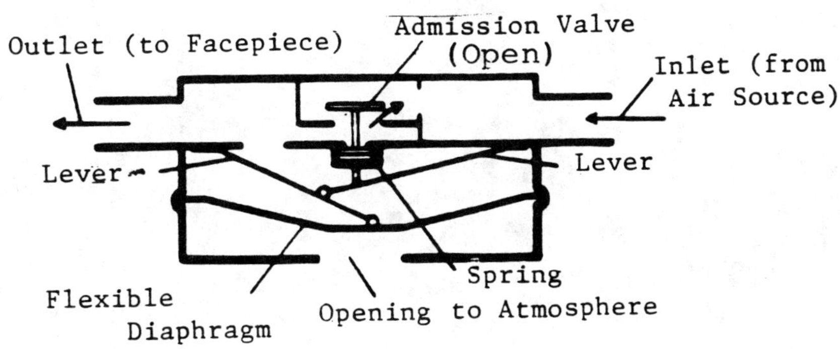

INHALATION. Low pressure created by inhalation pulls diaphragm inward. Resulting lever movement compresses spring and opens admission valve. Air flows through valve.

FIGURE 2-48. **Typical demand-type air flow regulator**

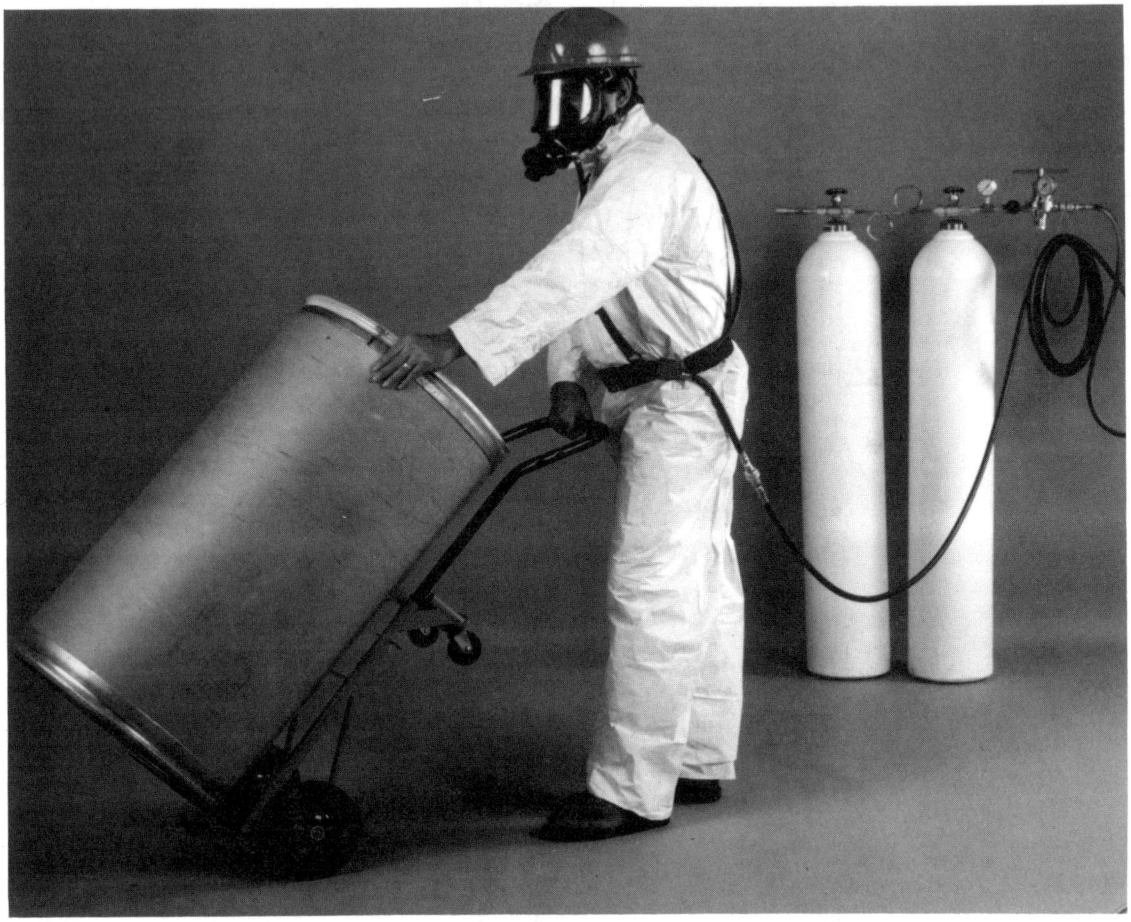

Photograph Courtesy of ISI

FIGURE 2-49. **Pressure-demand airline respirator**

a loose-fitting hood or helmet must be maintained at lowest air pressure and longest hose length specified. This means that by design, either the control valve cannot be closed completely, or a continually open bypass is provided to allow air to flow around the valve and maintain the required minimum rates.

Some special valves known as vortex tubes are available with some certified airline respirators. These valves fractionate the airstream into two high speed airflow components. One component becomes cool from adiabatic expansion while the other component becomes warm from adiabatic compression. Either component can be utilized in valve design to cool or heat the respirable air provided to the user for comfort and physiological support.

Figure 2-50 depicts a typical continuous-flow airline respirator with a tight-fitting facepiece. Notice the air-purifying element on the air-supply line. Figure 2-51 shows typical airline respirators, which may be obtained with half masks and full-facepieces. Figure 2-52 shows continuous-flow airline respirators with hoods.

Although addition of an air-purifying element in the supply line upstream of the air-supply hose attachment can help clean the air, other precautions also should be taken to ensure breathing air quality. The air supply to airline respirators is required to meet the requirements for Type I gaseous air (Grade D or higher quality) set forth by the Compressed Gas Association Commodity Specification for Air, G-7.1. Furthermore, OSHA requires that a breathing air compressor have certain safety devices to protect the air quality (see Chapter 3).

Airline respirators with special items to protect the wearer's head and neck from rebounding abrasive material may have facepieces, helmets, or hoods. Plastic, glass, and metal wire screen are used to protect the lenses of facepieces and the windows of helmets and hoods against the rebounding material. These respirators are known as abrasive-blasting airline respirators or Type "CE" supplied-air respirators.

Figure 2-53 shows Type "CE" respirators in use. Note the protective screen over the lens and the heavy apron on the abrasive- blasting hood.

Full suit airline respirators are available. They provide air not only for breathing but also to isolate the whole body from the surrounding atmosphere. They are used against substances that irritate or corrode the skin or which may penetrate the

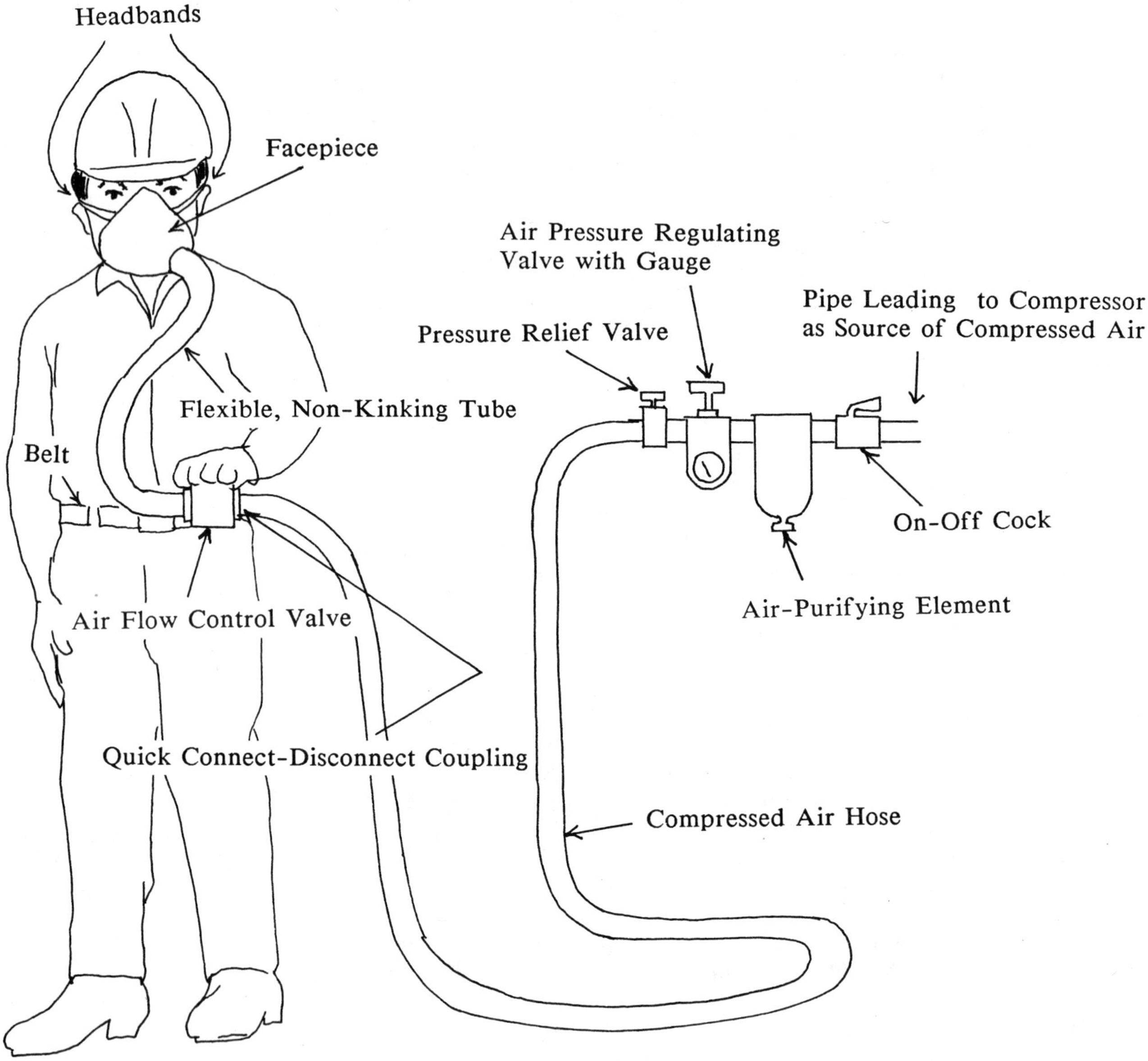

FIGURE 2-50. **Continuous-flow airline respirator**

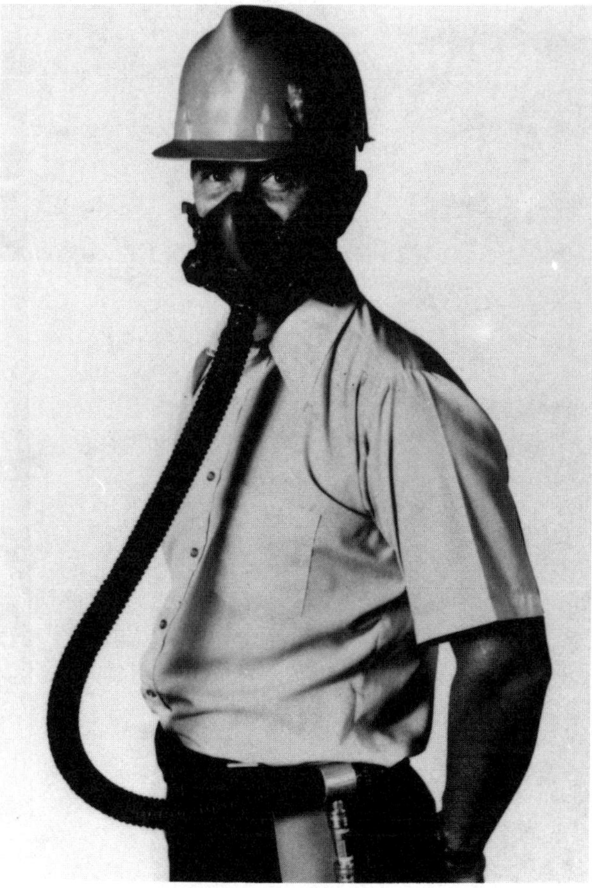

Photograph Courtesy of
U.S. Safety Service

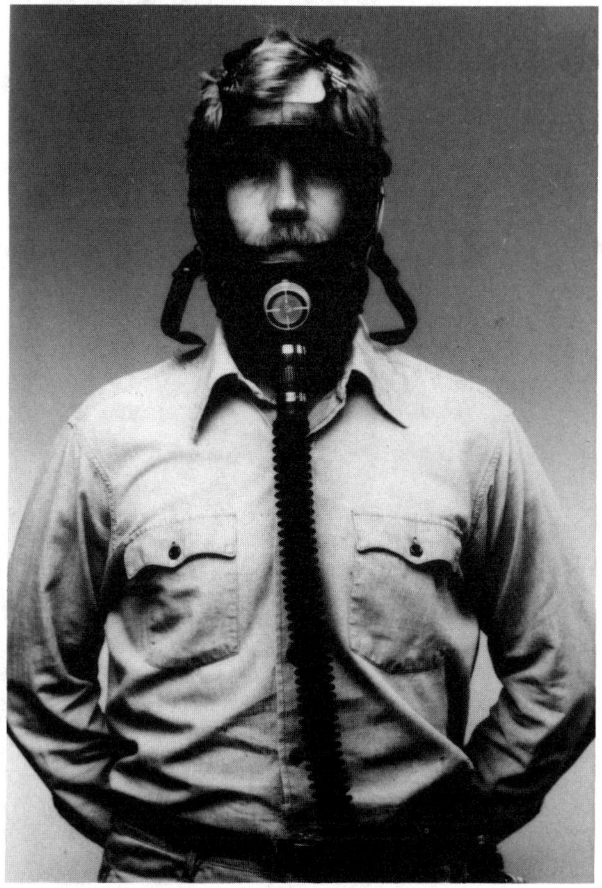

Photograph Courtesy of
Willson Safety Products

FIGURE 2-51. **Half mask and full-facepiece continous flow airline respirators**

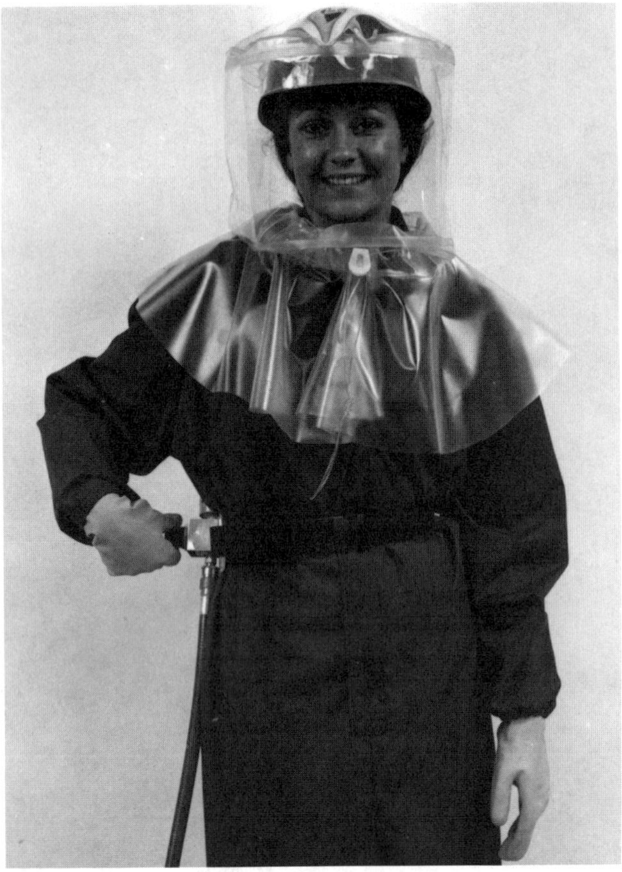

Photograph Courtesy of
Standard Safety Equipment

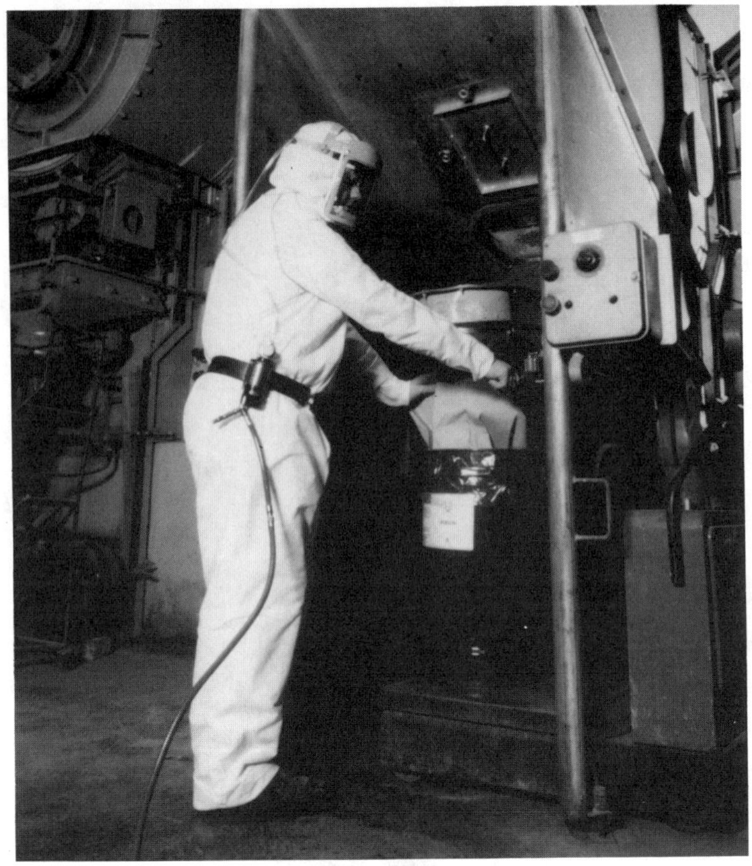

Photograph Courtesy of
Safety Products Limited

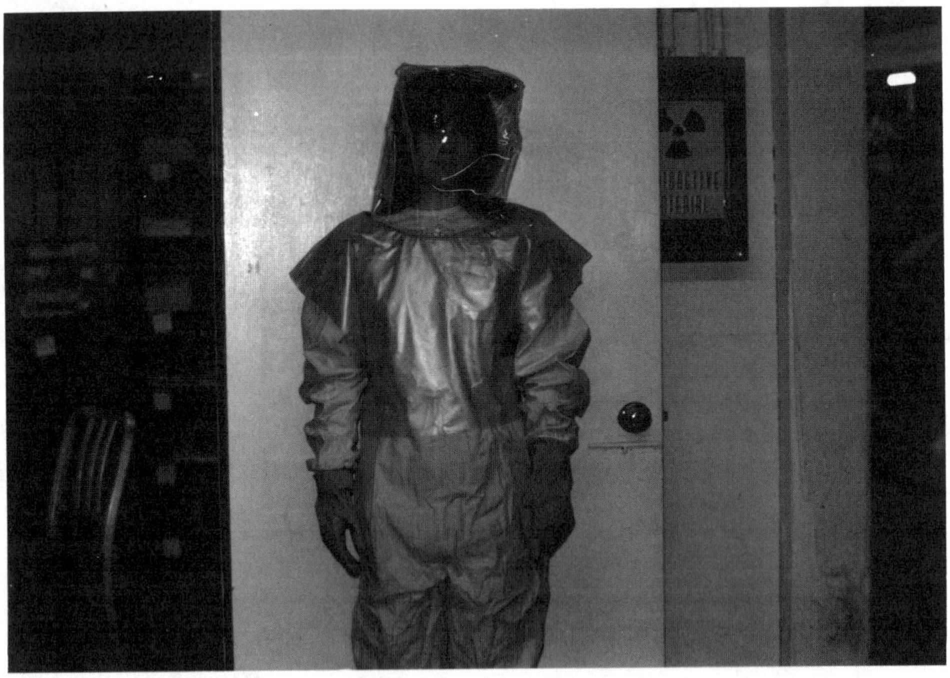

Photograph Courtesy of Mohawk Industries

FIGURE 2-52. **Continuous flow airline respirators with hoods**

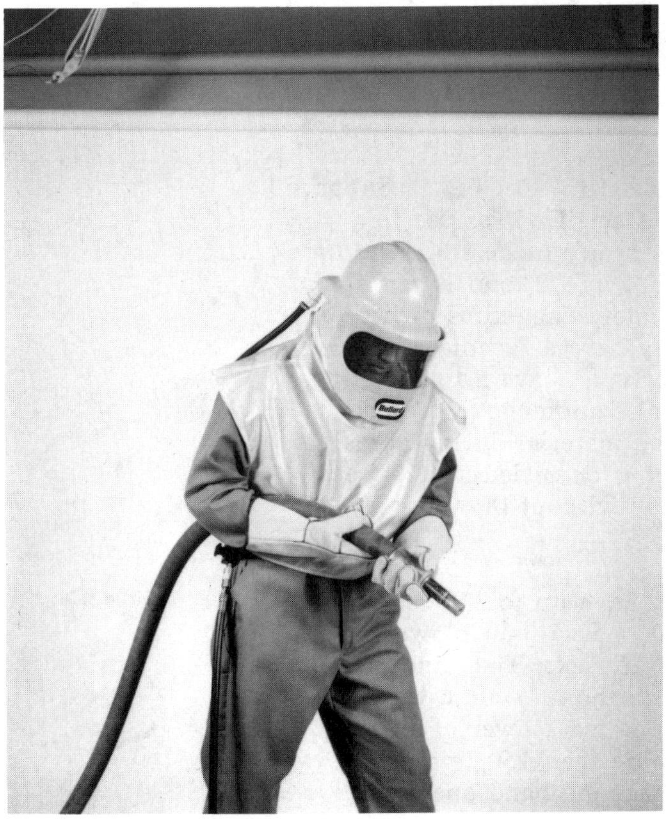

Photograph Courtesy of Bullard

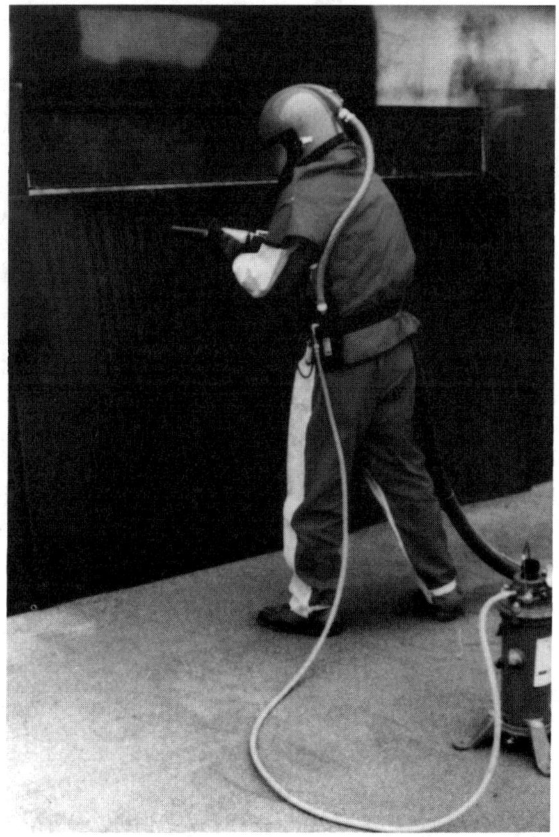

Photograph Courtesy of Clemco

***FIGURE 2-53.* Typical Type CE abrasive-blast airline respirator**

skin to produce toxic effects. Presently, 30 CFR 11 does not provide for certification of airline suits.

2. Hose Masks

Hose masks supply air from an uncontaminated source through a strong, large diameter hose to a respiratory inlet covering. Two types are available. One has a hand or motor operated air blower that pushes low pressure air through the hose to the respiratory inlet covering. The blower is designed so that air flows freely through it when it is not in operation. Therefore, if the blower fails, the wearer can still inhale respirable air by normal breathing. The other type of hose mask has no blower and requires the wearer to inhale through the hose.

The hose mask with a blower is categorized by 30 CFR 11 Subpart J as a Type "A" supplied-air respirator and is certified for use in atmospheres not immediately dangerous to life or health. The hose mask without a blower is categorized as Type "B" and is certified for use only in atmospheres not immediately dangerous to life or health. The hose mask with blower may have a facepiece, helmet, or hood, but the hose mask without blower must have a tight fitting facepiece. Hose masks may have special equipment to protect the wearer's head and neck from rebounding material during abrasive blasting. Such a hose mask with blower is classified as a Type "AE" supplied-air respirator, and the one without blower is classified as Type "BE."

A certified hose mask with blower may have up to 300 feet of air supply hose in multiples of 25 feet, but one without blower may have only up to 75 feet in multiples of 25 feet. The hand or motor operated blower must deliver air through the maximum length of hose at not less than 50 Lpm. The motor operated blower of a device with 50 feet of hose must deliver no more than 150 Lpm. However, no maximum air flow rate is specified for the hand operated blower.

Currently there are only three hose masks certified. They are not widely used in industrial applications. They are heavy, cumbersome and offer only a very low protection factor.

C. Combination Respirators

MSHA/NIOSH may certify respirators assembled from two or more types of respirators in combination as prescribed in 30 CFR 11.63(b).

To date MSHA/NIOSH have certified several types of air-purifying units or SCBA in combination with the Type C supplied-air respirator.

1. Combination Supplied-Air/Air-Purifying Respirator

One type of combination respirator that MSHA/NIOSH has certified is the Type C supplied-air and air-purifying respirator as shown in Figure 2-54. These devices are certified under the class of the air-purifying element since it is the component in the combination which provides the least protection to the user. This type of respirator consists of facepiece; regulator or control valve, if necessary; breathing tube, if necessary; belt or harness; supplied-air hose; and air-purifying element. The air-purifying element may be a canister, chemical cartridge, or particulate filter. It is mounted either directly on the facepiece or on an adapter which is worn on the belt.

The supplied-air portion of the respirator can be either Type C continuous-flow or pressure-demand.

An advantage of this type of respirator is that the wearer has respiratory protection while entering (in some cases) and leaving without being connected to an airline. The air-purifying element weighs less than a self-contained breathing apparatus cylinder. The disadvantage is that they have the limitations of the air-purifying element, and therefore, can be used only for specific conditions. Depending upon the specific respirator, the air-purifying element will have one of the following restrictions (consult the certification label of the respirator to determine which applies):

a. no restrictions

b. air-purifying element can be used only to: (1) enter prior to connecting to air supply, (2) egress after disconnecting or loss of air, or (3) to move from one air supply to another

c. escape only after loss of air.

2. Combination Supplied-Air/SCBA Respirator

To be usable in an IDLH atmosphere, an airline respirator must have an auxiliary air supply to protect against potential failure of the primary supply. This is provided by adding a self-contained cylinder of high pressure compressed air to a Type "C" or "CE" airline respirator. The auxiliary air supply may be certified for 3-, 5-, or 10-minute service time, or for 15 minutes or longer (see Figure 2-55). The certification tests for these combination devices are found in 30 CFR 11, Subpart H, "Self-Contained Breathing Apparatus." The devices shown in Figure 2-55 are only representative of this general class; designs vary widely.

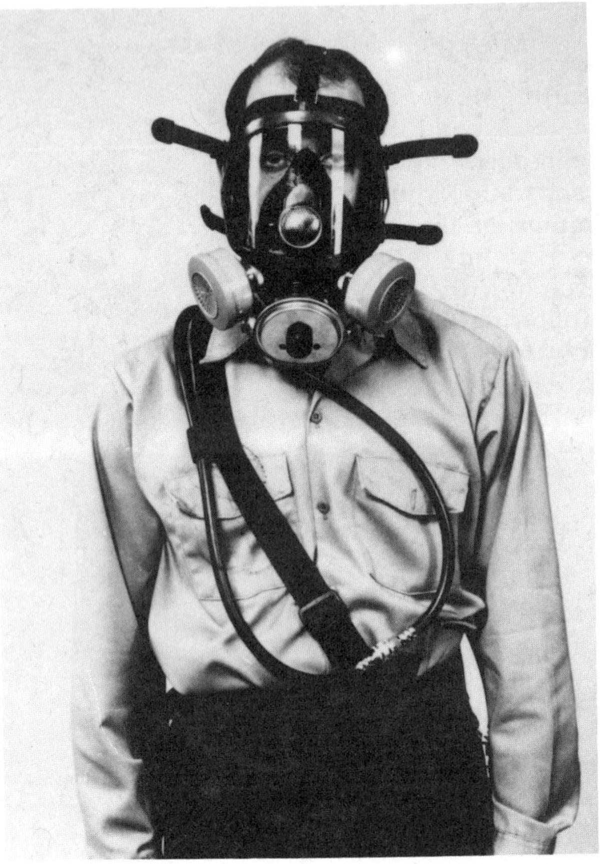

Photograph Courtesy of North Safety Products, Inc.

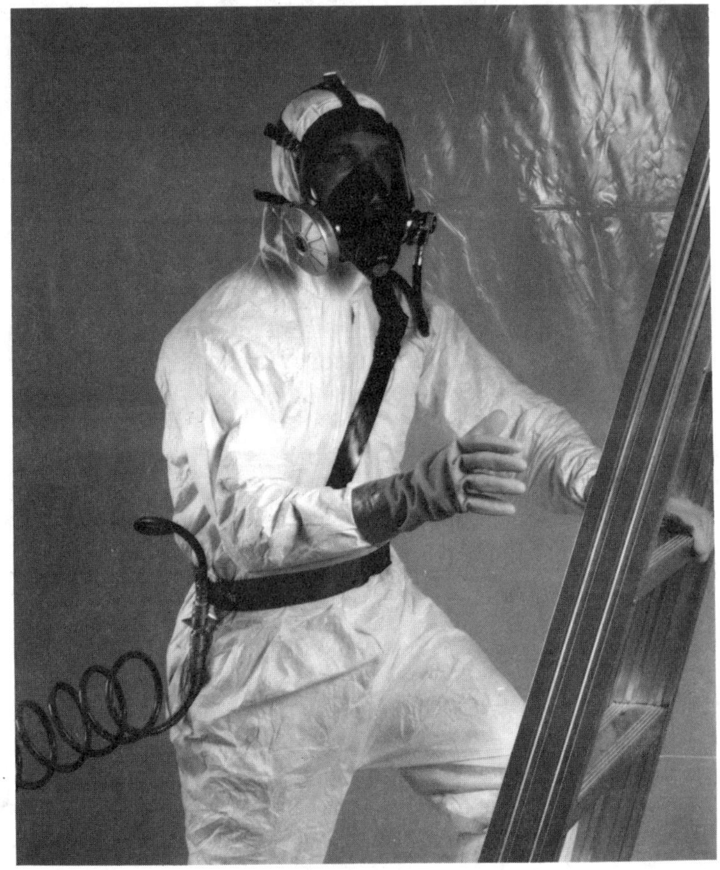

Photograph Courtesy of Racal Airstream

***FIGURE 2-54.* Combination supplied-air respirator with escape only high efficiency filter**

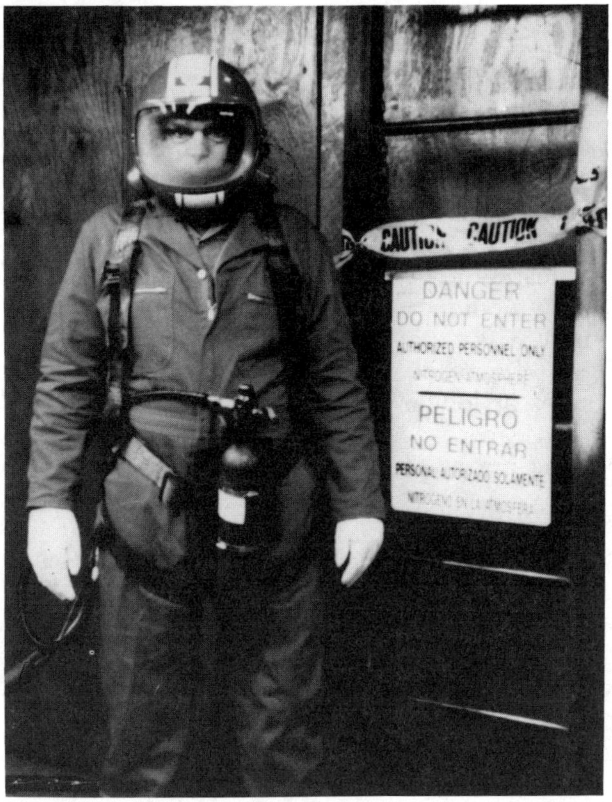
CAUTION CAUTION
DANGER
DO NOT ENTER
AUTHORIZED PERSONNEL ONLY
PELIGRO
NO ENTRAR
PERSONAL AUTORIZADO SOLAMENTE

Photograph Courtesy of Powermaster, Inc.

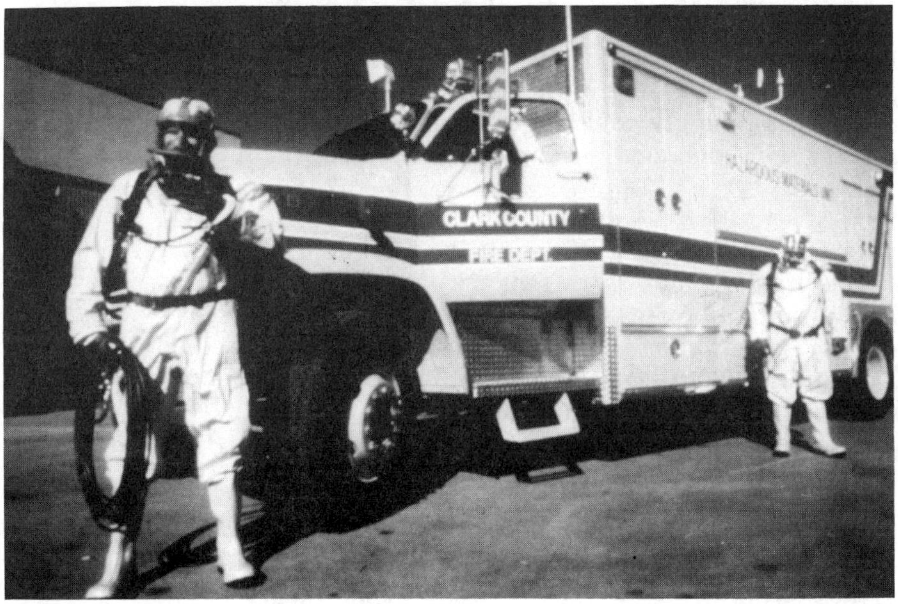

Photograph Courtesy of Interspiro

FIGURE 2-55. **Combination supplied-air/SCBA**

Because of the short service time of the self-contained breathing air supply, combination units generally are used for emergency entry into and escape from IDLH atmospheres. The self-contained portion of the device is used only when the airline portion fails and the wearer must escape, or when it may be necessary to disconnect the air line temporarily while changing locations. A combination airline and SCBA may be used for emergency entry into a hazardous atmosphere (to connect the airline), if the SCBA part is classified for 15 minutes or longer service and not more than 20% of the air supply's rated capacity is used during entry. It is seldom used as a routine means of protection, as the open-circuit SCBA might be.

D. Advantages and Disadvantages of Atmosphere-Supplying Respirators

1. Airline Respirators

A great advantage of the airline respirator is that it may be used for long continuous periods. Other advantages are minimal breathing resistance and discomfort, light weight, low bulk, moderate initial cost, and relatively low operating cost.

The biggest disadvantage of supplied-air respirators is that loss of the source of respirable air supplied to the respiratory inlet covering eliminates any protection to the wearer. Such loss may be caused by cutting, burning, kinking, or crushing the supply air hose, by air compressor failure, or by depletion of the respirable air in a storage tank. Possible loss of respirable air supports the NIOSH recommendation against airline respirator use in IDLH atmospheres. However, an airline respirator with an auxiliary self-contained air supply could be used in such atmospheres because the auxiliary self-contained air supply always can be used in escape.

The trailing air supply hose of the airline respirator severely restricts the wearer's mobility. This may make the airline respirator unsuitable for those who move frequently between widely separated work stations. A combination airline and self-contained breathing apparatus may be suitable if the supply of self-contained breathing air is adequate for the time required to move from place to place. A coiled airline hose provided with some MSHA/NIOSH certified devices will further promote wearer mobility at the worksite.

Airline respirators that operate in the demand mode have negative air pressure inside the respiratory inlet covering during inhalation which permits the contaminated atmosphere to leak into the respiratory inlet covering if it fits poorly. However, airline respirators that operate in the pressure-demand mode are designed to have positive air pressure inside the respiratory inlet covering which helps to ensure that contaminated air will not leak in. Thus, an airline respirator operating in the pressure-demand mode provides much better protection than one that operates in the demand mode.

2. *Hose Masks*

Advantages of the hose mask without blower are its theoretically long use periods and its simple construction, low bulk, easy maintenance, and minimal operating cost. An advantage of the hose mask with blower is its minimal resistance to breathing.

Obviously, air pressure inside the respiratory inlet covering of the hose mask with no blower is negative during inhalation, so contaminated air may leak in if the covering fits poorly. Therefore, hose masks, with and without blower, are certified only for use in non-IDLH atmospheres.

The trailing air supply hose of the hose mask also severely limits mobility, so it may be unsuitable for those who move frequently among widely separated work stations.

A severe restriction of the hose mask without blower is that it is limited to a maximum hose length of only 75 ft. Also, it requires the wearer to inhale against the resistance to air flow offered by the air hose which may become significant during heavy work. Inhaling against this resistance strains the wearer and may cause fatigue.

3. *Self-Contained Breathing Apparatus*

Because the SCBA wearer carries his own supply of respirable air, he is independent of the surrounding atmosphere. A great advantage of such apparatus is that it allows comparatively free movement over an unlimited area.

The bulk and weight of most SCBAs make them unsuitable for strenuous work or use in a constricted space. The limited service life makes them unsuitable for routine use for long continuous periods. The short service life of open-circuit type devices may limit them to use where the wearer can go conveniently and quickly from a hazardous atmosphere to a safe atmosphere to change the tank of supply air.

Open-circuit SCBA are normally less expensive to purchase and use than closed-circuit SCBA. Additionally, the open-circuit SCBA requires less maintenance and fewer inspections.

The demand-type open-circuit SCBA and most closed-circuit SCBA have negative air pressure inside the respiratory inlet covering during inhalation so contaminated air can leak in if they fit poorly. The pressure-demand type open-circuit SCBA and those closed-circuit SCBA that are positive pressure devices provide very good protection because the air inside the respiratory inlet covering is normally at positive pressure which helps to keep the contaminated atmosphere from leaking in.

CHAPTER 3

RESPIRATOR SELECTION

I. Regulatory Requirements

The selection, use, and maintenance of respirators in the United States is presently regulated by several Federal agencies. The agencies, the acts which authorize their activities, and the current regulations relating to selection, use, and maintenance of respirators, are as follows:

Act	Agency	Regulation(s)
Federal Mine Safety and Health Act of 1977	Mine Safety and Health Administration; Department of Labor	Title 30 CFR Parts 11 , 70
	National Institute for Occupational Safety and Health, Centers for Disease Control, Department of Health and Human Services	Title 30 CFR Part 11
Occupational Safety and Health Act of 1970	Occupational Safety and Health Administration, Department of Labor	Title 29 CFR Part 1910
Toxic Substances Control Act	Environmental Protection Agency	Title 40 CFR Part 750
Title II of the Energy Reorganization Act of 1974	Nuclear Regulatory Commission	Title 10 CFR Part 20

The Federal regulations cited above and Guidelines issued in accordance with those regulations, with few exceptions, call for selection and use of respirators that have been certified by MSHA and NIOSH. Exceptions to that principle include the MSHA allowance of use of certain Bureau of Mines-approved mine rescue breathing apparatus, the OSHA acceptance of cylinder interchange and "buddy breathing systems" for use by fire fighters in 29 CFR 1910.156, and the NRC acceptance of supplied-air suits tested by Los Alamos National Laboratory.

Since 1972, with promulgation of Title 30 CFR 11, MSHA and NIOSH have tested and certified various types of respiratory protective devices. The present regulations in Part 11 are the result of amendment of the 1972 regulation. NIOSH currently recognizes that certain requirements of Part 11 are inadequate and incomplete, and a proposed revision of Part 11 has been published for public comment as a Notice of Proposed Rulemaking 42 CFR Part 84. Final publication is expected following a public hearing and further revision of Part 84.

II. General Selection Information

NIOSH recommends that respirators only be used when engineering controls are not feasible or effective, while controls are being installed or repaired, or for emergency and other temporary (intermittent) situations. Respirator selection is very complex and should be performed by an Industrial Hygienist or other professional knowledgeable in respiratory protective devices.

In 1975, NIOSH and the Occupational Safety and Health Administration (OSHA) as part of the Standards Completion Program developed a Respirator Decision Logic. That Logic incorporated fit factor data developed by the Los Alamos National Laboratory (LANL) under contract to NIOSH and incorporated requirements from 30 CFR 11.

The Decision Logic was modified by NIOSH in 1987 to include:

1. the NIOSH respirator carcinogen policy,

2. respiratory protective devices developed since 1975, and

3. a revision of assigned protection factors for those respirators for which valid workplace protection factor studies had been performed.

The selection of a specific respirator should be made by individuals knowledgeable of the limitations associated with each class of respirator (see Chapter 2), and familiar with the actual work environment including job tasks to be performed. For example, mobility of the worker and temperature and humidity of the work environment should all be considered in making an adequate respirator selection.

III. NIOSH Respirator Decision Logic

The NIOSH Respirator Decision Logic is reproduced as part of Appendix E of this document. This Logic contains a set of questions which will lead the user to the proper respirator selection table and identifies the criteria necessary to determine the classes of respirators which will provide adequate protection.

IV. NIOSH Certified Equipment List

The ***NIOSH Certified Equipment List*** (NCE) is published annually and lists the coal mine dust personal sampler units and respirators certified by NIOSH as well as provides updated information on the products, certifications, respirator complaints and problems, and NIOSH respirator policy.

In 1985, the format of this publication was modified. Respirators are now listed by specific certification class. General cautions and limitations for each certification class are listed (see page 84). However, these limitations are by no means all inclusive. The respirator manufacturer may also identify further limitations or cautions for their respirators. In addition, regulatory agencies may also place a limit on the use of respirators in their standards. An example of the listing for entry into and escape open-circuit SCBA is given on page 85.

Single, complimentary copies of the NCE will be provided by NIOSH while the supply lasts. Multiple copies can be ordered from the Government Printing Office (GPO). Requests for single copies should be sent to:

Publication Dissemination, DSDTT
NIOSH
4676 Columbia Parkway
Cincinnati, Ohio 45226-1998

EXAMPLE OF LISTING FROM NIOSH CERTIFIED EQUIPMENT LIST

A. Self-contained Breathing Apparatus

1. Entry Into and Escape

a. Open circuit pressure demand

Approval

Certified as approved for respiratory protection during entry into or escape from oxygen deficient atmospheres, gases and vapors.

Limitations

Use only for temperatures above the temperature listed on approval label.

Approved only when compressed air reservoir is fully charged with air meeting the requirements of the Compressed Gas Association Specification G-7.1 for Type 1, Grade D air, or equivalent specifications.

The air container shall meet applicable DOT specifications.

Use adequate skin protection when worn in gases or vapors that poison by skin absorption.

Refer to certification label and instruction and maintenance manuals for additional information on use and maintenance of these respirators.

In making renewals and repairs, parts identical with those furnished by the manufacturer under the pertinent approval shall be maintained.

Demand mode shall be used only when donning apparatus.

This respirator shall be selected, fitted, used and maintained in accordance with Mine Safety and Health Administration and other applicable regulations.

Recommendations

NIOSH recommends that SCBA be inspected weekly if stored and immediately before use, if used regularly, for breathing gas pressure.

SCBA ENTRY INTO AND ESCAPE OPEN CIRCUIT PRESSURE DEMAND

Approval Number TC-13-F-	Approval Issued to	Model Number(s)	Service Life (min.)	Facepiece Type	Regulator Position
30	MSA	95069 96338 461696 461704 461946 461947 463814 463815 463831 463833 466209 470444 470445 470448 470449	30	FF	Bm
40	Scott	900014-00 900014-01/05/06/12/30/31/39/50/51 900214-00/01/05/06/50/51	30	FF	Bm
42	Scott	900015-00 900015-01/05/06	15	FF	Bm
45	USD	9038-20* 9038-22*/70*/72* 9838-22/70*/72* 9848-20/22 9849-20*/22* U9038-00 U9838-00/02 M9838-20*	30	FF	Bm
47	MSA	95063 460262 461697 461703	15	FF	Bm

CHAPTER 4

RESPIRATOR USE

I. Federal Regulatory Requirements

OSHA 1910.134 states that when effective engineering controls are not feasible, or while they are being instituted, appropriate respirators shall be used pursuant to the following requirements:

- o respirators shall be provided by the employer when such equipment is necessary to protect the health of the employee
- o the employer shall provide the respirators which are applicable and suitable for the purpose intended
- o the employer shall be responsible for the establishment and maintenance of a respiratory protection program.

The respirator protection program prescribed by OSHA contains provisions for the following:

- o written standard operating procedures
- o respirators selected on basis of hazards
- o instruction and training of user
- o cleaning and disinfection
- o storage
- o inspection
- o surveillance of work area conditions
- o evaluation of respirator protection program
- o medical review
- o use of certified respirators.

II. The Respiratory Protection Program

A. Employer Responsibility

1. Determination of Wearer's Exposure to Hazards

Appropriate surveillance of work area conditions and of worker exposure to respiratory hazards should be carried out using good industrial hygiene practices. This means that the concentration of the respiratory hazard to which workers are exposed should be determined periodically, using NIOSH sampling methods where available, and records should be kept. The monitoring should cover conditions throughout a full work shift as activities in the work area vary during the shift and change the hazard concentration. The time-weighted average concentration and ceiling (peak) concentration of the hazard during the work shift should be determined. Preferably, the air in the work area should be sampled in the workers' breathing zones.

2. Fit Testing Before Use

In order to obtain adequate respiratory protection, there should be a proper match between respirator and wearer. To assure selection of the best fitting respirator, the wearer should be fit tested using a quantitative fit test procedure. Quantitative fit testing procedures are included in Appendix B of this document.

Respirator facepieces should be tested for fit each time they are worn. The wearer can make either the positive or the negative-pressure test before entering a hazardous atmosphere, but a qualitative check using either isoamyl acetate or irritant fume is much preferred. Qualitative fit testing procedures are included in Appendix B of this document.

3. Random Inspection

Respirators in use should be randomly inspected frequently to ensure that those selected for the job are being used and that they are in good condition. Respiratory protection is no better than the respirator in use. Periodic monitoring of respirator use should include:

- o determination that the proper respirators are being used

- o determination that respirators are being worn properly

o consultation with wearers about:

-discomfort
-resistance to breathing
-fatigue
-interference with vision
-interference with communications
-restriction of movement
-interference with job performance
-confidence in the respirator.

In addition to general assessment of overall respiratory protection, specific evaluations should also be conducted of cleaning, inspection, maintenance and storage. Problems discovered during the inspections should be rectified.

B. Employee Responsibility

Proper supervision of respirator use should ensure that each worker understands that he/she has certain responsibilities. Each worker should:

o check the respirator fit after each donning as instructed

o use the respirator as instructed

o guard against damaging the respirator

o go immediately to an area having respirable air if the respirator fails to provide proper protection

o report any respirator malfunction to a person responsible for the respirator program.

III. Program Elements

A. Program Administration

Providing suitable respirators to workers seems simple, but issue of an unsuitable respirator may result in worker injury or death, so the matter cannot be treated lightly. The person responsible for issuing respirators should be adequately trained to make sure that the correct respirator is provided for each job. The respirator program administrator should have the technical and professional background in order to make sound judgments based on hazard evaluation input from the workplace.

Without a definite chain of supervision, there is no assurance that written standard operating procedures will be followed. Therefore, responsibility for the entire respirator program should be assigned to one person.

The large user may find it practical and economical to have a staff of personnel involved in the respirator program, each with his own area of responsibility. Each of these people should report to the one administrator who has overall responsibility for the program. The administrator's technical and professional background should enable him or her to make sound judgments based on hazard evaluation input from the workplace. The Administrator may be a safety engineer, industrial hygienist, health physicist, or physician. The Administrator should have the full support of higher level management; without it, an effective respirator program is difficult to initiate and maintain.

Respirator purchasing should be controlled by the program administrator for good reasons. Several respirator manufacturers produce a wide variety of devices for protection against specific hazards. Although most manufacturers today produce several size facepieces to choose from, not all workers may be able to receive an adequate fit if only one brand of respirator is purchased. However, if more than one brand of respirator is purchased, thus providing a variety of facepiece sizes, it is possible to fit most of a working population. Sometimes more than one type of respirator may be adequate against a particular hazard. The program administrator should select what he/she considers to be the best types of devices, considering comfort and worker acceptance, and ensure that they are purchased. It is unwise to select a respirator on the basis of price alone. A program administrator, with comprehensive knowledge, should have a strong influence on, if not absolute control over, respirator purchases.

Small volume respirator users often feel they cannot afford (and may not need) to involve several people specifically in a respirator program. However, they have to meet the same requirements as the program administrator for the large user because the hazards do not differentiate between large and small volume users. In a small firm, where only a few workers wear respirators for protection against one or very few different hazards, the program administrator may be a foreman or other supervisor. Where only one or two workers wear respirators, the entire program may be the responsibility of the company owner. In an extremely small operation, the entire program may be the responsibility of the worker.

The administrator should keep the respirator program as flexible as possible. Although the written operating procedures meet today's situation, they may not meet tomorrow's. New hazards are continually being identified, and allowable exposure limits often are revised as more knowledge becomes available. The program administrator should stay abreast of these changes by subscribing to pertinent publications, and should not hesitate to modify the program to meet changing conditions.

Thus, the administrator, of a large or small program, should establish a respirator program that meets current needs, ensure that it is carried out satisfactorily, and ensure that it remains effective by continual examination and modification to meet changing conditions.

In summary, the program administrator can be a highly trained professional who oversees several employees responsible for specific phases of the respirator program, or a single employee responsible for the employee's own respirator. Like the written operating procedures, the exact administration of the respirator program should be tailored to the individual situation.

B. Program Components

Unfortunately, respirators can be misused or taken too much on faith, primarily because of lack of knowledge. Such misuse can be avoided by establishing written procedures for respirator selection and use and through proper supervision of all aspects of the respirator program. Following are detailed methods for ensuring that a respirator program remains effective.

1. Written Standard Operating Procedures

The importance of written standard operating procedures is emphasized in OSHA 29 CFR Part 1910.134 which gives the first requirement for a "minimal acceptable (respirator) program" as establishment of "written standard operating procedures governing the selection and use of respirators." Part 1910.134, which is currently undergoing revision, does not provide any guidance on preparation of these procedures and does not differentiate between large and small users. However, the general content of written procedures has been established, and from that information as provided by NIOSH and others, any user, large or small, can formulate procedures.

The written standard operating procedures should contain all information needed to maintain an effective respirator program to meet the user's individual requirements. They should be written so as to be useful to those directly involved in the respirator program, the program administrator, those fitting the respirators and training the workers, respirator maintenance workers, and the supervisors responsible for overseeing respirator use on the job. It is not necessary that the operating procedures be written for the wearer, although in a very small program it may be desirable to direct their content to the wearer. Only analysis of the individual program will show to what extent information for the wearer should be included.

The procedures should contain all information needed to ensure proper respiratory protection of a specific group of workers against a specific hazard or several particular hazards. The hazard(s) should have been assessed thoroughly; otherwise the written procedures will have only limited validity. Generally, the procedures should contain the following:

- o guidance for selection of the approved respirator(s) for protection against particular hazard(s)

- o detailed instructions for training workers in proper use of the respirator(s), including respirator fitting

- o detailed maintenance procedures for:

  -cleaning and disinfection
  -drying
  -inspection
  -repair or replacement of worn or defective components
  -storage

- o administrative procedures for:

  -purchase of approved or accepted respirator(s)
  -control of inventory of spare parts, new respirators, and respirators ready for reissue after maintenance
  -issuance of respirators to ensure use of the proper one for a given hazard
  -guidance of supervisory personnel in continued surveillance of respirator use and determination of workers' exposure to respiratory hazards

- o instructions for respirator use during emergencies, including fire, which can create an atmosphere immediately hazardous to life or health

- o guidelines for medical surveillance of workers, including pre-employment physical examinations to eliminate those physically or psychologically unfit to wear respirators, and periodic physical examinations to review the overall effectiveness of the respirator program on the basis of physiological factors

- o procedures for evaluating the respirator program's effectiveness

Obviously, the above essentially restates the OSHA requirements for a minimal acceptable respirator program. The point is that all the information needed to establish and maintain an adequate respirator program should be written down.

The exact format of written standard operating procedures may vary widely. The large user who has many workers wearing respirators and, perhaps, several respiratory hazards to consider, may formulate separate procedures for selection and use of respirators for each hazard. For a small user, who has only a few workers to protect from only one or very few hazards, a much simplified document may serve; but it must cover the same subjects. In general, the complexity of the procedures increases as respirator use increases. The procedures also become more extensive as the toxicity of the respiratory hazard(s) increases, demanding better and more reliable protection. It is better to be overly detailed in developing written operating procedures than not detailed enough.

Some firms have developed an elaborate system wherein each wearer is issued a card that specifies what type of respirator the wearer can be issued for protection against a particular hazard. The wearer is required to show this card to the issuer, who can issue only the type of respirator listed. Often, such a card lists a particular brand of respirator on the basis of fitting tests.

When practical, a respirator should be assigned to each worker for exclusive use, and should be permanently marked to indicate to whom it is assigned. Care should be taken to ensure that the marking does not affect the respirator performance. If possible, records should be kept on the issuance and use of each respirator. To do so, each should be permanently identified. Records should include the date of initial issue, the dates of reissue, and a listing of repairs.

Particularly important are procedures for respirator use during emergencies such as fire, large spillage of toxic material, accidental release of a potentially lethal substance, or failure of a ventilation system. All possible emergencies should be considered in advance and prepared for in the written procedure. In the stress of an emergency, memories may be faulty. Furthermore, these emergency procedures should be used in training emergency response teams. A sample of and a check list for a respirator standard operating procedure are included in Appendix A.

2. Medical Surveillance

OSHA 29 CFR 1910.134 states that no one should be assigned a task requiring use of respirators unless found physically able to do the work while wearing the respirator. In addition, some regulatory standards for specific substances and occupations may also contain requirements for medical examinations. Both types of standards declare that a physician should determine what health and physical conditions are pertinent, and that respirator wearers' medical status should be reviewed periodically.

Pre-placement medical examinations should screen out those who are physically or psychologically unfit to wear respirators. As another part of this examination, medical tests pertinent to the respiratory hazards that workers may encounter should be made to get baseline data against which to assess physiological changes in respirator wearers. In addition, the workers' previous medical and employment history should also be considered.

The types of information which should be obtained from the worker include:

a. History of respiratory disease--identifies workers with a history of asthma, emphysema, or chronic lung disease. These people may be at risk when wearing a respirator.

b. Work history--identifies workers who have been exposed to asbestos, silica, cotton dust, beryllium, etc., within the past ten years, or workers who have worked in occupations or industries where such exposure was probable. If past exposures are identified, medical tests can be obtained for comparison. Some of the specific items of information which might be obtained include:

- o previous occupations
- o problems associated with breathing during normal work activities
- o past problems with respirator use.

c. Any other medical information -which might offer evidence of the worker's ability or inability to wear and use respirators, such as:

- o psychological problems or symptoms including claustrophobia
- o any known physical deformities or abnormalities, including those which may interfere with respirator use
- o past and current usage of medication
- o tolerance to increased heart rate, which can be produced by heat stress.

Periodic routine medical examinations should be made to determine whether respirator wearers have been exposed to harmful levels of respiratory hazards. Examination frequency should be tailored to particular situations and in accordance with specific substance standards. Tests to determine whether harmful amounts of hazardous substances have been taken into the body should be used. The results of the periodic examinations should be compared with those of the pre-employment examinations and previous periodic examinations to determine whether the respirators used are adequate. If possible, periodic biochemical tests should be made to measure respirator wearers' exposures to respiratory hazards.

3. *Training*

a. *Elements of an adequate training program*

Selecting the respirator appropriate to a given hazard is important, but equally important is using the selected device properly. Proper use can be ensured by carefully training both supervisors and workers in selection, use, and maintenance of respirators. This implies that there should be a training program.

Like the overall respirator program, the content of the training program can vary widely, depending on circumstances. However, OSHA 29 CFR 1910.134 requires that training of both workers and supervisors include the following, no matter what the circumstances:

- an opportunity to handle the respirator
- proper fitting
- test of facepiece-to-face seal, and
- a long familiarizing period of wear in normal air.

Furthermore, OSHA requires that the wearer receive fitting instructions including demonstrations and practice in wearing, adjusting, and determining the fit of the respirator.

Training of supervisors and workers also should include:

- discussion of the engineering and administrative controls in use and why respirators also are needed
- explanation of the nature of the respiratory hazard and what happens if the respirator is not used properly
- explanation of why a particular type of respirator has been selected, and
- discussion of how to recognize and handle emergencies.

These training requirements apply to large and small organizations, with no differentiation to meet individual needs. The training the supervisor needs may differ from that for the individual worker, and both may differ markedly from that needed by members of emergency response teams. This chapter summarizes methods for satisfying the OSHA requirements and suggests ways that respiratory protection training may be tailored to individual needs based on job function.

The exact format of the training program will vary widely, depending upon the organization. The large user may need a full-time professional instructor. At the other extreme is the very small user who may be forced into a do it yourself training program. Respirator training courses are available from NIOSH and others. It must be emphasized again, however, that the OSHA requirements apply to large and small users alike.

b. Supervisor Training

Supervisors, at least those who oversee the daily activities of one or more workers who wear respirators frequently, should have a reasonably comprehensive knowledge of respirators and respiratory protection practices. Their training should include, but not necessarily be limited to, knowledge of the following:

- worker training and instruction
- basic respiratory protection practices
- selection and use of respirators to protect each worker against every respiratory hazard to which the worker may be exposed
- the nature and extent of the respiratory hazards to which the workers may be exposed
- the structure and operation of the entire respirator program, and
- the legal requirements pertinent to use of respirators in their respective situations.

The supervisor should understand the responsibility to facilitate functioning of the program, including maintenance that the worker may be expected to do, issuance of respirators, control of their use, and evaluation of the program's effectiveness.

These suggestions obviously apply to the large organization. A smaller organization may have to combine the supervisor training with that of the workers. This benefits the workers as they receive more comprehensive training.

c. *Worker Training*

The extent and frequency of the workers' training depends primarily on the complexity of the respirator, nature and extent of the hazard. Training for respiratory protection against highly toxic chemicals may need to be more stringent than for less toxic chemicals. If the hazard is a nuisance particulate, for example, the danger from misuse of the respirator is not likely to be as serious as with a highly toxic particulate where a single misuse may have serious consequences. The same holds true, of course, for gases and vapors. If the respirator is to be used in an emergency, training in its use should be very thorough and complete. In any case, the worker should be given some instruction in respiratory protection practices.

As a bare minimum, both worker and supervisor should be trained in basic respiratory protection practices. Also, each should be trained in use of the respirators selected for a particular situation. Because proper respirator use depends especially upon the wearer's motivation, it is important that the need for the respirator be explained fully. ANSI Standard Z88.2 (1969), Section 7.4 lists the following points to be included in a minimal acceptable respirator program:

> "(1) Instruction in the nature of the hazard, whether acute, chronic, or both, and an honest appraisal of what may happen if the respirator is not used.
> (2) Explanation of why more positive control is not immediately feasible. This shall include recognition that every reasonable effort is being made to reduce or eliminate the need for respirators.
> (3) A discussion of why this is the proper type of respirator for the particular purpose.
> (4) A discussion of the respirator's capabilities and limitations.
> (5) Instruction and training in actual use of the respirator (especially a respirator for emergency use) and close and frequent supervision to assure that it continues to be properly used.
> (6) Classroom and field training to recognize and cope with emergency situations.
> (7) Other special training as needed for special use."

A major thrust in this training is toward explaining as much as possible about the need and reasons for wearing a respirator. This, of course, is to motivate the user to accept the fact that protection is necessary, and to instill the desire to wear and maintain a respirator properly. Just handing a respirator to a worker with orders to wear it because OSHA says so is one of the easiest ways to ensure its misuse.

At best, a respirator may cause discomfort and inconvenience, so there is a natural resistance toward wearing it conscientiously. Much of this natural resistance can be overcome by taking the time and effort to inform the wearer as thoroughly as possible why the respirator is necessary. This effort will create acceptance of respirators and contribute to correct use.

4. Fitting

All the care that goes into the design, manufacture and certification of a respirator to ensure its maximum efficiency will not protect the wearer if there is an improper match between facepiece and wearer or improper wearing practices. The problem is twofold. Assuming that more than one brand of a particular type of facepiece is available, the first problem is to determine which fits best. The second problem is to ensure that the user knows when the respirator fits properly. Both problems can be solved by use of some sort of fitting test, which is one of the OSHA requirements.

Determination of facepiece fit should involve both qualitative and quantitative tests. A qualitative test relies on the wearer's subjective response. A quantitative test uses some other means of detecting facepiece leakage. The general advantages and disadvantages of each are as follows:

Advantages of Qualitative Tests:

Usually, qualitative tests are fast, require no complicated, expensive equipment, and are easily performed in the field.

Disadvantages of Qualitative Tests:

Most qualitative tests rely on the wearer's subjective response, so they may not be entirely reliable.

Advantages of Quantitative Tests:

The greatest advantage of a quantitative test is that it does not rely on a subjective response. The quantitative test is recommended when facepiece leakage must be minimized for work in highly toxic atmospheres or those immediately dangerous to life or health.

Disadvantages of Quantitative Tests:

Quantitative fitting tests require expensive equipment that can be operated only by highly trained personnel. Each test respirator must be equipped with a sampling probe to allow removal of a continuous air sample from the facepiece, so the same facepiece cannot be worn in actual service.

In addition, recent NIOSH studies have indicated that the sampling bias for the current quantitative fit tests technique is unsatisfactory. NIOSH is performing research into probe location and probe design in an effort to decrease this sampling bias (see Chapter 6).

Selection of a qualitative and/or quantitative fitting test depends upon circumstances such as the severity and extent of the respiratory hazard and the size of the organization. Ideally, both qualitative and quantitative tests should be used. A quantitative test can be used in selecting the best respirator for each worker during training. To supplement the periodic quantitative fitting, a qualitative test can be used before each entry into a contaminated atmosphere. Again, this is only a suggested procedure that can be modified on the basis of an objective professional evaluation of the circumstances.

Quarter- and half-masks, and full-facepieces have inherently different fitting characteristics. Moreover, several brands of each are marketed, each having slightly different fitting characteristics. Although every manufacturer designs facepieces to fit as broad a section of the working population as possible, no respirator marketed will fit everyone. Therefore, more than one brand of a given type of respirator should be purchased to take advantage of the different fitting characteristics of each. In this way, the chances of properly fitting all workers are increased. Having more than one facepiece to choose from also gives the worker a better chance of finding a respirator that is reasonably comfortable while providing good protection. It is in this process of matching the respirator to the individual user that the fitting test, particularly the quantitative test, has the greatest impact.

Respirator fit testing procedures are included in Appendix B.

5. *Respirator Inspection, Cleaning, Maintenance, and Storage*

Scrupulous respirator maintenance should be made an integral part of the overall respirator program. Manufacturers' instructions for inspection, cleaning, and maintenance of respirators should be followed to ensure that the respirator continues to function properly. Wearing poorly maintained or malfunctioning respirators may be more dangerous than not wearing a respirator at all. The worker wearing a defective device may falsely assume that protection is being provided. Emergency escape and rescue devices are particularly vulnerable to inadequate inspection and maintenance, although they generally are used infrequently, and then in the most hazardous and demanding circumstances. The possible consequences of wearing a defective emergency escape and rescue device are lethal.

The OSHA standards strongly emphasize the importance of an adequate maintenance program, but permit its tailoring to the type of plant, working conditions, and hazards involved. However, all programs are required to include at least:

- inspection for defects (including a leak check)
- cleaning and disinfecting
- repair, and
- storage.

A proper maintenance program ensures that the worker's respirator remains as effective as when it was new.

a. Inspection for Defects

Probably the most important part of a respirator maintenance program is frequent inspection of the devices. If conscientiously performed, inspections will identify damaged or malfunctioning respirators before they can be used. The OSHA requirements outline two primary types of inspection, that while the respirator is in use and that while it is being cleaned. In a small operation, where workers maintain their own respirators, the two types of inspection become essentially one and the same. In a large organization with a central respirator maintenance facility, the inspections differ. A sample respirator inspection record is included in Appendix A.

b. Frequency of Inspection

OSHA requires that "all respirators be inspected before and after each use," and that those not used routinely, i.e. emergency escape and rescue devices, "shall be inspected after each use and at least monthly..." NIOSH, however, recommends that all stored SCBA be inspected weekly. In one case, the respirator is to be inspected both before and after each use, in the other case, only after use. However, it is highly unlikely that anyone needing a respirator in a hurry, as during an emergency, is going to inspect it. In fact, it could be dangerous to take time to do so.

c. Inspection Procedures

Inspection procedures differ depending upon whether air-purifying or atmosphere-supplying devices are involved, and whether the inspection is to be conducted in the field during use, or during routine cleaning.

The OSHA standards require that respirator inspection include:

- o a check of the tightness of the connections,
- o a check of the facepiece, valves, connecting tube, canisters, and
- o a check of the regulator and warning devices on SCBA for proper functioning.

d. Field inspection of air-purifying respirators

Routinely used air-purifying respirators should be checked as follows before and after each use:

i. Examine the facepiece for:

- o excessive dirt
- o cracks, tears, holes, or distortion from improper storage
- o inflexibility (stretch and massage to restore flexibility)
- o cracked or badly scratched lenses in full-facepieces
- o incorrectly mounted full-facepiece lens or broken or missing mounting clips, and
- o cracked or broken air-purifying element holder(s), badly worn threads, or missing gasket(s) (if required).

ii. Examine the headstraps or head harness for:

- o breaks
- o loss of elasticity
- o broken or malfunctioning buckles and attachments, and
- o excessively worn serrations on the head harness which might permit slippage (full-facepieces only).

iii. After removing its cover, examine the exhalation valve for:

- o foreign material, such as detergent residue, dust particles, or human hair under the valve seat
- o cracks, tears, or distortion in the valve material
- o improper insertion of the valve body in the facepiece
- o cracks, breaks, or chips in the valve body, particularly in the sealing surface
- o missing or defective valve cover, and
- o improper installation of the valve in the valve body.

iv. Examine the air-purifying elements for:

- o incorrect cartridge, canister, or filter for the hazard
- o incorrect installation, loose connections, missing or worn gaskets, or cross-threading in holder
- o expired shelf-life date on cartridge or canister
- o cracks or dents in outside case of filter, cartridge, or canister, and
- o evidence of prior use of sorbent cartridge or canister, indicated by absence of sealing material, tape, foil, etc., over inlet.

v. If the device has a corrugated breathing tube, examine it for:

- o broken or missing end connectors, gaskets, or o-rings
- o missing or loose hose clamps, and
- o deterioration, determined by stretching the tube and looking for cracks.

vi. Examine the harness of a front- or back-mounted gas mask for:

- o damage to wear to the canister holder which may prevent its being held securely in place, and
- o broken harness straps or fastenings.

e. Field Inspection of Atmosphere-Supplying Respirators

For a routinely used atmosphere-supplying device, use the following procedures.

i. If the device has a tight-fitting facepiece, use the procedures outlined above for air-purifying respirators, except those pertaining to the air-purifying elements.

ii. If the device is a hood, helmet, blouse, or full suit, use the following procedures:

- o Examine the hood, blouse, or full suit for rips and tears, seam integrity, etc.
- o Examine the protective headgear, if required, for general condition, with emphasis on the suspension inside the headgear.
- o Examine the protective faceshield, if any, for cracks or breaks or impaired vision due to rebounding abrasive particles.
- o Make sure that the protective screen is intact and secured correctly over the faceshield of abrasive blasting hoods and blouses.

iii. Examine the air supply system for:

- o integrity and good condition of air supply lines and hoses, including attachments and end fittings, and
- o correct operation and condition of all regulators, valves, or other air-flow regulators.

On SCBA, determine that the high pressure cylinder of compressed air or oxygen is sufficiently charged for the intended use, preferably fully charged (mandatory on an emergency device). On closed circuit SCBA, make sure that a fresh canister of CO_2 sorbent is installed before use, or in accordance with manufacturers instructions. On open-circuit SCBA, recharge the cylinder if less than 80% of the useful service time remains. However, it is much preferred that an open-circuit SCBA be fully charged before use.

When an air-purifying or atmosphere-supplying device is used nonroutinely, all the above procedures should be followed after each use. OSHA requires that devices for emergency use be inspected once a month and that "a record shall be kept of inspection dates and findings for respirators maintained for emergency use." NIOSH recommends that such inspections be conducted at least weekly, because of the hazard that undetected loss of breathing gas from emergency SCBA will present to the wearer.

If defects are found during any field inspection, two remedies are possible. If the defect is minor, repair and/or adjustment may be made on the spot as in Figure 4-1. If it is major, the device should be removed from service until it can be repaired. **UNDER NO CIRCUMSTANCES SHOULD A DEVICE THAT IS KNOWN TO BE DEFECTIVE BE USED OR STORED FOR FUTURE USE.**

f. Inspection during cleaning

Because respirator cleaning usually involves some disassembly, it presents a good opportunity to examine each respirator thoroughly. Figure 4-2 shows inspection of the valve. The procedures outlined above for a field inspection should be used, but only after the respirator is cleaned and reassembled prior to returning it to service.

During this inspection, the respirator should be leak checked, as OSHA requires. The exact meaning of "leak check" has been much discussed, but no universal definition has emerged. Generally, a "leak check" is an examination of the freshly cleaned and reassembled respirator to determine that the complete assembly is gastight.

Several methods could be devised for meeting this requirement. One is worthy of mention as it is being used in several existing respirator programs. The respirator facepiece is placed over a machined metal head form with an inflated sealing surface. The straps are fastened down, and the inflatable seal built into the headform is pressurized to provide gastight seal between the headform and the facepiece. A continuous air sample is withdrawn from inside the facepiece, through the headform, and is passed through an aerosol detector like that described in Appendix B. An aerosol stream is directed through a small diameter tube around the potential leak points in the facepiece. Any leaks are shown by the penetration meter or recorder of the aerosol analyzing system, if it is set on the most sensitive scale.

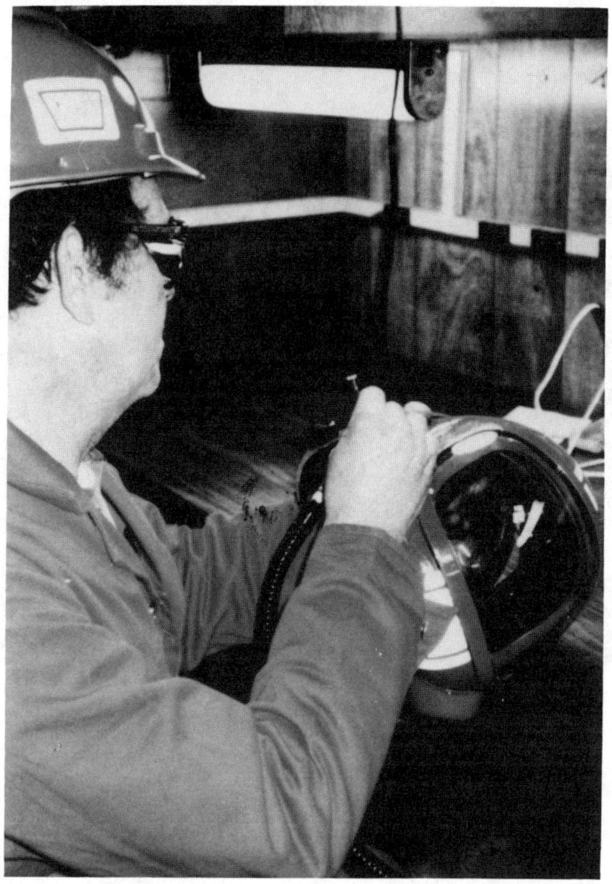

Photograph Courtesy of Powermaster, Inc.

***FIGURE 4-1.* Repair of a Helmet**

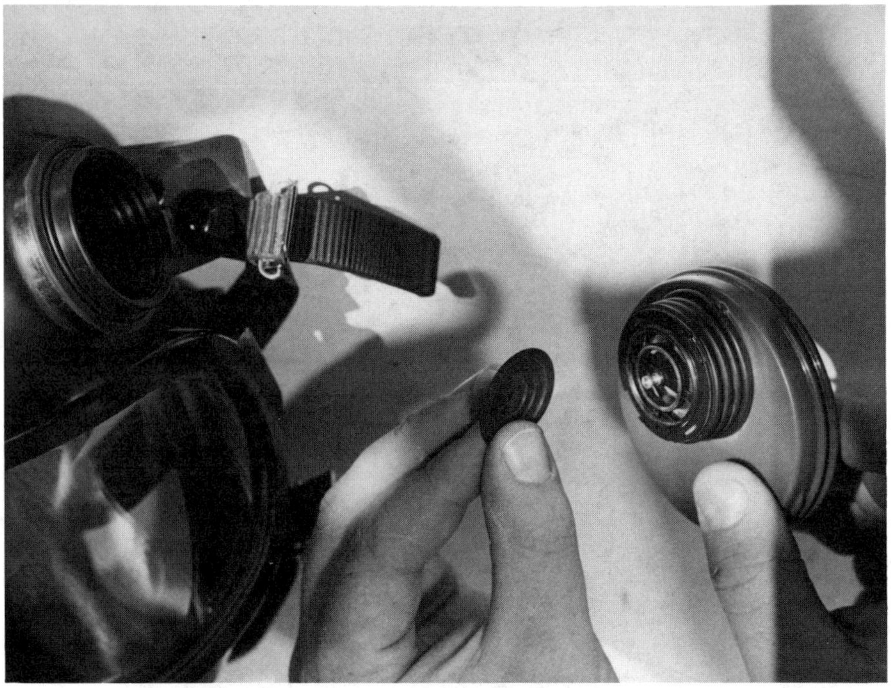

Photograph Courtesy of ISI

FIGURE 4-2. **Inspection of the Valve**

This procedure will detect leak sources and indicate the magnitude of the leak. However, it must be considered a qualitative, rather than quantitative, test. Some users have built a small test chamber around the headform. Instead of the aerosol being passed around the facepiece, the chamber contains an aerosol-laden atmosphere that permits actual quantitative determination of leakage in a manner similar to a quantitative fitting test.

This test requires use of the expensive aerosol system which is practical only for large organizations. The small respirator user is in the difficult position of not being able to afford this sophisticated equipment, although bound by the same requirements as the larger user. The best advice for the small user is to use ingenuity and devise a method that will satisfy the basic purpose of the leak check without adversely affecting the filter element, and assure that the reassembled respirator is leak free.

g. Cleaning and disinfecting

The OSHA requirements in 29 CFR 1910.134 are not specific about cleaning and disinfecting procedures, stating that "routinely used respirators shall be collected, cleaned, and disinfected as frequently as necessary to insure that proper protection is provided." and that emergency use respirators "shall be cleaned and disinfected after each use."

In a large respirator program in which respirators are used routinely, they should be exchanged daily for cleaning and inspection. In a small program involving only occasional respirator use, this period could be weekly or monthly. Each worker who maintains a respirator should be thoroughly briefed on cleaning and disinfecting it. Although a worker may not be required to maintain the respirator, briefings on the cleaning procedure will encourage acceptance of the respirator by providing assurance that the worker will receives a clean, disinfected, properly maintained device. This is particularly important where respirators are not individually assigned. Where respirators are individually assigned, they should be durably identified to ensure that the worker always receives the same device. Identification markers should neither penetrate the facepiece nor block filters, cartridge ports, or exhalation valves.

In a small respirator program, or where workers clean their own respirators, washing with detergent in warm water using a brush, thorough rinsing in clean water, and air drying in a clean place is generally accepted as sound procedure. Precautions should be taken to prevent damage from rough handling during this procedure. Precautions should also be taken to prevent exposure of the person cleaning the respirator to the contaminant in the respirator and to cleaning agents.

In a large program, there may be a centralized cleaning and maintenance facility with specialized equipment and personnel trained in respirator maintenance. Figure 4-3 shows a typical, hypothetical, large respirator maintenance facility. Good features are the separate areas for disassembly of used respirators and assembly of freshly cleaned and maintained devices which ensure that the clean respirators do not become contaminated. Also, there is ample storage space for the clean respirators, and spare parts (filters, exhalation valves, headbands, etc.) are readily available. There is also a test bench for checking the operation of SCBA regulators as well as a leak test system. A facility of this type would take up about 500 ft^2.

In the following discussion of cleaning and maintenance procedures, reference to Figure 4-3 should help in understanding the overall process.

h. Disassembly

The used respirators are collected and deposited in a central location, (A) of Figure 4-3. They are taken to an area (C) where the filters, cartridges, or canisters are removed and discarded. Canisters and cartridges should be intentionally damaged to prevent reuse. If the facepieces are equipped with reusable dust filters, they may be cleaned with compressed air in a hood (B) that prevents dust from getting into the room and affecting the maintenance personnel. The air tanks from SCBA are removed and connected to the charging station (J), and the rest of the unit is sent to the SCBA test bench (I) where the regulator is tested. SCBA facepieces are cleaned like air-purifying respirator facepieces.

CAUTION: Improper disposal of an oxygen-generating canister from a closed circuit SCBA is dangerous. Mine Safety Appliances Company suggests the following procedure for disposing of their "Chemox" oxygen generating canister:

"Punch a hole in the front, back, and bottom of the canister, and gently place it in a bucket of clean water deep enough to cover it by at least 3 inches. When bubbling stops, any residual oxygen has been dissipated and the canister is expended. Pour the water, which is caustic, down a drain or dispose of it in any other suitable manner." This procedure is safe. Not following this procedure recommended by the manufacturer, particularly, can cause a violent explosion.

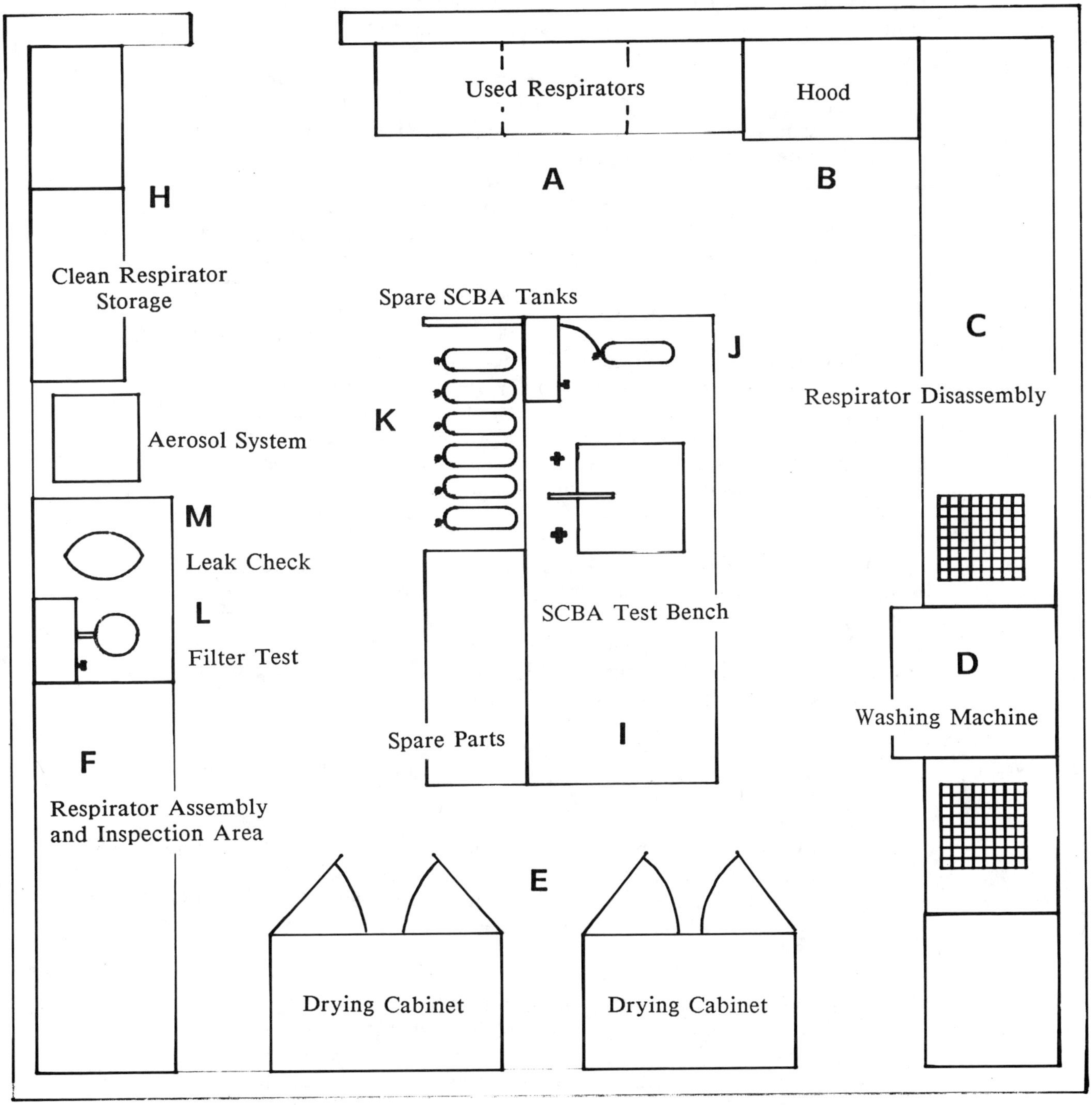

FIGURE 4-3. **Typical Large Respirator Maintenance Facility**

i. Cleaning and sanitizing

The Manufacturer's instructions should be followed for cleaning and sanitizing respirators, especially in regard to maximum temperatures.

The actual cleaning may be done in a variety of ways. In Figure 4-3, it is assumed that a commercial dishwasher (D) is used. A standard domestic type clothes washer also may be used if a rack is installed around the agitator to hold the facepieces in fixed positions. If the facepieces are placed loose in a washer, the agitator may damage them. A standard domestic dishwasher also may be used, but it is not preferred because it will not immerse the facepieces.

Any good detergent may be used, but cleaner and sanitizer solutions that clean effectively and contain a bactericide are available. The bactericide is generally a quaternary ammonium compound, which has some disadvantages, because its concentration must be adjusted to the composition of the local water to provide a constant degree of disinfection. Also, there is a possibility of dermatitis if the quaternary ammonium salts are not completely rinsed from the respirator.

An alternative is to wash the respirators in detergent, followed by a disinfecting rinse. Disinfection is not absolutely necessary if the respirator is reused by the same worker. However, where individual issue is not practiced, disinfection is strongly recommended. Reliable, effective disinfectants may be made from readily available household solutions, including:

- Hypochlorite solution (50 ppm of chlorine) made by adding approximately 2 ml of hypochlorite (laundry) bleach to 1 liter of water. A 2-minute immersion disinfects the respirators.

- Aqueous solution of iodine (50 ppm of iodine) made by adding approximately 0.8 ml tincture of iodine per liter of water. The iodine is approximately 7% ammonium and potassium iodide, 45% alcohol, and 48% water. Again, a 2-minute immersion is sufficient.

If the respirators are washed by hand, a separate disinfecting rinse may be provided. If a washing machine is used, the disinfectant should be added to the rinse cycle, and the amount of water in the machine at that time will have to be measured to determine the correct amount of disinfectant.

To avoid damaging the rubber and plastic in the respirator facepieces, the cleaner and disinfectant temperatures should not exceed 140°F, but they should not be less than 120°F to ensure adequate cleaning.

j. Rinsing

The cleaned and disinfected respirators should be rinsed thoroughly in clean water (140°F maximum) to remove all traces of detergent, cleaner and sanitizer, and disinfectant. This is very important to prevent dermatitis.

k. Drying

The respirators may be allowed to dry by themselves on a clean surface. They also may be hung from a horizontal wire, like drying clothes, but care must be taken not to damage the facepieces. A better method is to use a commercially available, electrically heated steel storage cabinet, Figure 4-3(E), with a built-in circulating fan, and replacing the solid shelves with steel mesh, if necessary.

l. Reassembly and Inspection

The clean dry respirator facepieces should be reassembled and inspected in an area, Figure 4-3(F), separate from the disassembly area to avoid contamination. The inspection procedures have been discussed, but there may be more things to look for because of the cleaning. The most common is detergent or soap residue left by inadequate rinsing. This appears most often under the seat of the exhalation valve, and can cause valve leakage or sticking.

At this time, the respirators should be thoroughly inspected and all defects corrected. New or retested filters, or new cartridges and canisters should be installed, and the completely reassembled respirator should be tested for leaks, Figure 4-3(M).

The facepiece of a SCBA can now be combined with the tested regulator from (I) and a full charged cylinder from the storage rack (K), and an operational check can be performed.

m. Maintenance and Repair

The OSHA standards state that "replacement or repairs shall be done by experienced persons with parts designed for the respirator." Besides being contrary to OSHA requirements, substitution of parts from a different brand or type of respirator invalidates MSHA/NIOSH certification of the device. Therefore, the user would be wearing an uncertified device, in violation of the OSHA requirement.

Maintenance personnel should be thoroughly trained. They should be aware of their limitations and never try to replace components or make repairs and adjustments beyond manufacturer's recommendations, unless they have been specially trained by the manufacturer.

These restrictions apply primarily to maintenance of the more complicated devices, especially closed and open circuit SCBA, and even more specifically their reducing or admission valves (regulators) which "... shall be returned to the manufacturer or to a trained technician for adjustment or repair." Figure 4-4 shows a complicated inspection being performed at the factory prior to delivery of the respirator to a user. There should be no problems in repairing and maintaining most other respirators, particularly the most commonly used air-purifying types.

An important aspect of any maintenance program is having enough spare parts on hand. Only continual surveillance of replacement rate will determine what parts in what quantities should be kept in stock. It is desirable to have some sort of recordkeeping system to indicate spare parts usage and the inventory on hand.

n. Storage

All the care that has gone into cleaning and maintenance of a respirator can be negated by improper storage. OSHA requires that respirators be stored to protect against:

- o dust
- o sunlight
- o heat
- o extreme cold
- o excessive moisture, and
- o damaging chemicals.

What is omitted, though implied in a later statement, is protection against mechanical damage. Leaving a respirator unprotected, as on a workbench, or in a tool cabinet or tool box among heavy wrenches, etc., may damage it.

It is strongly recommended that freshly cleaned respirators be placed in heat-sealed or reusable plastic bags until reissue. They should be stored in a clean, dry location away from direct sunlight. They should be stored in a single layer with the facepiece and exhalation valve in a more or less normal position to prevent the rubber or plastic from taking a permanent distorted "set."

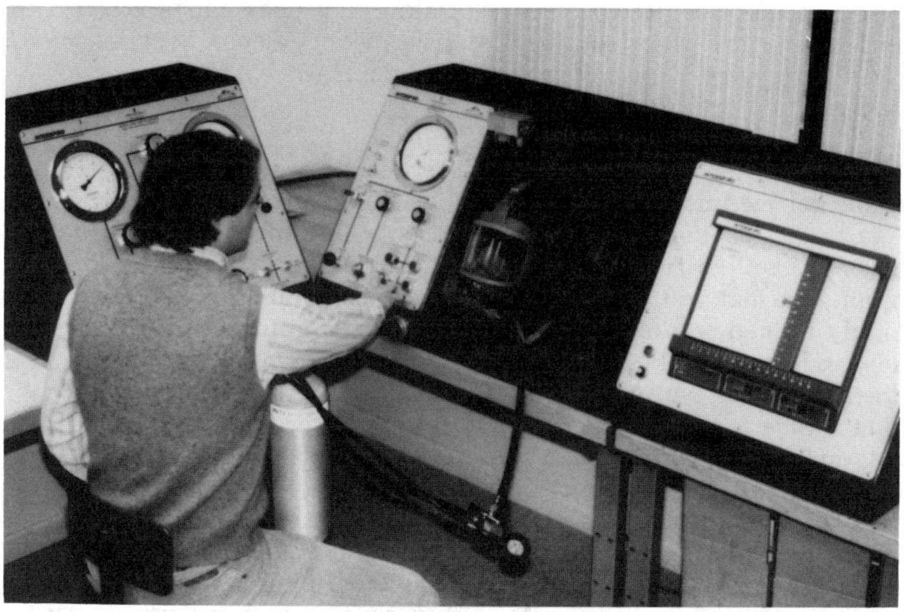

Photograph Courtesy of Interspiro

FIGURE 4-4. **Inspection at the Factory**

Air-purifying respirators kept ready for nonroutine or emergency use should be stored in a cabinet in individual compartments. A steel wall-mounted cabinet, with six compartments is shown in Figure 4-5. Note that each compartment is clearly labeled with the user's name and that the respirators are in plastic bags. Note also that the respirator in the lower right compartment is stored improperly. Another acceptable method of storage in a standard steel storage cabinet is shown in Figure 4-5. Note that the respirators are stored in a single layer.

The storage cabinet should be readily accessible, and all workers should be made aware of its location, as is done for fire extinguishers. Avoidance of serious injury from inhalation of a toxic substance may depend entirely on how quickly workers can get to the emergency respirators. This type of storage should be encouraged for routinely used respirators if it does not interfere with the normal work routine. A little inconvenience here is justified to prevent use of a respirator damaged by improper storage.

A chest or wall mounted case, Figure 4-6, may be purchased from the respirator manufacturer for storing a SCBA for use in emergencies. Again, the locations of SCBA should be well known and clearly marked. Unlike fire extinguishers, however, they should be located in an area that will predictably remain uncontaminated. Even highly trained workers take 30 seconds to 1 minute to put on these devices. In a highly contaminated atmosphere such as might be created by massive release of a toxic material, this may be too long a time to stay safely in the area. Therefore, the first reaction should be to escape to an uncontaminated area, then put on the SCBA which should be located there and re-enter the hazardous area for whatever task must be done. There are undoubtedly exceptions to this general rule, and only thorough evaluation of the potential hazard, taking into account the physical configuration of the work area, will permit a final decision about the correct storage location for a SCBA.

Routinely used respirators may be stored in a variety of ways if they are protected against the substances and conditions listed at the beginning of this section. This means that when a respirator is not in use, it should be stored in a plastic bag inside a rigid container. The OSHA requirements suggest that respirators be stored in the cartons in which they came, but these usually provide only minimal protection from mechanical damage.

The adequately trained worker should develop a respect for respirators which will automatically provide incentive to protect it from damage. Besides providing better assurance of adequate protection, this training will lower maintenance costs because of decreased damage.

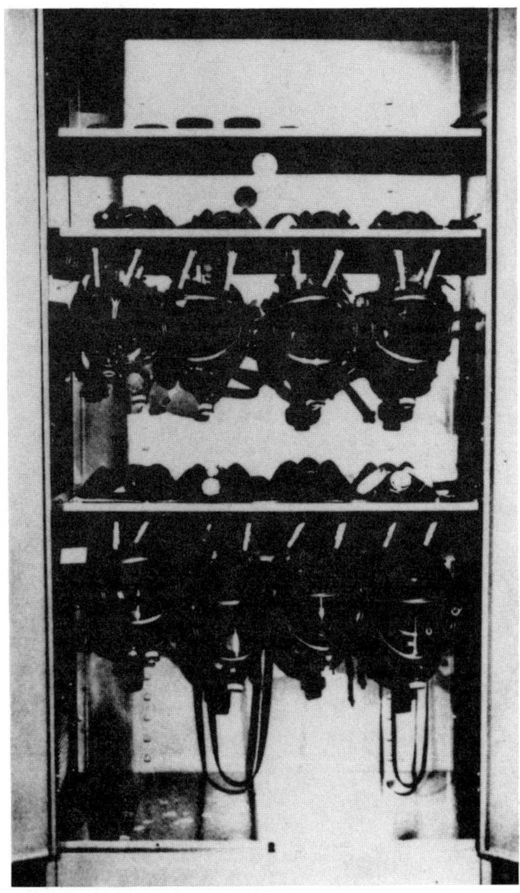

FIGURE 4-5. **Storage Cabinet for Facepieces**

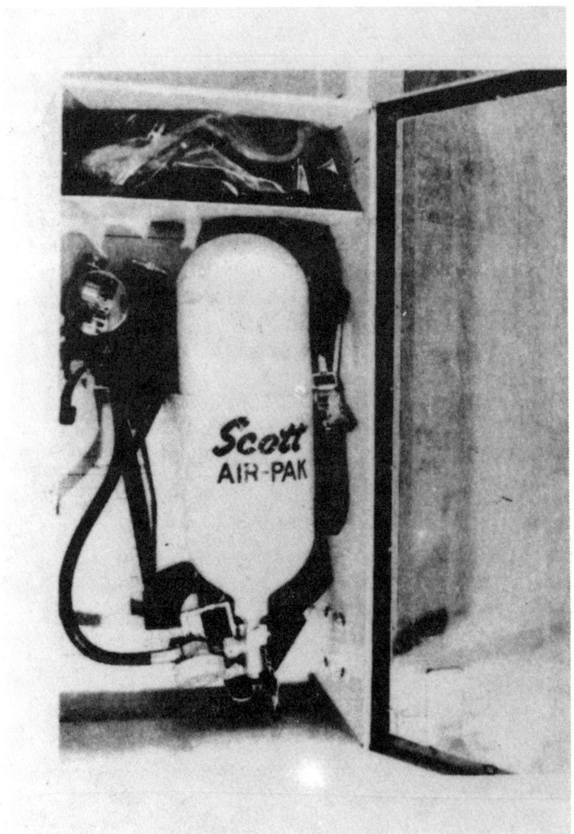

FIGURE 4-6. **Wall-mounted Storage Cabinet for SCBA**

6. Surveillance of Work Area Conditions and Worker Exposure

OSHA 29 CFR 1910.134 states, "appropriate surveillance of work area conditions and degree of employee exposure or stress shall be maintained." This necessitates periodic monitoring of the air contaminant concentration to which the respirator wearer is exposed. Many things such as changes in the operation or process, air movement, temperature, or humidity, affect the concentration of a substance in the work area atmosphere. Therefore, the air contaminant should be sampled. Preferably, sampling should be in the respirator wearer's breathing zone. Both the time-weighted average and peak concentrations of the contaminant should be determined. Comparing the measured time-weighted average concentration with the maximum use concentration determined for the type of respirator being used is a means of checking that the proper respirator has been selected.

7. Respirator Program Evaluation

OSHA 29 CFR 1910.134 states, "There shall be regular inspection and evaluation to determine the continued effectiveness of the program." Periodic monitoring is necessary to ensure that workers are adequately protected. The program should be evaluated at least annually, and the written operating procedures should be modified to reflect the evaluation results if necessary. A sample respirator program and checklist are included in Appendix A.

Frequent inspection of respirator use will determine whether the correct respirators are being used and worn properly. Examination of respirators in use and in storage will indicate how well they are maintained. Wearers should be consulted periodically about their acceptance of respirators, including the discomfort, resistance to breathing, fatigue, interference with vision and communication, restriction of movement, and interference with job performance, and their confidence in the respirator's effectiveness.

The results of periodic inspections of respirator use, consultations with wearers, measurements of hazard levels in work areas, and medical surveillance of wearers should be reviewed, studied, and analyzed to determine the effectiveness of the respirator program. Evidence of excessive exposure to hazards should be followed up to determine why inadequate protection was provided, and action should be taken to remedy the problem. The results of the program evaluation should be presented in a written report that lists plans to correct faults and the target dates for their implementation.

CHAPTER 5

RESPIRATOR USE UNDER SPECIAL CONDITIONS

The following are special problems which may be encountered in the wearing and use of respiratory protective equipment:

A. Facial Hair

Facial hair that lies along the sealing area of the respirator, such as beards, sideburns, moustaches, or even a few days growth of stubble, should not be permitted on employees who are required to wear respirators that rely on a tight facepiece fit to achieve maximum protection. Facial hair between the wearer's skin and the sealing surfaces of the respirator will prevent a good seal. A respirator that permits negative air pressure inside the facepiece during inhalation may allow leakage and, in the case of positive pressure devices, will either reduce service time or waste breathing air. A worker should not enter a contaminated work area when conditions prevent a good seal of the respirator facepiece to the face.

B. Eye Glasses

Ordinary eye glasses should not be used with full-facepiece respirators. Eye glasses with temple bars or straps that pass between the sealing surface of a full-facepiece and the worker's face will prevent a good seal, and should not be used. Special corrective lenses can be mounted inside a full-facepiece respirator and are available from all manufacturers of full-facepiece respirators. To ensure good vision, comfort, and proper sealing of the facepiece, these corrective lenses should be mounted by an individual designated by the manufacturer as qualified to install accessory items.

Eye glasses or goggles may interfere with the half facepieces. When interference occurs, a full-facepiece with special corrective lenses should be provided and worn.

C. Contact Lenses

Several factors may restrict or even prohibit the use of contact lenses while wearing any type of respiratory device. This is especially true of atmosphere-supplying respirators. With full-facepieces, incoming air directed toward the eye can cause discomfort from dirt, lint, or other debris lodging between the contact lens and the pupil.

OSHA is considering a change in their respiratory standard, with regard to use of contact lenses under respirators. Data generated by Lawrence Livermore National Laboratory is being taken into consideration.

D. Facial Deformities

Facial deformities, such as scars, deep skin creases, prominent cheekbones, severe acne, and the lack of teeth or dentures, can prevent a respirator from sealing properly.

E. Communications

Talking while wearing a respirator equipped with a facepiece may break the seal of the facepiece. When communication is necessary within a contaminated area, it should be done with the help of special communicating equipment obtained from the manufacturer of the respirator.

F. In Dangerous Atmospheres

Written procedures should be prepared for safe respirator use in IDLH atmospheres that may occur in normal operations or emergencies. Personnel should be familiar with these procedures and respirators. At least one standby person, equipped with proper rescue equipment including an SCBA should be present in the nearest safe area for emergency rescue of those wearing respirators in an IDLH atmosphere. Communications (visual, voice, signal line, telephone, radio, or other suitable type) should be maintained among all persons present (those in the IDLH atmosphere and the standby person or persons). The respirator wearers should be equipped with safety harnesses and safety lines to permit their removal from the IDLH atmosphere if they are overcome.

Confined spaces are enclosures that are difficult to get out of, such as storage tanks, tank cars, boilers, sewers, tunnels, pipelines, pits, and tubs. The atmospheres in a confined space may be immediately dangerous to life or health because of toxic air contaminants or lack of oxygen. Before anyone enters a confined space, tests should be made to determine the presence and concentration of any flammable vapor or gas, or any toxic airborne particulate, vapor, or gas, and to determine the oxygen concentration.

The confined space should be force-ventilated to keep the concentration of a flammable substance at a safe level. No one should enter if a flammable substance exceeds the lower explosive limit. No one should enter without wearing the proper type of respirator if any air contaminant exceeds the established permissible exposure limit or if there is an oxygen deficiency. Even if the contaminant concentration is below the established breathing time-weighted average limit and there is enough oxygen, the safest procedure is to ventilate the entire space continuously and to monitor the contaminant and oxygen concentrations continuously if people are to work in the confined space without respirators.

Airline and hose mask type supplied-air respirators or appropriate air-purifying respirators may be worn in a confined space only if tests show that the atmosphere contains adequate oxygen and that air contaminants are below levels immediately dangerous to life or health. While people wearing these types of respirators are in a confined space, its atmosphere should be monitored continuously.

If the atmosphere in a confined space is immediately dangerous to life or health owing to a high concentration of air contaminant or oxygen deficiency, those who must enter the space should wear a pressure-demand SCBA or a combination pressure-demand airline and self-contained breathing apparatus that always maintains positive air pressure inside the respiratory inlet covering. This is the best safety practice for confined spaces.

While personnel are in a confined space, at least one standby person with proper rescue equipment, including an SCBA, should be present outside for emergency rescue. Communications (visual, voice, signal line, telephone, radio, or other suitable type) should be maintained with those inside. Also, those inside the space should be equipped with safety harnesses and safety lines to allow their removal in case they are overcome.

G. In Low and High Temperatures

Low temperatures may fog respirator lenses. Coating the inner surface of the lens with the anti-fogging compound normally available from the respirator manufacturer should prevent fogging down to 32°F, but severe fogging may occur below 0°F. Full facepieces with nose cups that direct the warm, moist exhaled air through the exhalation valve without its touching the lens, are available. They should provide satisfactory vision at as low as -30°F. At very low temperatures, exhalation valves may freeze due to moisture. Dry respirable air should be used with airline respirators and with the type of SCBA that has an air cylinder when they are used in low temperatures.

NIOSH performs cold temperature testing on SCBA. The minimum temperature that the SCBA has been tested to and approved for is listed on the approval label.

A person working in high temperature air is under stress. Wearing a respirator causes additional stress which should be minimized by using a light-weight respirator with low breathing resistance. In atmospheres that are not immediately dangerous to life or health the airline type supplied-air respirator is recommended. Such a respirator used in low or high temperature atmospheres may be equipped with a vortex tube to either warm or cool the air supplied.

H. Physiological Response of Respirator Use

Wearing any respirator, alone or in conjunction with other types of protective equipment, will impose some physiological stress on the wearer. Weight of the equipment, for example, increases the energy requirement for a given task. Selection of respiratory protective devices should be based on the breathing resistance, weight of the respirator, the type and amount of protection needed as well as the individual's tolerance of the given device.

Use of respirators in conjunction with protective clothing can greatly affect the human response and endurance, especially in hot environments. Normally, in hot environments or during heavy work, the body relies a great deal on heat loss through the evaporation of sweat. With impermeable clothing, the heat loss by water evaporation is not possible. Additionally, the weight of the respirator (up to 35 pounds for an SCBA) adds to the metabolic rate of workers, increasing the amount of heat the body produces. The net effect is one of heat stress.

NIOSH studies of workers wearing chemical protective clothing (CPC) and firefighters' ensembles have indicated that heat stress is a serious consideration. Significant physiological stress was observed, even at low work intensities (30% of maximum work capacity--level walking at 3.4 miles per hour) in a neutral environment (23°C and 55% R.H.). With the chemical protective (CPC) ensemble, worker tolerance time was reduced by 56% as compared to light work clothing only. Elevated rectal temperatures (in excess of 39.0°C) were observed in three of the nine subjects. With the heavier firefighters' ensemble, tolerance time was reduced by 84% as compared to light work clothing only and heart rates averaged 25-50 beats per minute higher than with lightweight work clothing. At higher work intensities (60% of maximum), tolerance time was decreased by as much as 96%.

Based upon this limited research, the following recommendations are made:

1. Select the lightest weight protective ensembles and respiratory protective devices that adequately protect the worker. This will minimize the physiological demands placed on the worker by carrying the weight of this equipment.

2. If available, select protective clothing made of material that will allow evaporation of water vapor, while providing skin protection from the contaminant.

3. Reduce work rate by:

  a. adjusting the work/rest schedules,

  b. using automated procedures and/or mechanical assistance where possible, and

  c. minimizing the work intensity,

4. Educate workers on the symptoms and prevention of heat illness and schedule periodic fluid replacement breaks,

5. Reduce heat stress by scheduling work at night or early morning or by providing external cooling, where possible (either through cooling garments and/or by providing cool respirable breathing air through pressure-demand air supplied respirators), and

6. When conducting pipe/boiler lagging removal, ensure that steam lines are cool to minimize heat exposure from these sources.

CHAPTER 6.

NEW DEVELOPMENTS AT NIOSH

While conducting the MSHA/NIOSH-certification program for respirators, NIOSH has been actively interested in new developments in respiratory protection. To support such development work, which is dedicated toward improvement of worker protection, NIOSH has funded respirator research through contracts and grants, has sponsored meetings and workshops on respirator research, and has conducted in-house research projects. Most of the NIOSH respirator research projects have been directed toward improving the performance of respirators through development of new and more severe requirements for 30 CFR 11. However, some fundamental research projects in respiratory physiology, filtration mechanics, sorption technology, and quantitative respirator efficiency testing, have been undertaken.

A. Respiratory Physiology

To develop guidelines for workers wearing respirators and associated protective clothing, NIOSH has undertaken several research projects examining physiological response and worker tolerance at a variety of work rates and temperatures. The initial studies examined the effects of wearing four types of clothing/respirator ensembles while the subjects were performing at 30 and 60 percent of their individual aerobic capacity. Thermal, cardiovascular, respiratory, and subjective parameters were measured. Further work has recently been conducted examining responses at 10, 20 and 30 degrees Centigrade. Additional types of protective ensembles have also been studied. Preliminary results show that significant stress occurs with workload and temperature. These factors, as well as type of ensemble should be considered in determining safe work practices.

B. Filtration Mechanics

Research projects are underway and are planned to study the effects of several parameters, such as particle size, particle weight, particle shape, and material, on the efficiency of various filter materials. A study with a lead aerosol indicated that particle weight had no significant effect on filter efficiency. A study of fibrous aerosols is beginning. A filtration study with variably sized latex spheres is nearly complete.

C. Sorption Technology

In addition to conducting tests of MSHA/NIOSH-certified respirator cartridges against a variety of organic vapors, to determine the relation of the service times and resistances to the carbon tetrachloride test now in 30 CFR 11, NIOSH is studying the applicability of the Jonas Kinetic Model for predicting organic vapor permeation. Test data indicate that sorbents tested against carbon tetrachloride have above average service life, in comparison with other organic vapors tested thus far.

D. Quantitative Respirator Efficiency Testing

NIOSH is presently conducting research studies to evaluate published assigned protection factors and to determine the causes of known variability in quantitative fit testing. Quantitative workplace fit tests of powered air-purifying respirators have demonstrated that the previously assigned protection factors for that type of respirator were too high. The lower assigned protection factors for powered air-purifying respirators, prescribed in this publication, reflect this research. A similar study of pressure-demand self-contained breathing apparatus during firefighting operations has been initiated in 1987. NIOSH has determined that several factors variously affect the magnitude of a respirator leak, during quantitative fit testing, both in the laboratory and in workplace studies. The greatest effects have been found to be from leak site and probe location.

E. Certification of New Types of Respirators

Acting in accordance with the authority in 30 CFR 11 Section 11.30 (b), which permits MSHA/NIOSH to certify other types of respirators not described in 30 CFR 11, NIOSH has issued a number of special minimum requirements documents which permit the testing and certification of special respirators. NIOSH issues such requirements only after thorough investigation of the respirators and their use, and after extensive discussion and review by users, regulatory agencies and respirator manufacturers.

Other types of respirators which have been or may be certified under these special requirements include vinyl chloride, formaldehyde and other chemical cartridge respirators, and combination high-efficiency filter and supplied-air respirators.

On November 18, 1985, a Federal Register Notice was published detailing the requirements for certification of positive pressure closed-circuit self-contained breathing apparatus. Basically, there are two types which may be certified: (1) apparatus which use a breathing gas of pure oxygen, and (2) apparatus which use a breathing gas in which the oxygen concentration is not greater than 30 percent by volume. The following requirements, limitations, and cautions apply under present 30 CFR 11 Federal regulations:

Requirements for Certification of Positive-Pressure Closed-Circuit Self-Contained Breathing Apparatus

1. Where the apparatus uses a breathing gas (other than pure oxygen) the breathing gas will be respirable and not contain more than 30 percent by volume of oxygen.

2. The positive pressure closed-circuit self-contained breathing apparatus will meet all applicable requirements of 30 CFR 11 as prescribed for closed-circuit self-contained breathing apparatus, including those designed as demand flow devices.

3. The positive pressure closed-circuit self-contained breathing apparatus will maintain a positive pressure in the facepiece during all pressure and flow tests.

Certification Label Specifications

The following minimum limitations and conditions apply to positive pressure closed-circuit self-contained breathing apparatus and will appear on the certification label for each device:

Limitations

1. Do not use this apparatus where there is direct exposure to open flames or in high radiant heat. (This limitation applies to 100 percent oxygen apparatus only.)

2. Provide proper care, training, and maintenance of the apparatus as specifically described in the manufacturer's instructions and maintenance manuals.

3. After each use of this apparatus, a fully charged breathing gas container and a recharge of carbon dioxide scrubber shall be installed.

4. Thorough cleaning and disinfecting of facepiece, breathing tube, and breathing bag must be done in accordance with the manufacturer's instructions.

Cautions

1. Keep exposed hair to a minimum when using apparatus near open flames or in high radiant heat.

2. A good facepiece seal is important since facepiece leakage will seriously reduce service time.

3. Use of pure oxygen or oxygen enriched air increases flammability and lowers the ignition temperature of most materials.

In addition, presently available information indicates that the use of pure oxygen during direct exposure to open flames and/or high radiant heat should not be permitted. Further, NIOSH has determined that until it has been demonstrated satisfactorily that these devices can be worn safely under such conditions they should be presently limited to use which do not involve exposure to open flames or high radiant heat. Therefore, the oxygen concentration in a mixed gas system is limited to between 23 and 30 percent for use under these conditions. These limitations are based on what is physiologically safe for the necessary oxygen level at the lower end and on the effects of increased oxygen concentrations on both combustion and ignition temperatures at the upper end. These requirements are in addition to those presently listed in 30 CFR 11, both of which must be met by the SCBA prior to certification.

Consequently, when positive pressure closed-circuit breathing apparatus become available as certified devices, then the present closed circuit limitations and recommendations will be expanded to give users more selection guidance for safe application. That is, apparatus selection could become more performance oriented versus design oriented as present considerations and practices require.

F. NIOSH Respirator Problem Investigation

Since July 1, 1982, NIOSH has been investigating reports of problems with MSHA/NIOSH-certified respirators. These reports are from NIOSH audits of certified respirators, and from regulatory agencies and users and manufacturers of respirators. As of August 1, 1987, a total of 215 reports were received. The total includes 15 fatalities of employees who were wearing self-contained breathing apparatus at the time of their deaths.

The goals of the program are to increasingly justify the user's reliance on the MSHA/NIOSH respirator certification program and to indicate to respirator manufacturers that NIOSH is sincere in its desire to increase the safety and reliability of certified respirators.

During the last year of the program, NIOSH has noted that more manufacturers are receiving and directly investigating reports of problems on their own. They are advising NIOSH of the receipt of each problem and are providing NIOSH with follow-up information concerning the investigation and resolution of each problem. NIOSH regards this as an advantageous development, since it promotes more prompt response to and resolution of problems, increases customer satisfaction, and offers the manufacturer opportunities to learn about users' needs and wishes on a first-hand basis.

NIOSH will continue this program and encourages users to contact respirator manufacturers and NIOSH concerning problems with MSHA/NIOSH-certified respirators.

REFERENCES

Janpuntich, DA. (1984) Respiratory Particulate Filtration. **J. Ind. Soc. Respir. Prot.** 2(1):137-169.

NIOSH. (1976) *A Guide to Industrial Respiratory Protection*, DHEW (NIOSH) Pub. No. 76-189. Cincinnati: U.S. Department of Health, Education, and Welfare, Public Health Service, Centers for Disease Control, National Institute for Occupational Safety and Health.

Code of Federal Regulations, Title 30, Part 11, revised July 1, 1986.

American National Standards Institute, Inc. (1984) *American National Standard for Respirator Protection-Respirator Use-Physical Qualifications for Personnel*, ANSI Z88.6-1984. New York: ANSI, Inc.

NIOSH. (1987) *NIOSH Certified Equipment List as of October 1, 1986*, DHHS (NIOSH) Pub. No. 87-102. Cincinnati: U.S. Department of Health and Human Services, Public Health Service, Centers for Disease Control, National Institute for Occupational Safety and Health.

Myers WR, Peach MJ, Cutright K, and Iskander W. (1984) Workplace Protection Factor Measurements on Powered Air-Purifying Respirators at a Secondary Lead Smelter: Results and Discussion. **Am. Ind. Hyg. Assoc. J.** 45(10):681-688.

Myers WR, Peach MJ, and Cutright K. (1984) Field Test of Powered Air-Purifying Respirators at a Battery Manufacturing Facility. **J. of the Int. Soc. for Resp. Prot.** 4(1):62-89.

Lenhart SW. and Campbell DL. (1984) Assigned Protection Factors for Two Respirator Types Based Upon Workplace Performance Testing. **Ann. Occup. Hyg.** 28(2):173-182.

Myers WR, and Peach MJ III. (1983) Performance Measurements on a Powered Air-Purifying Respirator Made During Actual Field Use in a Silica Bagging Operation. **Ann. Occup. Hyg.** 27(3):251-259.

Dixon SW, and Nelson TJ. (1984) Workplace Protection Factors for negative Pressure Half-Mask Facepiece Respirators. **J. of the Int. Soc. for Resp. Prot.** 2(4):347-361.

Dixon SW, Nelson TJ, and Wright JE. (1984) Program Protection Factor Study on the 3M W316 Airhat. Presented at the American Industrial Hygiene Conference, May 22, 1984, Detroit, Michigan. E. I. duPont deNemours and Company.

daRoza RA, and Weaver W. (1985) *Is it Safe to Wear Contact Lenses with a Full-Facepiece Respirator?* Lawrence Livermore National Laboratory manuscript UCRL-53653.

NIOSH. (1978) *NIOSH Pocket Guide to Chemical Hazards*, DHEW (NIOSH) Pub. No. 78-210. Cincinnati: U.S. Department of Health, Education, and Welfare, Public Health Service, Centers for Disease Control, National Institute for Occupational Safety and Health.

NIOSH. (1985) *NIOSH Pocket Guide to Chemical Hazards*, DHHS (NIOSH) Pub. No. 85-114. Cincinnati: U.S. Department of Health and Human Services, Public Health Service, Centers for Disease Control, National Institute for Occupational Safety and Health.

Code of Federal Regulations, Title 29, Part 1910, Section 134, revised July 1, 1986.

Compressed Gas Association, Inc. (1966) *Commodity Specification for Air* CGA, G-7.1-1966. New York: CGA.

Code of Federal Regulations, Title 30, Part 70, revised July 1, 1986.

Code of Federal Regulations, Title 40, Part 750, revised July 1, 1986.

American National Standards Institute, Inc. (1973) *American National Standard for Identificaton of Air Purifying Respirator Canisters and Cartridges*, ANSI K13.1-1973. New York: ANSI.

Public Law 91-173, U.S. Congress: *Coal Mine Health and Safety Act of 1969.* 30 U.S. Code; secs. 301(a) and 302(a).

Public Law 95-164, U.S. Congress: *Federal Mine Health and Safety Act of 1977.* 30 U.S. Code; sec. 508.

Noonan GP, Linn HI, and Reed LD. (1986) *A Guide to Respiratory Protection for the Asbestos Abatement Industry*, EPA publication no. DW75932235-01-1. Washington, D.C.: U.S. Environmental Protection Agency, Office of Pesticide and Toxic Substances.

American National Standards Institute, Inc. (1969) *American National Standard for Practices for Respiratory Protection*, ANSI Z88.2-1969. New York: ANSI.

American National Standards Institute, Inc. (1980) *American National Standard for Practices for Respiratory Protection*, ANSI Z88.2-1980. New York: ANSI.

APPENDIX A

SAMPLE RESPIRATOR PROGRAM

RESPIRATOR PROGRAM EVALUATION CHECK LIST

The following is a sample respirator program:

A B C COMPANY

RESPIRATOR PROGRAM

Purpose:

The purpose of this operating procedure is to ensure the protection of all employees from respiratory hazards, through proper use of respirators. Respirators are to be used only where engineering control of respirator hazards is not feasible, while engineering controls are being installed, or in emergencies.

Responsibility

The company Safety Officer is ____ ____. He/she is solely responsible for all facets of this program and has full authority to make necessary decisions to ensure success of this program. This authority includes hiring personnel and equipment purchases necessary to implement and operate the program. The Safety Officer will develop written detailed instructions covering each of the basic elements in this program, and is the sole person authorized to amend these instructions.

The ABC Company has expressly authorized the Safety officer to halt any operation of the company where there is danger of serious personal injury. This policy includes respiratory hazards.

Program Elements

1. The Safety Officer will develop detailed written standard operating procedures governing the selection and use of respirators, using the NIOSH Respirator Decision Logic as a guideline. Outside consultation, manufacturer's assistance, and other recognized authorities will be consulted if there is any doubt regarding proper selection and use. These detailed procedures will be included as appendices to this respirator program. Only the Safety Officer may amend these procedures.

2. Respirators will be selected on the basis of hazards to which the worker is exposed. All selections will be made by the Safety Officer. Only MSHA/NIOSH-certified respirators will be selected and used.

3. The user will be instructed and trained in the proper use of respirators and their limitations. Both supervisors and workers will be so instructed by the Safety Officer. Training should provide the employee an opportunity to handle the respirator, have it fitted properly, test its facepiece-to-face seal, wear it in normal air for a long familiarity period, and finally to wear it in a test atmosphere. Every respirator wearer will receive fitting instructions, including demonstrations and practice in how the respirator should be worn, how to adjust it, and how

to determine if it fits properly.

Respirators should not be worn when conditions prevent a good face seal. Such conditions may be a growth of beard, sideburns, a skull cap that projects under the facepiece, or temple pieces on glasses. No employees of A B C, who are required to wear respirators, may wear beards. Also the absence of one or both dentures can seriously affect the fit of a facepiece. The worker's diligence in observing these factors will be evaluated by periodic checks. To assure proper protection, the facepiece fit will be checked by the wearer each time the wearer puts on the respirator. This will be done by following the manufacturer's facepiece-fitting instructions.

4. Where practicable, the respirators will be assigned to individual workers for their exclusive use.

5. Respirators will be regularly cleaned and disinfected. Those issued for the exclusive use of one worker will be cleaned after each day's use, or more often if necessary. Those used by more than one worker will be thoroughly cleaned and disinfected after each use. The Safety Officer will establish a respirator cleaning and maintenance facility and develop detailed written cleaning instructions.

6. The central respirator cleaning and maintenance facility will store respirators in a clean and sanitary location.

7. Respirators used routinely will be inspected during cleaning. Worn or deteriorated parts will be replaced. Respirators for emergency use such as self-contained devices will be thoroughly inspected at least once a month and after each use. Inspection for SCBA breathing gas pressure will be performed weekly.

8. Appropriate surveillance of work area conditions and degree of employee exposure or stress will be maintained.

9. There will be regular inspection and evaluation to determine the continued effectiveness of the program. The Safety Officer will make frequent inspections of all areas where respirators are used to ensure compliance with the respiratory protection programs.

10. Persons will not be assigned to tasks requiring use of respirators unless it has been determined that they are physically able to perform the work and use the equipment. The ABC Company physician will determine what health and physical conditions are pertinent. The respirator user's medical status will be reviewed annually.

11. Certified respirators will be used.

John Doe
President, ABC Company

The following is a sample respirator program evaluation checklist:

Respirator Program Evaluation Checklist

In general, the respirator program should be evaluated for each job or at least annually, with program adjustments, as appropriate, made to reflect the evaluation results. Program function can be separated into administration and operation.

A. Program Administration

_________ (1) Is there a written policy which acknowledges employer responsibility for providing a safe and healthful workplace, and assigns program responsibility, accountability, and authority?

_________ (2) Is program responsibility vested in one individual who is knowledgeable and who can coordinate all aspects of the program at the jobsite?

_________ (3) Can feasible engineering controls or work practices eliminate the need for respirators?

_________ (4) Are there written procedures/statements covering the various aspects of the respirator program, including:

_________ designation of an administrator;
_________ respirator selection;
_________ purchase of MSHA/NIOSH certified equipment;
_________ medical aspects of respirator usage;
_________ issuance of equipment;
_________ fitting;
_________ training;
_________ maintenance, storage, and repair;
_________ inspection;
_________ use under special condition; and
_________ work area surveillance?

B. Program Operation

(1) Respiratory protective equipment selection

_________ Are work area conditions and worker exposures properly surveyed?

_________ Are respirators selected on the basis of hazards to which the worker is exposed?

_________ Are selections made by individuals knowledgeable of proper selection procedures?

_________ (2) Are only certified respirators purchased and used; do they provide adequate protection for the specific hazard and concentration of the contaminant?

_________ (3) Has a medical evaluation of the prospective user been made to determine physical and psychological ability to wear the selected respiratory protective equipment?

_________ (4) Where practical, have respirators been issued to the users for their exclusive use, and are there records covering issuance?

(5) Respiratory protective equipment fitting

_________ Are the users given the opportunity to try on several respirators to determine whether the respirator they will subsequently be wearing is the best fitting one?

_________ Is the fit tested at appropriate intervals?

_________ Are those users who require corrective lenses properly fitted?

_________ Are users prohibited from wearing contact lenses when using respirators?

_________ Is the facepiece-to-face seal tested in a test atmosphere?

_________ Are workers prohibited from wearing respirators in contaminated work areas when they have facial hair or other characteristics may cause faceseal leakage?

(6) Respirator use in the work area

_________ Are respirators being worn correctly (i.e., head covering over respirator straps)?

_________ Are workers keeping respirators on all the time while in the work area?

(7) Maintenance of respiratory protective equipment

Cleaning and Disinfecting

_________ Are respirators cleaned and disinfected after each use when different people use the same device, or as frequently as necessary for devices issued to individual users?

_________ Are proper methods of cleaning and disinfecting utilized?

Storage

_________ Are respirators stored in a manner so as to protect them from dust, sunlight, heat, excessive cold or moisture, or damaging chemicals?

_________ Are respirators stored properly in a storage facility so as to prevent them from deforming?

_________ Is storage in lockers and tool boxes permitted only if the respirator is in a carrying case or carton?

Inspection

_________ Are respirators inspected before and after each use and during cleaning?

_________ Are qualified individuals/users instructed in inspection techniques?

_________ Is respiratory protective equipment designated as "emergency use" inspected at least monthly (in addition to after each use)?

_________ Are SCBA incorporating breathing gas containers inspected weekly for breathing gas pressure?

_________ Is a record kept of the inspection of "emergency use" respiratory protective equipment?

Repair

_________ Are replacement parts used in repair those of the manufacturer of the respirator?

_________ Are repairs made by manufacturers or manufacturer-trained individuals?

(8) Special use conditions

_________ Is a procedure developed for respiratory protective equipment usage in atmospheres immediately dangerous to life or health?

_________ Is a procedure developed for equipment usage for entry into confined spaces?

(9) Training

_________ Are users trained in proper respirator use, cleaning, and inspection?

_________ Are users trained in the basis for selection of respirators?

_________ Are users evaluated, using competency-based evaluation, before and after training?

SAMPLE RESPIRATOR INSPECTION RECORD

1. TYPE____________________________________ 2. NO. __________

3. DEFECTS FOUND:

A. Facepiece____________________________________

B. Inhalation Valve________________________________

C. Exhalation Valve Assembly__________________________

D. Headbands____________________________________

E. Cartridge Holder________________________________

F. Cartridge/Canister ______________________________

G. Filter ______________________________________

H. Harness Assembly_______________________________

I. Hose Assembly ________________________________

J. Speaking Diaphragm _____________________________

K. Gaskets_____________________________________

L. Connections___________________________________

M. Other Defects_________________________________

APPENDIX B

FIT TESTING PROCEDURES

APPENDIX B.1. PROCEDURES FOR FIT CHECKING

The seal of a respirator should be tested prior to entering a contaminated atmosphere by procedures recommended by the manufacturer or by the following fit checks.

Irritant or Odorous Chemical Agent

The wearer is exposed to an irritant smoke, isoamyl acetate vapor, or other suitable test agent easily detectable by irritation, odor, or taste. An air-purifying respirator must be equipped with the appropriate air-purifying element. If the wearer is unable to detect penetration of the test agent, the respirator is probably tight enough.

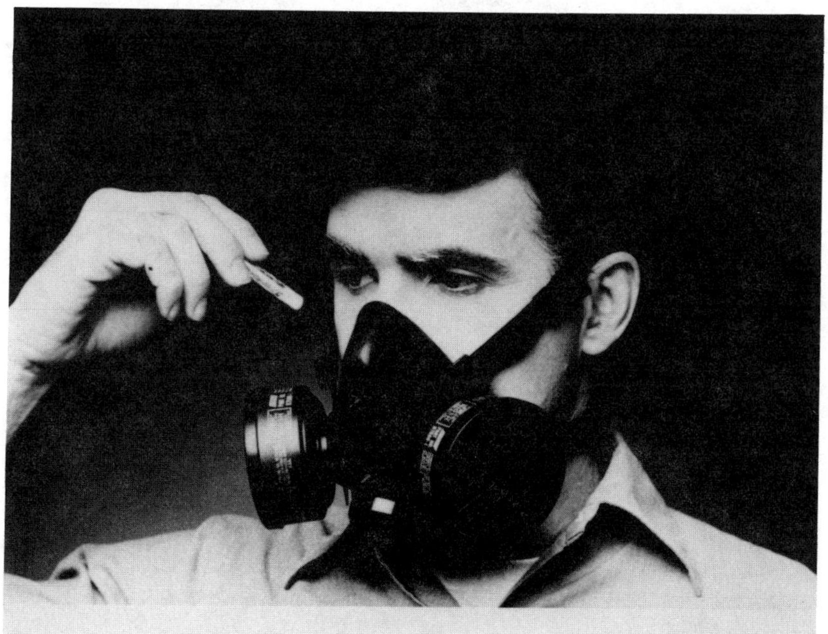

FIGURE B-1. **Odorous vapor check test**

Negative Pressure Test

The wearer can perform this test by himself in the field. The wearer should use this test (Figure B-1) just before entering any toxic atmosphere. It consists merely of closing off the inlet of the canister, cartridge(s), or filter(s) by covering with the palm(s) or replacing the seal(s), or of squeezing the breathing tube so that it does not pass air; inhaling gently so that the facepiece collapses slightly; and holding the breath for 10 seconds. If the facepiece remains slightly collapsed and no inward leakage is detected, the respirator is probably tight enough. This test, of course, can be used only on respirators with tight fitting facepieces.

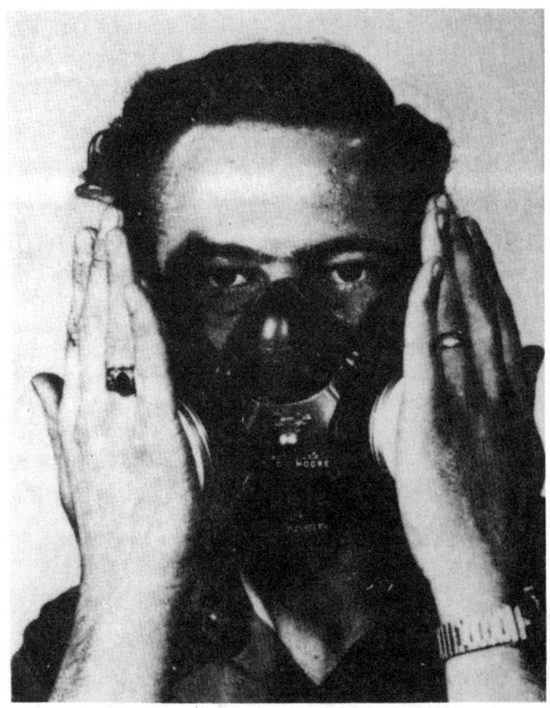

FIGURE B-2. **Negative pressure test**

Positive Pressure Test

This test is very like the negative pressure test, and it has the same advantages and limitations. It is conducted by closing off the exhalation valve and exhaling gently into the facepiece. The fit is considered satisfactory if slight positive pressure can be built up inside the facepiece without any evidence of outward leakage. For some respirators, this method requires that the wearer remove the exhalation valve cover and then carefully replace it after the test, often a difficult task. Removing and replacing the exhalation valve cover often disturbs the respirator fit even more than does the negative pressure test. Therefore, this test should be used sparingly if it requires removing and replacing a valve cover. The test is easy for respirators whose valve cover has a single small port that can be closed by the palm or a finger. The wearer should perform this test (Figure B-2) just before entering any hazardous atmosphere.

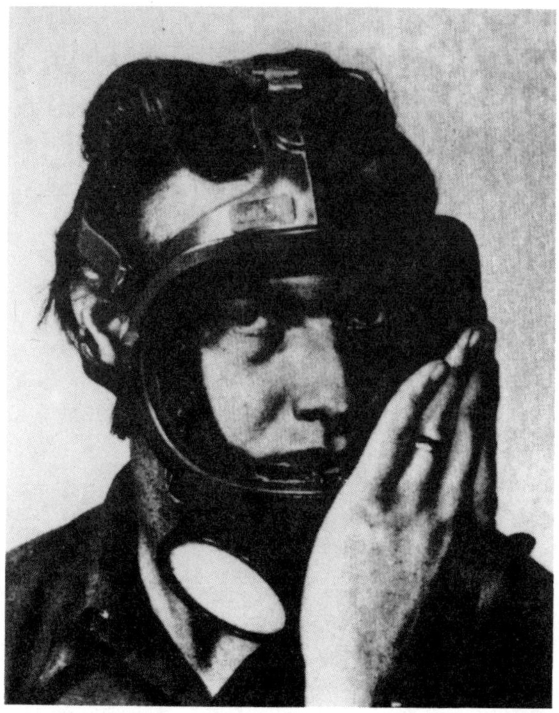

FIGURE B-3. **Positive pressure test**

APPENDIX B.2. QUALITATIVE FIT TEST PROCEDURES

[Note: The following procedures are found in the OSHA Lead Standard (29 CFR 1910.1025) Appendix D.]

This appendix specifies the only allowable qualitative fit test protocols permissible for compliance with paragraph (f)(3)(ii).

I. Isoamyl Acetate Protocol

A. Odor Threshold Screening

1. Three 1-liter glass jars with metal lids (e.g. Mason or Bell jars) are required.

2. Odor-free water (e.g. distilled or spring water) at approximately 25°C shall be used for the solution.

3. The isoamyl acetate (IAA) (also known as isopentyl acetate) stock solution is prepared by adding 1 cc of pure IAA to 800 cc of odor free water in a 1-liter jar and shaking for 30 seconds. The solution shall be prepared new at least weekly.

4. The screening test shall be conducted in a room separate from the room used for actual fit testing. The two rooms shall be well ventilated but may not be connected to the same recirculating ventilation system.

5. The odor test solution is prepared in a second jar by placing 4 cc of the stock solution into 500 cc of odor free water using a clean dropper or pipette. Shake for 30 seconds and allow to stand for two to three minutes so that the IAA concentration above the liquid may reach equilibrium. This solution may be used for only one day.

6. A test blank is prepared in a third jar by adding 500 cc of odor free water.

7. The odor test and test blank jars shall be labeled 1 and 2 for jar identification. If the labels are put on the lids they can be periodically dried off and switched to avoid people thinking the same jar always has the IAA.

8. The following instructions shall be typed on a card and placed on the table in front of the two test jars (i.e. 1 and 2):

"The purpose of this test is to determine if you can smell banana oil at a low concentration. The two bottles in front of you contain water. One of these bottles also contains a small amount of banana oil. Be sure the covers are on tight, then shake each bottle for two seconds. Unscrew the lid of each bottle, one at a time, and sniff at the mouth of the bottle. Indicate to the test conductor which bottle contains banana oil."

9. The mixtures used in the IAA odor detection test shall be prepared in an area separate from where the test is performed, in order to prevent olfactory fatigue in the subject.

10. If the test subject is unable to correctly identify the jar containing the odor test solution, the IAA QLFT may not be used.

11. If the test subject correctly identifies the jar containing the odor test solution he may proceed to respirator selection and fit testing.

B. Respirator Selection

1. The test subject shall be allowed to select the most comfortable respirator from a large array of various sizes and manufacturers that includes at least three sizes of elastomeric half facepieces and units of at least two manufacturers.

2. The selection process shall be conducted in a room separate from the fit test chamber to prevent odor fatigue. Prior to the selection process, the test subject shall be shown how to put on a respirator, how it should be positioned on the face, how to set strap tension and how to assess a "comfortable" respirator. A mirror shall be available to assist the subject in evaluating the fit and positioning of the respirator. This may not constitute his formal training on respirator use, only a review.

3. The test subject should understand that he is being asked to select the respirator which provides the most comfortable fit for him. Each respirator represents a different size and shape and, if fit properly, will provide adequate protection.

4. The test subject holds each facepiece up to his face and eliminates those which are obviously not giving a comfortable fit. Normally, selection will begin with a half-mask and if a fit cannot be found here, the subject will be asked to go to the full-facepiece respirators. (A small percentage of users will not be able to wear any half-mask.)

5. The more comfortable facepieces are recorded; the most comfortable mask is donned and worn at least five minutes to assess comfort. Assistance in assessing comfort can be given by discussing the points in #6 below. If the test subject is not familiar with using a particular respirator, he shall be directed to don the mask several times and to adjust the straps each time, so that he becomes adept at setting proper tension on the straps.

6. Assessment of comfort shall include reviewing the following points with the test subject:

   o Chin properly placed.
   o Positioning of mask on nose.
   o Strap tension.
   o Fit across nose bridge.
   o Room for safety glasses.
   o Distance from nose to chin.
   o Room to talk.
   o Tendency to slip.
   o Cheeks filled out.
   o Self-observation in mirror.
   o Adequate time for assessment.

7. The test subject shall conduct the conventional negative and positive-pressure fit checks (e.g. see ANSI Z88.2-1980). Before conducting the negative-or positive-pressure checks, the subject shall be told to "seat" his mask by rapidly moving the head side-to-side and up and down, taking a few deep breaths.

8. The test subject is now ready for fit testing.

9. After passing the fit test, the test subject shall be questioned again regarding the comfort of the respirator. If it has become uncomfortable, another model of respirator shall be tried.

10. The employee shall be given the opportunity to select a different facepiece and be retested if during the first two weeks of on-the-job wear the chosen facepiece becomes unacceptably uncomfortable.

C. *Fit test.*

1. The fit test chamber shall be substantially similar to a clear 55 gallon drum liner suspended inverted over a 2 foot diameter frame, so that the top of chamber is about 6 inches above the test subject's head. The inside top center of the chamber shall have a small hook attached.

2. Each respirator used for the fitting and fit testing shall be equipped with organic vapor cartridges or offer protection against organic vapors. The cartridges or masks shall be changed at least weekly.

3. After selecting, donning, and properly adjusting a respirator himself, the test subject shall wear it to the fit testing room. This room shall be separate from the room used for odor threshold screening and respirator selection, and shall be well ventilated, as by an exhaust fan or lab hook, to prevent general room contamination.

4. A copy of the following test exercises and rainbow (or equally effective) passage shall be taped to the inside of the test chamber:

   Test Exercises

   i. Normal breathing

   ii. Deep breathing. Be certain breaths are deep and regular.

   iii. Turning head from side-to-side. Be certain movement is complete. Alert the test subject not to bump the respirator on the shoulders. Have the test subject inhale when his head is at either side.

   iv. Nodding head up-and-down. Be certain motions are complete and made about every second. Alert the test subject not to bump the respirator on the chest. Have the test subject inhale when his head is in the fully up position.

   v. Talking. Talk aloud and slowly for several minutes. The following paragraph is called the Rainbow Passage. Reading it will result in a wide range of facial movements, and thus be useful to satisfy this requirement. Alternative passages which serve the same purpose may also be used.

Rainbow Passage

When the sunlight strikes raindrops in the air, they act like a prism and form a rainbow. The rainbow is a division of white light into many beautiful colors. These take the shape of a long round arch, with its path high above, and its two ends apparently beyond the horizon. There is, according to legend, a boiling pot of gold at one end. People look, but no one every finds it. When a man looks for something beyond reach, his friends say he is looking for the pot of gold at the end of the rainbow.

vi. Normal breathing.

5. Each test subject shall wear his respirator for at least 10 minutes before starting the fit test.

6. Upon entering the test chamber, the test subject shall be given a 6 inch by 5 inch piece of paper towel or other porous absorbent single ply material, folded in half and wetted with three-quarters of one cc of pure IAA. The test subject shall hang the wet towel on the hook at the top of the chamber.

7. Allow two minutes for the IAA test concentration to be reached before starting the fit test exercises. This would be an appropriate time to talk with the test subject, to explain the fit test, the importance of his cooperation, the purpose for the head exercises, or to demonstrate some of the exercises.

8. Each exercise described in No. 4 above shall be performed for at least one minute.

9. If at any time during the test, the subject detects the banana-like odor of IAA, he shall quickly exit from the test chamber and leave the test area to avoid olfactory fatigue.

10. Upon returning to the selection room, the subject shall remove the respirator, repeat the odor sensitivity test, select and put on another respirator, return to the test chamber, etc. The process continues until a respirator that fits well has been found. Should the odor sensitivity test be failed, the subject shall wait about 5 minutes before retesting. Odor sensitivity will usually have returned by this time.

11. If a person cannot be fitted with the selection of half-mask respirators, include full-facepiece models in the selection process. When a respirator is found that passes the test, its efficiency shall be demonstrated for the subject by having him break the face seal and take a breath before exiting the chamber.

12. When the test subject leave the chamber he shall remove the saturated towel, returning it to the test conductor. To keep the area from becoming contaminated, the used towels shall be kept in a self-sealing bag. There is no significant IAA concentration buildup in the test chamber from subsequent tests.

13. Persons who have successfully passed this fit test may be assigned the use of the tested respirator in atmospheres with up to 10 times the PEL of airborne lead. In other words this IAA protocol may be used to assign a protection factor no higher than 10.

II. SACCHARIN SOLUTION AEROSOL PROTOCOL

A. Taste Threshold Screening.

1. Threshold screening as well as fit testing employees shall use an enclosure about the head and shoulders that is approximately 12 inches in diameter by 14 inches tall with at least the front portion clear and that allows free movement of the head when a respirator is worn. An enclosure substantially similar to the 3M hood assembly of part #FT 14 and FT 15 combined is adequate.

2. The test enclosure shall have a three-quarter inch hole in front of the test subject's nose and mouth area to accommodate the nebulizer nozzle.

3. The entire screening and testing procedure shall be explained to the test subject prior to the conduct of the screening test.

4. The test subject shall don the test enclosure. For the threshold screening test, he shall breathe through his open mouth with tongue extended.

5. Using a DeVilbiss Model 40 Inhalation Medication Nebulizer, the test conductor shall spray the threshold check solution into the enclosure. This nebulizer shall be clearly marked to distinguish it from the fit test solution nebulizer or equivalent.

6. The threshold check solution consists of 0.83 grams of sodium saccharin, USP in water. It can be prepared by putting 1 cc of the test solution (see C6 below) in 100 cc of water.

7. To produce the aerosol, the nebulizer bulb is firmly squeezed so that it collapses completely then released and allowed to fully expand.

8. Ten squeezes are repeated rapidly and then the test subject is asked whether the saccharin can be tasted.

9. If the first response is negative, ten more squeezes are repeated rapidly and the test subject is again asked whether the saccharin is tasted.

10. If the second response is negative, ten more squeezes are repeated rapidly and the test subject is again asked whether the saccharin is tasted.

11. The test conductor will take note of the number of squeezes required to elicit a taste response.

12. If the saccharin is not tasted after 30 squeezes (Step 9), the test subject may not perform the saccharin fit test.

13. If a taste response is elicited, the test subject shall be asked to take note of the taste for reference in the fit test.

14. Correct use of the nebulizer means that approximately 1 cc of liquid is used at a time in the nebulizer body.

15. The nebulizer shall be thoroughly rinsed in water, shaken dry, and refilled at least each morning and afternoon or at least every four hours.

B. Respirator Selection.

Respirators shall be selected as described in section IB above, except that each respirator shall be equipped with a particular filter cartridge.

C. Fit Test.

1. The fit test uses the same enclosure described in B1 and B2 above.

2. Each test subject shall wear his respirator for at least 10 minutes before starting the fit test.

3. The test subject shall don the enclosure while wearing the respirator selected in section A above. This respirator shall be properly adjusted and equipped with a particular filter cartridge.

4. The test subject may not eat, drink (except plain water), or chew gum for 15 minutes before the test.

5. A second DeVilbiss Model 40 Inhalation Medication nebulizer is used to spray the fit test solution into the enclosure. This nebulizer shall be clearly marked to distinguish it from the screening test solution nebulizer or equivalent.

6. The fit test solution is prepared by adding 83 grams of sodium saccharin to 100 cc of warm water.

7. As before, the test subject shall breathe through the open mouth with tongue extended.

8. The nebulizer is inserted into the hole in front of the enclosure and the fit test solution is sprayed into the enclosure using the same technique as for the taste threshold screening and the same number of squeezes required to elicit a taste response in the screening. (See B10 above).

9. After generation of the aerosol the test subject shall be instructed to perform the following exercise for one minute each:

    a. Normal breathing.

    b. Deep breathing. Be certain breaths are deep and regular.

    c. Turning head from side-to-side. Be certain movement is complete. Alert the test subject not to bump the respirator on the shoulders. Have the test subject inhale when his head is at either side.

    d. Nodding head up-and-down. Be certain motions are complete and made about every second. Alert the test subject not to bump the respirator on the chest. Have the test subject inhale when his head is in the fully up position.

e. Talking. Talk aloud and slowly for several minutes. The following paragraph is called the Rainbow Passage. Reading it will result in a wide range of facial movements, and thus be useful to satisfy this requirement. Alternative passages which serve the same purpose may also be used.

Rainbow Passage

When the sunlight strikes raindrops in the air, they act like a prism and form a rainbow. The rainbow is a division of white light into many beautiful colors. These take the shape of a long round arch, with its path high above, and its two ends apparently beyond the horizon. There is, according to legend, a boiling pot of god at one end. People look, but no one every finds it. When a man looks for something beyond reach, his friends say he is looking for the pot of gold at the end of the rainbow.

10. Every 30 seconds, the aerosol concentration shall be replenished using one-half the number of squeezes as initially (C8).

11. The test subject shall so indicate to the test conductor if at any time during the fiat test the taste of saccharin is detected.

12. If the saccharin is detected the fit is deemed unsatisfactory and a different respirator shall be tried.

13. Successful completion of the test protocol shall allow the use of the tested respirator in contaminated atmospheres up to 10 times the PEL. In other words this protocol may be used to assign protection factors no higher than ten.

III. IRRITANT FUME PROTOCOL

A. Respirator Selection.

Respirators shall be selected as described in section 1B above, except that each respirator shall be equipped with high efficiency cartridges.

B. Fit Test.

1. The test subject shall be allowed to smell a weak concentration of the irritant smoke to familiarize him with its characteristic odor.

2. The test subject shall properly don the respirator selected as above, and wear it for at least 10 minutes before starting the fit test.

3. The test conductor shall review this protocol with the test subject before testing.

4. The test subject shall perform the conventional positive pressure and negative pressure fit checks. Failure of either check shall be cause to select an alternate respirator.

5. Break both ends of a ventilation smoke tube containing stannic oxychloride, such as the MSA part No. 5645, or equivalent. Attach a short length of tubing to one end of the smoke tube. Attach the other end of the smoke tube to a low pressure air pump set to deliver 200 milliliters per minute.

6. Advise the test subject that the smoke can be irritating to the eyes and instruct him to keep his eyes closed while the test is performed.

7. The test conductor shall direct the stream of irritant smoke from the tube towards the faceseal area of the test subject. He shall begin at least 12 inches from the facepiece and gradually move to within one inch, moving around the whole perimeter of the mask.

8. The following exercises shall be performed while the respirator seal is being challenged by the smoke. Each shall be performed for one minute.

   a. Normal breathing

   b. Deep breathing. Be certain breaths are deep and regular.

   c. Turning head from side-to-side. Be certain movement is complete. Alert the test subject not to bump the respirator on the shoulders. Have the test subject inhale when his head is at either side.

   d. Nodding head up-and-down. Be certain motions are complete and made about every second. Alert the test subject not to bump the respirator on the chest. Have the test subject inhale when his head is in the fully up position.

   e. Talking--slowly and distinctly, count backwards from 100.

f. Normal breathing

9. If the irritant smoke produces an involuntary reaction (cough) by the test subject, the test conductor shall stop the test. In this case the test respirator is rejected and another respirator shall be selected.

10. Each test subject passing the smoke test without evidence of a response shall be given a sensitivity check of the smoke from the same tube to determine whether he reacts to the smoke. Failure to evoke a response shall void the fit test.

11. Steps B4, B7, B8 of this protocol shall be performed in a location with exhaust ventilation sufficient to prevent general contamination of the testing area by the irritant smoke.

12. Respirators successfully tested by the protocol may be used in contaminated atmospheres up to ten times the PEL. In other words this protocol may be used to assign protection factors not exceeding ten.

APPENDIX B.3. QUANTITATIVE FIT TEST PROCEDURES

Except for procedures peculiar to instrument operation and calibration, quantitative respirator fitting tests are practically identical. The following is a suggested procedure for use in all types of test systems.

I. PRELIMINARY CHECKOUT PROCEDURES

A. Start up and calibrate the test system according to manufacturer's instructions. Be sure that the system is stable and that the aerosol or gas concentration in the enclosure has reached equilibrium.

B. Inspect all respirators to be used in the tests for defects and cleanness according to the procedures described in this guide.

II. QUANTITATIVE FITTING TEST PROCEDURES

A. Recheck the respirator before handing it to the test subject, paying particular attention to the sampling probe and line attached to the facepiece.

B. Describe the test to the subject, making sure that the subject fully understands its purpose, the procedures, and the actions expected.

C. If the subject is not familiar with wearing respirators, demonstrate correct wearing procedures. The subject's level of expertise usually becomes apparent as the subject puts on the respirator. The untrained or poorly trained subject will put the respirator on incorrectly or be hesitant in movements.

D. Have the subject put on the respirator, according to manufacturer's instructions. Be sure the subject does not tighten the headstraps to the point of discomfort. Remember that this test should approximate working conditions in which the subject might have to wear the respirator continuously for an hour to two at a time.

In testing a half- or quarter-mask, check its compatibility with safety glasses. If the subject's safety glasses interfere, try other brands of respirators of the same type. The subject may have to wear a full-facepiece, which provides eye protection, if a half- or quarter-mask compatible with safety glasses cannot be found.

E. Once it has been determined that the respirator is worn properly, the fit can be checked quickly using a qualitative fitting test. Make sure that the correct filter, cartridge, or canister for the particular test is installed in the respirator. Also make sure that the subject pinches off the sampling hose. If leakage is detected, try to determine its source and cause. If the leakage is from a poorly fitting facepiece, try another brand of the same type of respirator. In fact, several different brands of respirators should be made available so the subject can choose the most comfortable, a very important aspect of fitting respirators.

F. After the best possible qualitative fit has been obtained, the subject enters the test enclosure and connects the sampling hose. If necessary, and without disturbing the facepiece fit, replace the filter, cartridge, or canister used during the qualitative test with the air-purifying element required for the quantitative test. To minimize filter leakage, use high-efficiency particulate filters when the test agent is an aerosol. Allow enough time (2-3 minutes) at this point for the test enclosure concentration to stabilize. Then recheck the test system calibration.

G. In response to verbal instructions, the subject begins head and facial movements simulating those made during normal work.

(1) Normal breathing with head motionless for 1 minute;

(2) Deep breathing (simulating that during hard work) with head motionless for 30 seconds. Do not prolong this exercise because of the danger of hyperventilation;

(3) Turning head slowly up and down while breathing normally, pausing for at least two breaths before changing direction. Continue for at least 1 minute;

(4) Moving head slowly up and down while breathing normally, pausing for at least two breaths before changing direction. Continue for at least 1 minute;

(5) Reading from a prepared text, slowly and clearly, and loudly enough to be heard and understood by the test operator. Continue for 1 minute;

(6) Normal breathing with head motionless for at least 1 minute.

These exercises are more or less "standard" and have been found to provide a meaningful evaluation of respirator performance. Therefore, if they are used, the data can be compared with published information. The times suggested for each are minimal and may be extended if needed to obtain better data.

H. After the test, the subject leaves the test enclosure and removes the respirator. The operator should then ask about the respirator comfort and note any marks on the subject's face which indicate pressure points. If the test indicated a good fit, any discomfort may be due to a mismatch between the subject and the facepiece or to headstraps that are too tight. Every effort should be made to provide the most comfortable respirator possible.

I. The test results may be analyzed and the protection level determined by one of two methods. The first involves watching a meter during the test to determine that penetration does not exceed a certain value.

The second, much preferred, method is to record the entire test using a strip chart recorder operated at a chart speed of about 2 inches per minute.

The first information should uniquely identify the test by number, date, subject, and type of respirator. Next comes the test system calibrations after the subject has entered the test enclosure, to establish the maximum span of the penetration-measuring instrument ("100% calibration). This should be done at least twice to ensure that the calibration is correct.

Next follow the five exercises, separated by horizontal lines across the chart. As the penetration-measuring instrument has several ranges, the range should be shown next to the right margin of the chart. When it becomes necessary to change the penetration range, as in the example under turning head from side to side (TH), make a short mark where the change was made and indicate the new scale setting.

Each exercise should be identified by some notation. For example, the following notation could be used on the strip chart recording:

Normal Breathing	NB
Deep Breathing	DB
Turning Head from Side to Side	TH
Moving Head Up and Down	UD
Talking	T

These are suggested notations; others may be used, but they should be consistent.

All the above notations should be made during the test. However, it is neither necessary nor desirable to calculate the penetrations until later. The operator should pay full attention to running the equipment and noting the subject's actions during the test.

The cyclic nature of the recorder trace is a function of the subject's breathing cycle. As this example shows, in an air-purifying respirator with a half-mask, negative air pressure created in the facepiece during inhalation increases the leakage. Exhalation creates slightly positive air pressure, reducing the leakage. Also, the lungs absorb some of the test agent, especially if it is an aerosol, thus reducing the quantity of test agent in the exhaled breath. Consequently, the maximum penetration during inhalation indicates the fraction of ambient concentration which has penetrated the facepiece. Therefore respirator performance is based on the average of the peak penetrations.

After the test, the operator may analyze the recording. This is done, treating each exercise separately, by drawing a line through the inhalation peaks to approximate their average. The midpoint of each line is the "average peak penetration" for the exercise. This number should be entered on the chart for each exercise. Where the penetration changes abruptly, it is usually advantageous to split the data into more than one section and treat each separately.

For example, if five chart divisions under UD show a penetration of 2.55% and three show 3.75%, the average peak penetration for the entire exercise is calculated as follows:

5 divisions x 2.55 =	12.75
3 divisions x 3.75 =	11.25
8 divisions	24.00

24.00/8 = 3.00% peak average penetration.

After the average peak penetration has been calculated for each exercise, the data may be entered on a fitting test record. The record should include the information from the recorder chart which uniquely identifies the test. The record should indicate results of the qualitative pretest, the average peak penetrations calculated for each exercise, the test criterion expressed as the maximum allowable average peak penetration, the test average peak penetration obtained by averaging the average peak penetrations for each exercise, and whether the overall performance was satisfactory or not. This determination is based on the qualitative fit, compatibility with safety glasses, and average penetration.

The subject evaluation of the comfort of the particular respirator is based on the following criteria:

1. VERY COMFORTABLE

   Mask can be worn for an indefinite period without becoming unbearably bothersome or painful. No pain points: mask feels comfortable.

2. COMFORTABLE

   Mask can be worn for 2 to 4 hours without undue discomfort. Some pressure points with slight discomfort.

3. BARELY COMFORTABLE

   Mask can be worn for approximately 1/2 to 1 hour without intolerable discomfort. Some discomfort from pressure.

4. UNCOMFORTABLE

   Mask can be tolerated for the period of the test only.

5. INTOLERABLE

   Mask cannot be worn at all without discomfort.

All other factors being equal, final choice of a respirator should be based on comfort. A worker should not be required to wear a device he considers "uncomfortable" or "intolerable." He may wear a "barely comfortable" respirator if the proposed usage is intermittent for short periods.

In summary, the above is a suggested procedure for conducting a quantitative respirator fitting test, evaluating the results, and recording the data meaningfully, without laborious record keeping. Moreover, the data will be compatible with those from other work.

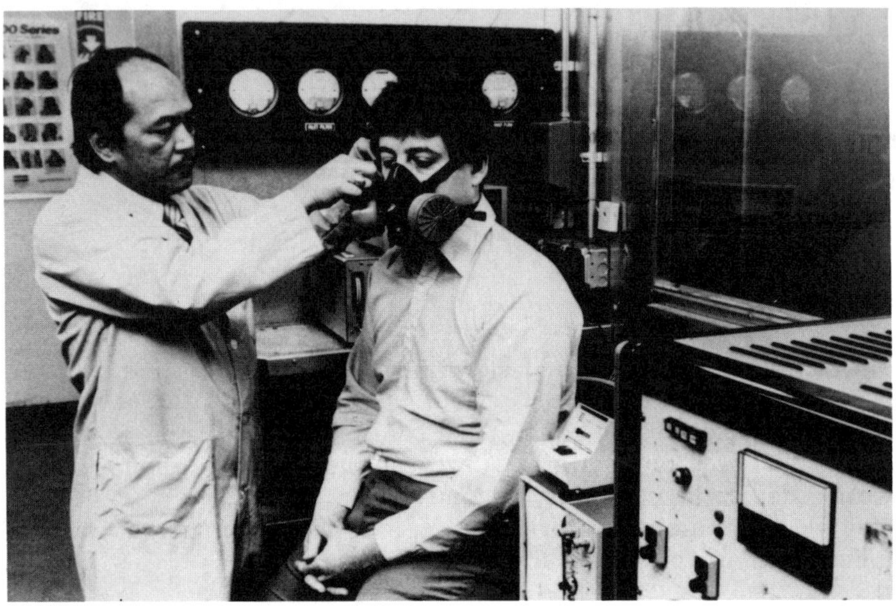

Photograph Courtesy of North Safety Products

FIGURE B-4. **Checking fit prior to doing quantitative fit testing**

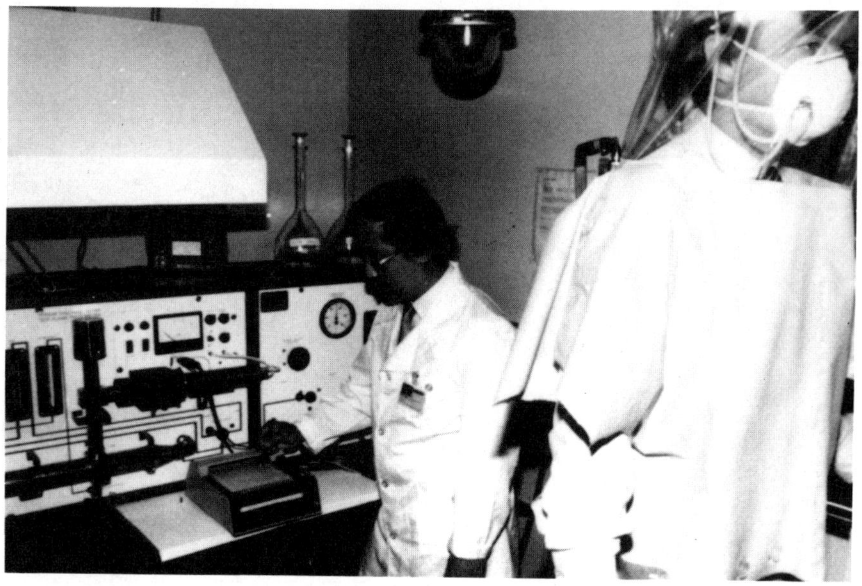

Photograph Courtesy of Gerson Co., Inc.

FIGURE B-5. **Quantitative fit testing of a single-use respirator**

APPENDIX C

SELECTED NIOSH RESPIRATOR USER NOTICES

DEPARTMENT OF HEALTH & HUMAN SERVICES

Public Health Service

Centers for Disease Control
National Institute for Occupational
Safety and Health – ALOSH
944 Chestnut Ridge Road
Morgantown, WV 26505

January 15, 1982

NIOSH EMERGENCY INFORMATION BULLETIN ON THE USE OF SELF-CONTAINED BREATHING APPARATUS IN LOW TEMPERATURES

Extreme caution should be exercised by all persons using open circuit self-contained breathing apparatus (SCBA) in hazardous environments during sub-freezing weather. SCBAs are widely used by fire fighters combatting winter fires. All users who wear SCBAs in cold temperatures should take particular note of the following important precautions:

1. Moisture in the air cylinders must be kept at an absolute minimum since small amounts of moisture in the air supply may freeze and result in failure of the breathing apparatus.

2. Always use a nosecup in the SCBA facepiece when temperatures are below freezing. Failure to use a nosecup under such circumstances can result in facepiece fogging and severely impaired vision. Chemical anti-fog agents may not perform adequately in low temperatures.

3. Carefully read the approval label on the respirator to determine if it is necessary to install special accessories prior to use of the SCBA in sub-freezing weather. Certain older U.S. Bureau of Mines approved SCBAs require such low temperature accessories (SCBAs approved prior to March 25, 1972).

4. When leaving an extremely hot environment, such as a fire scene, and entering cold air (below or near freezing), always place the SCBA facepiece in your turnout coat to keep it warm if it is to be quickly reused. SCBAs when not being actively breathed can freeze-up very quickly.

5. Use special care after washing SCBA facepieces and breathing tubes to remove all moisture to prevent water drainage and freeze-up of the regulator.

6. SCBA alarms can fail in low temperatures; therefore, visual checks of remaining service time should be made when SCBAs are used in sub-freezing conditions.

7. Be familiar with procedures on how to cope with exhalation valves which can freeze open or closed in low temperatures. (Contact the manufacturer or the State Fire Training Officer for specific instructions.)

8. SCBAs are NIOSH laboratory approved for use in temperatures down to -25° F. Therefore, if SCBAs are to be used in temperatures below -25° F, extreme caution should be used.

9. Also observe the following general precautions:

    a. Use G-7.1, Type I, Grade D air or air of equivalent specification.

    b. Follow all information listed on the NIOSH/ MSHA or BOM approval label for the specific SCBA in use.

    c. Follow the manufacturer's recommendations included in their instruction and maintenance manual accompanying the SCBA.

    d. Follow all applicable Federal, State, and Local regulations concerned with the use of SCBAs.

    e. Keep SCBAs in a warm location between uses.

James A. Oppold, Ph.D., PE
Director
Division of Safety Research

DEPARTMENT OF HEALTH & HUMAN SERVICES

Public Health Service

Centers for Disease Control
National Institute for Occupational
Safety and Health – ALOSH
944 Chestnut Ridge Road
Morgantown, WV 26505–2888

November 15, 1982

RESPIRATOR INFORMATION NOTICE
ON
MSA Powered Air Purifying Respirator
Mine Safety Appliance Company, Pittsburgh, PA
Model Numbers: 463354, 466607, 466608
Approval Number: TC-21C-186

On April 24, 1981, NIOSH issued a Respirator Information Notice which described the results of a NIOSH study of the MSA high efficiency powered air purifying respirator (PAPR) during use in a silica flour mill. The observed workplace protection factors (defined as the ratio of the concentration of contaminant outside the facepiece to the concentration of contaminant inside the facepiece measured while the respirator is worn) were significantly below the anticipated workplace protection factor of 1000. As a result, NIOSH stated that workers wearing the MSA PAPR may not receive the protection they anticipated. NIOSH stated further than the Institute had no evidence that the problem discovered in that study existed in other industries or situations of use. NIOSH also stated that the Institute would conduct further studies to evaluate the performance of the MSA PAPR against substances physically and chemically different from silica flour to determine whether results with silica flour were indicative of a problem associated with conditions of exposure or related to the malfunction of equipment.

Staff of NIOSH subsequently conducted a field evaluation of the half-mask MSA high efficiency PAPR at a primary lead smelter. The challenge aerosols contained predominantly lead dust and or lead fume. From this and other NIOSH studies, additional information has been developed and this Notice supersedes the Notice of April 24, 1981.

This field evaluation of the MSA PAPR produced the following preliminary results. The workplace protection factors associated with the respirator was found to be approximately lognormally distributed. The MSA PAPR produced a geometric mean workplace protection factor of 376 with a geometric standard deviation of 2.64 against lead fume and lead dust. Approximately 95% of the observed workplace protection factors for the MSA PAPR exceeded 77 while 84% of the observed workplace protection factors were below 1000. During this study no wearer of the MSA PAPR was exposed to concentrations of lead exceeding the permissible exposure limit (PEL).

Subsequent to issuance of the Respirator Information Notice of April 24, 1981, NIOSH and MSHA commenced proceedings to withdraw the certification of the MSA PAPR. That action was predicated upon the determination by

NIOSH that the MSA PAPR, during use in a silica flour mill, apparently did not provide the anticipated level of protection, i.e., a workplace protection factor of 1000. That action was subsequently voluntarily dismissed by the agencies pending the results of further studies. This study and additional studies of the PAPR class conducted by NIOSH indicate that the previously anticipated protection factor of 1000 expected of the entire class of PAPRs is inappropriately high. In view of this, the certification withdrawal proceedings against the MSA PAPR, which were previously dismissed will not be reinstituted. However, NIOSH recommends that users of PAPRs not rely upon them to consistently provide a workplace protection factor of 1000.

The results of the additional PAPR studies will be addressed in a subsequent Respirator Information Notice. For more information on this subject, contact the Testing and Certification Branch, Division of Safety Research, NIOSH, 944 Chestnut Ridge Road, Morgantown, West Virginia 26505, (304) 291-4331.

James A. Oppold, Ph.D., PE, CSP
Director
Division of Safety Research

DEPARTMENT OF HEALTH & HUMAN SERVICES Public Health Service

Centers for Disease Control
National Institute for Occupational
Safety and Health – ALOSH
944 Chestnut Ridge Road
Morgantown, WV 26505–2888

March 3, 1983

RESPIRATOR INFORMATION NOTICE

ON

3M Powered Air Purifying Respirator
3M, St. Paul, Minnesota
Model Number: W-344
Approval Number: TC-21C-246

Racal Powered Air Purifying Respirator
Racal Airstream, Inc., Frederick, Maryland
Model Number: AH3
Approval Number: TC-21C-212

In a Respirator Information Notice dated November 15, 1982, NIOSH recommended that powered air purifying respirators (PAPRs) with high efficiency filters not be relied upon to consistently provide a workplace protection factor of 1000. That recommendation was based upon the results of the two studies of PAPRs with tight fitting facepieces described in that Notice as well as the additional NIOSH study of helmeted PAPRs described in this Notice.

The NIOSH study of helmeted PAPRs with high efficiency filters was conducted by NIOSH on the 3M W-344 PAPR and the Racal AH3 PAPR at a secondary lead smelter. In this study the challenge aerosols contained lead dust and/or lead fume.

This study produced the following preliminary results. The workplace protection factors associated with both respirator models were found to be approximately lognormally distributed. The results of the t-tests indicate that there is no significant difference ($P < .05$) between the mean workplace protection factors of the 3M and Racal PAPRs under the particular circumstances of these studies. For both the 3M and Racal PAPRs, approximately 98% of the observed workplace protection factors were below 1000. Approximately 95% of the observed workplace protection factors for both the 3M and Racal PAPRs exceeded 33. The geometric mean workplace protection factor for 3M and Racal PAPRs was 182 with a geometric standard deviation of 3.2.

As stated in the November 15, 1982, Respirator Information Notice, the preliminary results of the NIOSH studies of the MSA, 3M and Racal PAPRs indicate that the protection factor expected from this class of respirators is inappropriately high.

For more information on this subject, contact Glendel J. Provost, Division of Safety Research, NIOSH, 944 Chestnut Ridge Road, Morgantown, West Virginia 26505. Commercial telephone number is (304) 291-4595 and the FTS number is 923-4595.

James A. Oppold, Ph.D., PE, CSP
Director
Division of Safety Research

DEPARTMENT OF HEALTH & HUMAN SERVICES

Public Health Service

Centers for Disease Control
National Institute for Occupational
Safety and Health – ALOSH
944 Chestnut Ridge Road
Morgantown, WV 26505–2888

December 16, 1983

RESPIRATOR USER'S NOTICE

Effects of Chemicals on Rubber and Plastic Parts of Self-contained Breathing Apparatus

The National Institute for Occupational Safety and Health (NIOSH) has received several reports of damage to parts of self-contained breathing apparatus that have apparently been exposed to concentrations of chemicals. These exposures have occurred during emergency response activities after accidental chemical vapor release and/or chemical discharge. The most recent report concerned a leak of dimethyl amine in Benicia, California, on August 12 and 13, 1983. Self-contained breathing apparatus and other equipment used during control of this leak were reportedly rendered unserviceable after exposure.

In view of these reports, fire fighting personnel who are engaged in emergency response activities should be equipped with proper chemical protective clothing in addition to respiratory protection. Information on the protective capabilities of such clothing should be obtained from the clothing manufacturer.

NIOSH is conducting a study of permeation of protective clothing materials by chemicals. Part of this study involves preparation of a data base of information on that subject. As part of this data base, NIOSH would appreciate receiving information on further cases of reported damage to self-contained breathing apparatus by chemicals. Reports should be addressed to the Testing and Certification Branch, Division of Safety Research, NIOSH, 944 Chestnut Ridge Road, Morgantown, WV 26505-2888. Reports should include the name of the chemical, Chemical Abstracts Service (CAS) Registry number, if known, identification and/or type of material damaged, extent of damage, and either the approximate concentration of the chemical or details of the exposure (e.g., exposure to liquid and/or vapor, temperature, wind conditions, and degree of enclosure of exposure).

Thomas C. Purcell

Thomas C. Purcell, Ph.D.
Acting Director,
Division of Safety Research

DEPARTMENT OF HEALTH & HUMAN SERVICES

Public Health Service

Centers for Disease Control
National Institute for Occupational
Safety and Health – ALOSH
944 Chestnut Ridge Road
Morgantown, WV 26505–2888

December 16, 1983

RESPIRATOR USER'S NOTICE

Effects of Heat and Flames on Rubber and Plastic
Parts of Self-contained Breathing Apparatus

The National Institute for Occupational Safety and Health (NIOSH) has received several reports of damage to parts of self-contained breathing apparatus that have apparently been exposed to excessive heat and/or flames during fire fighting activities. A preliminary investigation of these reports indicates that development of new turnout gear for fire fighters permits them to enter and remain in higher temperatures and flame exposures. These higher temperatures and flame exposures can apparently damage some presently-used rubber and plastic parts of self-contained breathing apparatus.

NIOSH is proposing to include requirements for high-temperature performance of self-contained breathing apparatus in Title 30, Code of Federal Regulations, Part 11 (30 CFR 11), the regulations governing approval of respirators. NIOSH has been advised by self-contained breathing apparatus manufacturers that they are developing new materials with greater resistance to heat and flames. NIOSH recommends that fire fighters avoid overexposure of breathing apparatus parts to high heat and/or flames, where possible.

NIOSH requests that fire fighting personnel and others report further incidents of heat and flame damage of self-contained breathing apparatus. Such reports should be sent to the Testing and Certification Branch, Division of Safety Research, NIOSH, 944 Chestnut Ridge Road, Morgantown, WV 26505-2888.

Thomas C. Purcell, Ph.D.
Acting Director,
Division of Safety Research

DEPARTMENT OF HEALTH & HUMAN SERVICES

Public Health Service

Centers for Disease Control
National Institute for Occupational
Safety and Health – ALOSH
944 Chestnut Ridge Road
Morgantown, WV 26505–2888

November 6, 1984

RESPIRATOR USERS' NOTICE

USE OF UNAPPROVED SUBASSEMBLIES

The National Institute for Occupational Safety and Health (NIOSH) has received many questions and complaints in regard to interchangeability of respirator subassemblies and unapproved modifications to MSHA/NIOSH certified respirators. Further, some problems reported to NIOSH have, upon investigation, been found to have been caused by user's modifying certified respirators which have resulted in the modified respirator failing to perform as anticipated, thus jeopardizing the respirator user.

MSHA/NIOSH respirator certification regulations, Title 30 Code of Federal Regulations Part 11 (30 CFR 11), state that approved respirators are ones that "are maintained in an approved condition and are the same in all respects as those respirators for which a certificate has been issued." [30 CFR 11, 11.2(b)] In addition, the regulations permit NIOSH/MSHA to only approve complete respirator assemblies and prohibit the approval of respirator subassemblies such as cylinders or air supply hoses. These requirements are intended to insure that one manufacturer has overall control and responsibility for the integrity of the approved respirator.

In some cases even minor modifications to respirators may make significant changes in the performance of the respirator. Manufacturers who modify certified respirators must test the modification to determine if the respirator continues to meet the minimum requirements of 30 CFR 11, and must submit the modifications to NIOSH. A user who modifies a certified respirator may not be able to determine whether a change will decrease respiratory protection. Several cases have been reported to NIOSH where unapproved modifications or use of an unapproved subassembly have resulted in respirator failures. Therefore, users of NIOSH/MSHA approved respirators are cautioned against interchanging subassemblies or making unapproved modifications to their respiratory protective devices.

John B. Moran
Director
Division of Safety Research

DEPARTMENT OF HEALTH & HUMAN SERVICES

Public Health Service

Centers for Disease Control
National Institute for Occupational
Safety and Health – ALOSH
944 Chestnut Ridge Road
Morgantown, WV 26505–2888

June 28, 1985

RESPIRATOR USERS NOTICE

Use and Maintenance of Pressure-demand Self-contained Breathing Apparatus

Since July 1, 1983, the Occupational Safety and Health Administration (OSHA) Fire Brigade Standard, Title 29, Code of Federal Regulations, Part 1910.156, has required that pressure-demand or other positive pressure self-contained breathing apparatus be worn by fire brigade members performing interior structural fire fighting. Although this standard is only applicable to all industrial fire brigades and to municipal fire departments in states with state-OSHA plans, other fire service organizations and industrial users of self-contained breathing apparatus (SCBA) have also recognized the superior protective capabilities of positive-pressure SCBA. As a result, there has been a steady change from demand to pressure-demand SCBA in the United States.

To provide the increased respiratory protection afforded by pressure-demand SCBA, it is generally necessary to increase the static pressure within the facepiece. The complex mechanics necessary to maintain this increased pressure and to control air flow when the facepiece is removed, together with the wearer's physiological response to the pressure-demand system, have presented problems to SCBA users.

Pressure demand SCBA requires more careful maintenance and different training, than is required for demand SCBA. Manufacturers have been providing maintenance and use instructions and training for purchasers of pressure-demand SCBA. The National Institute for Occupational Safety and Health (NIOSH) recommends that users of pressure-demand SCBA read those instructions, follow them carefully in apparatus use and maintenance, and take advantage of the manufacturer's training assistance. In addition to the manufacturers, training courses are offered by Fire Service organizations and by private organizations.

In the area of pressure-demand SCBA maintenance and repair, NIOSH strongly recommends that users have this service performed by a manufacturer-trained representative. This service is required to assure continued safe performance of pressure-demand SCBA.

Please advise NIOSH of any problems encountered in maintenance and use of pressure-demand self-contained breathing apparatus. Call the NIOSH Respirator Problem Coordinator, (304) 291-4595 (FTS 923-4595).

To assist you, NIOSH has prepared the following list of manufacturer's and fire service organization personnel who can provide further information on pressure-demand breathing apparatus training:

Clifton Precision
5100 State Road
Drexel Hill, PA 19026
Mr. Robert Gray (215) 622-1718

Globe Safety Equipment, Inc.
P.O. Box 7248
Dayton, OH 45407
Mr. Steven Bates (513) 224-7468

International Safety Instruments, Inc.
P.O. Box 846
Lawrenceville, GA 30246
Mr. Donald Dawson (404) 962-2552

MSA
600 Penn Center Boulevard
Pittsburgh, PA 15235
Mr. Jay Mears (412) 273-5145

North Safety Equipment
2000 Plainfield Pike
Cranston, RI 02920
Mr. Richard T. Flynn (401) 943-4400

Rexnord
45 Great Valley Parkway
Malvern, PA 19355
Mr. Justin Mills (215) 647-7200 *

Scott Aviation
225 Erie Street
Lancaster, NY 14086
Mr. Dennis Browner (716) 683-5100

U.S.D.
3323 West Warner Avenue
Santa Ana, CA 92702
Mr. Brian Miller (714) 241-4601

National Draeger, Inc.
P.O. Box 120
Pittsburgh, PA 15230
Mr. Les Boord/Ms. Karen Cox/Mr. Richard Weaver (412) 787-8383

International Association of Fire Chiefs
1329 18th Street, NW
Washington, DC 20036
Mr. Jan Thomas (202) 833-3420

International Association of Fire Fighters
1750 New York Avenue, NW
Washington, DC 20006
Mr. Richard Duffy (202) 737-8484

International Society of Fire Service Instructors
20 Main Street
Ashland, MA 01721
Mr. Ed McCormack (617) 881-5800

John B. Moran
Director
Division of Safety Research

* New contact for reporting respirator problems (replaced Mr. John Moffa)

DEPARTMENT OF HEALTH & HUMAN SERVICES

Public Health Service

Centers for Disease Control
National Institute for Occupational Safety and Health – ALOSH
944 Chestnut Ridge Road
Morgantown, WV 26505–2888

January 17, 1986

RESPIRATOR USERS NOTICE

Inspection of Certain Aluminum Cylinders for Breathing-gas Pressure

The light weight and high charging pressure of aluminum cylinders have resulted in their widespread acceptance and use with self-contained breathing apparatus (SCBA). The National Institute for Occupational Safety and Health (NIOSH) estimates that more than half of the SCBA of 30- and 60-minute duration in regular use today are equipped with aluminum cylinders.

Since first receiving reports of defective fiber-glass wrapped aluminum cylinders in 1983, NIOSH has advised users of potential hazards associated with use of certain fiber-glass wrapped aluminum cylinders. At this time, NIOSH believes there is sufficient evidence to warrant issuance of this NOTICE regarding inspection of fiber-glass wrapped aluminum cylinders.

The presently available evidence indicates that fiber-glass wrapped aluminum cylinders manufactured under Department of Transportation (DOT) exemptions DOT-E 7235 and DOT-E 8059 (including 2216 and 4500 psi) may, upon aging, develop neck cracks and may leak breathing gas during storage and use. This may result in significant loss of breathing gas from an unattended cylinder. If undetected, this loss of breathing gas could be dangerous to the user.

Based on this, NIOSH recommends that where SCBA are equipped with fiber-glass wrapped aluminum cylinders, inspection for cylinder pressure should be made at least weekly, for stored units. When used on a daily basis, as in fire fighting, cylinder pressure should be checked daily and immediately before use.

If a leak is suspected, the cylinder and cylinder valve should be tested as prescribed in American National Standard, Z88.5-1981, Practices for Respiratory Protection for the Fire Service, Section 6.2.4.2.

Leaks in cylinders should be reported to the SCBA manufacturer who will, in turn report them to the cylinder manufacturer. The numbers and charging pressures of leaking cylinders should also be reported to DOT (Mr. Art Mallen, DOT Office of Hazardous Materials, 400 7th St. SW, Washington, DC 20590) and to NIOSH (Mr. John Moran at the address shown at the top of this letter).

Aluminum cylinders used with SCBA, with exemption numbers other than DOT-E 7235 and DOT-E 8059 are not covered in this notice. Self-contained self rescuers used in mines are also not included.

MORE

REMINDER

January 17, 1986

Manufacturers of MSHA/NIOSH-approved SCBA Incorporating DOT-E 7235 4500 Fiber-glass Wrapped Aluminum Cylinders

The following manufacturers incorporate DOT-E 7235 4500 cylinders in their MSHA/NIOSH-approved SCBA:

- o Bendix
- o Clifton Precision
- o Draeger
- o Siebe Gorman
- o Scott
- o U.S.D. (SurvivAir)

DOT-E 7235 4500 cylinders must be retrofitted by Luxfer (Telephone: 714-684-5110) with steel neck rings, to prevent explosive rupture. DOT regulations prohibit charging of any DOT-E 7235 4500 cylinder that has not been fitted with a steel neck ring. Any apparatus utilizing a DOT-E 7235 4500 cylinder without a neck ring, is considered unapproved by MSHA/NIOSH.

Change in Address of Manufacturer's Contact

The following address change has been reported to NIOSH for manufacturer's personnel who are responsible for handling reports of problems with MSHA/NIOSH-approved respirators:

Clifton Precision:	New Address:	750 West Sproul Road, Springfield, PA 19064-4084
	Contact:	Mr. Martin Ziegler

John B. Moran
Director, Division of Safety Research

APPENDIX D

SAMPLE MSHA/NIOSH APPROVAL LABELS

Figure 1. Sample MSHA/NIOSH Approval Label for Pressure Demand SCBA.

PERMISSIBLE

30 Minute
Self Contained Pressure Demand
Compressed Air Breathing Apparatus

United States Department of Labor
MSHA
Mine Safety and Health Administration

U.S. Department of Health and Human Services
Centers for Disease Control
NIOSH
National Institute for Occupational Safety and Health

MINE SAFETY AND HEALTH ADMINISTRATION
NATIONAL INSTITUTE FOR OCCUPATIONAL SAFETY AND HEALTH

APPROVAL NO. TC-13F-000

ISSUED TO

ABC Company
Anywhere, USA

SAMPLE

LIMITATIONS

Approved for respiratory protection during the entry into or escape from oxygen deficient atmospheres, gases and vapors at temperatures above -22°F. Approved only when compressed air reservoir is fully charged with air meeting the requirements of the Compressed Gas Association Specification G-7-1 for Type 1, Grade D air or equivalent specifications. The container shall meet applicable DOT specifications. Demand mode shall be used only when donning aparatus. At temperatures above 32°F use without nosecup is permitted.

CAUTION

Use adequate skin protection when worn in gases or vapors that poison by skin absorption (for example, hydrocyanic adic gas). In making renewals and repairs, part identical with those furnished by the manufacturer under the pertinent approval shall be maintained. This respirator shall be selected, fitted, used, and maintained in accordance with Mine Safety and Health Administration, and other applicable regulations.

SAMPLE

MSHA — NIOSH Approval TC-13F-000

Issued to ABC Co., February 31, 2000

The approved assembly consists of the following part numbers:

000-000
000-000
etc.

Figure 2. Sample MSHA/NIOSH Approval Label for Pressure-Demand SAR

PERMISSIBLE

Combination Ten Minute Self-Contained Compressed Air Breathing Apparatus for Escape Only Pressure Demand Type C Supplied Air Respirator

United States Department of Labor
MSHA
Mine Safety and Health Administration

U.S. Department of Health and Human Services
Centers for Disease Control
NIOSH
National Institute for Occupational Safety and Health

MINE SAFETY AND HEALTH ADMINISTRATION
NATIONAL INSTITUTE FOR OCCUPATIONAL SAFETY AND HEALTH

APPROVAL NO. TC-13F-000

ISSUED TO

ABC Company
Anywhere, U.S.A.

SAMPLE

LIMITATIONS

Approved for respiratory protection during entry and escape from oxygen deficient atmospheres, gas, and vapors, when using air-line air supply. Approved for escape only, when using self-contained air supply. Approved for use at temperatures above -25°F.

Approved only when compressed air reservoir is fully changed with air meeting the requirements of the Compressed Air Gas Association Specifications G-7-1 for type 1, Grade D air, or equivalent specifications. The containers shall meet applicable DOT specifications.

This approval applies only when the device is supplied with respirable breathing air through 12.5 to 300 feet of hose at air pressures between 78 and 80 pounds per square inch gage or from self-contained air supply. If the supplied-air fails, open cylinder valve and proceed to fresh air immediately.

CAUTION

Use with adequate skin protection when worn in gases and vapors that poison by skin absorption (for example: hydrocyanic-acid gas). In making renewals and repairs, parts identical with those furnished by the manufacturer under the pertinent approval shall be maintained. This respirator shall be selected, fitted, used, and maintained in accordance with Mine Safety and Health Administration, and other applicable regulations.

SAMPLE

MSHA — NIOSH Approval TC-13F-000

Issued to ABC Company, February 31, 2000

The approval assembly consists of the following part numbers:

000-000
000-000
etc.

APPENDIX E

NIOSH RESPIRATOR DECISION LOGIC

NIOSH RESPIRATOR DECISION LOGIC

U.S. DEPARTMENT OF HEALTH AND HUMAN SERVICES
Public Health Service
Centers for Disease Control
National Institute for Occupational Safety and Health
Division of Standards Development and Technology Transfer

May 1987

DISCLAIMER

Mention of the name of any company or product does not constitute endorsement by the National Institute for Occupational Safety and Health.

DHHS (NIOSH) Publication No. 87-108

FOREWORD

The initial Respirator Decision Logic was developed in 1975 as part of the National Institute for Occupational Safety and Health/Occupational Safety and Health Administration (NIOSH/OSHA) Standards Completion Program and was updated in 1978. Due to technical advances in respirator design and research, NIOSH has again revised the Respirator Decision Logic.

This revision retains many aspects of the original Respirator Decision Logic, but it differs in five areas: odor warning properties with respect to air-purifying cartridge/canister respirators, recognition of the problems in assigning protection factors, changes in protection factors for certain respirator classes, respirator recommendations for carcinogens, and medical recommendations.

The recognition of wide variation among workers in their sensitivities for detection of odors has led to the recommendation that employers not rely solely on currently published data on odor thresholds to ensure that workers who wear air-purifying cartridge or canister respirators are capable of smelling the contaminant at the applicable exposure limit. Recent research on in-plant respirator testing suggests that some previously assigned protection factors based on data from laboratory fit testing may not be valid. This revised Respirator Decision Logic has incorporated assigned protection factors based on data from recent in-plant research for some powered air-purifying respirators (PAPR) and some similar respirators, such as loose-fitting and tight-fitting continuous flow air-line respirators. Since NIOSH maintains that there is no safe exposure to carcinogens, only the most protective respirators should be used to protect workers from exposure to carcinogens in the workplace. Finally, specific medical recommendations are included to assist physicians in determining an individual's fitness to wear a respirator.

J. Donald Millar, M.D., D.T.P.H. (Lond.)
Assistant Surgeon General
Director, National Institute for
Occupational Safety and Health
Centers for Disease Control

ACKNOWLEDGMENTS

This Respirator Decision Logic was prepared by a subcommittee of the NIOSH Respiratory Protection Committee, Sheldon H. Rabinovitz, Ph.D., Chairman. The Committee consists of members of each Division of NIOSH. The subcommittee consisted of the following individuals:

Warren R. Myers, Ph.D., Chairman, DSR
Nancy J. Bollinger, DSR
Thomas K. Hodous, M.D., DRDS
Nelson A. Leidel, Sc.D., OD
Sheldon H. Rabinovitz, Ph.D., DSDTT
Laurence D. Reed, DSR

The document was reviewed by the following experts in respiratory protection:

Earle Shoub, Consultant
Robert A. daRoza, Chairman, ANSI Z88 Committee
Mark Nicas, California Division of Occupational Safety and Health
Christopher C. O'Leary, Chairman, American Industrial Hygiene Association, Respiratory Protection Committee
Robert C. Spear, Ph.D., Professor and Director, Northern California Occupational Health Center, University of California, Berkeley

In addition, appreciation is extended to the following persons for their assistance in preparing this document:

R. Schutz for technical review; C. Browning, R. Grubbs, E. Kuempel, and H. Linn for editorial review; and J. Curless, L. DeVor, B. Ellis, J. Hamons, D. Hill, C. Klinker, N. Morgan, and A. Ritchey for typing.

CONTENTS

TABLES

FIGURE

I. INTRODUCTION

A. Background and Scope

The National Institute for Occupational Safety and Health (NIOSH) routinely makes recommendations regarding the use of respirators for workers exposed to workplace environments that contain hazardous concentrations of airborne contaminants and/or oxygen-deficient atmospheres. Such recommendations are made only when engineering controls are not technically feasible, while controls are being installed or repaired, or when emergency and other temporary situations arise. Respirators are the least preferred method of worker protection from respiratory hazards because they can be unreliable if an adequate respiratory protection program is not established by the employer and because they require worker cooperation. The intent of this decision logic is to provide industrial hygienists and other professionals knowledgeable in respirator selection with a procedure for selecting suitable classes of respirators for particular concentrations of specific contaminants. In this decision logic, concerns are raised about limitations of the data used to set protection factors for several classes of respirators.

To ensure uniformity and adherence to proper respirator usage, NIOSH recommendations have been based on the Respirator Decision Logic developed jointly in 1975 by NIOSH and the Occupational Safety and Health Administration (OSHA) as part of the Standards Completion Program and updated in June 1978. That decision logic incorporated requirements contained in 30 CFR 11 and fit factor data developed by the Los Alamos National Laboratory (LANL). NIOSH has now modified that decision logic to reflect new developments that include increased use of respirators to control exposure to carcinogens in the workplace, introduction of new respiratory equipment, and reporting of field research data on workplace protection factors (WPF's).

This modified decision logic identifies the criteria necessary to determine the classes of respirators that will provide a known degree of respiratory protection for a given work environment, assuming that the respirators are used correctly. The degree of protection is related in part to protection factors. Many of the assigned protection factors (APF's) that appear in this decision logic are based on laboratory studies and should be regarded as approximate.

The selection of a specific respirator must be made by individuals knowledgeable about the limitations associated with each class of respirators and familiar with the actual workplace environment, including the job task(s) to be performed. The correct use of a respirator is just as important as the selection process if adequate worker protection is to be achieved. Without a complete respiratory protection program, workers will not receive the degree of protection anticipated from a respirator, even if it is a correct choice for the situation. Training, motivation, medical evaluation, fit testing, and a respirator maintenance program are critical elements for the successful use of a respirator. As a minimum, compliance with 29 CFR 1910.134 is mandatory whenever respirators are used by workers, whether on a required or voluntary basis.

B. Cautionary Statements

NIOSH concerns about the use of respirators are discussed further in various parts of the document and are summarized in the following six cautionary statements:

- **Assigned Protection Factors**

  In general, the assigned protection factors (APF's) that appear in this decision logic are not based on measurements of actual field (workplace) performance. As noted in the footnotes accompanying Tables 1, 2, and 3, in only a few instances are the APF's based on any workplace performance testing; the majority of the APF's have no workplace performance basis at all. APF's based solely on laboratory fit testing should be viewed and applied with particular caution, even when the laboratory testing involves a simulated work regimen. To date, no relation has been demonstrated between laboratory fit factors and measured workplace performance. As more performance testing of respirators is undertaken in the workplace by NIOSH and others, NIOSH may find it necessary to revise the APF's upward or downward. For the present, APF's should not be considered reliable predictors of performance levels that will be achieved during actual use, since APF's are not based on a sufficient amount of workplace testing.

- **Fit Testing**

  No qualitative or quantitative fit tests have been demonstrated to be capable of effectively identifying inadequately fitting respirators (i.e., respirator-wearer combinations that provide less protection than the APF). The presently used fit tests (e.g., ANSI-recommended, OSHA-approved) may fail to identify individual wearers with inadequate respiratory protection. Thus fit tests should be used with caution and with recognition of their possible deficiencies. As appropriate, periodic evaluations of the effectiveness of each respirator during use in the workplace should be conducted to ensure that each wearer is being provided with adequate respiratory protection.

- **QNFT Fit Factor Screening Levels**

  Regarding quantitative fit testing (QNFT), no studies are available to indicate what fit factor value (i.e., screening level) will ensure a high probability of identifying inadequately fitting respirators. That is, there are no studies demonstrating what fit factor values are adequate accept/reject criteria for QNFT fit screening. When QNFT is used for fit screening, the fit factor screening level should be chosen with caution and with recognition of the uncertainty of its effectiveness. As appropriate, periodic evaluation of the effectiveness of each respirator during use in the workplace should be conducted to ensure that each wearer is being provided with adequate respiratory protection.

- **Adequate Warning Properties**

  No physiological effects in humans (e.g., odor, taste, eye irritation, respiratory irritation) have been demonstrated as being capable of consistently providing respirator wearers with timely, consistent, persistent, and reliable warning of hazardous airborne concentrations inside a respirator. Individual wearers may be unable to detect the warning effect when necessary and may fail to take action necessary to protect themselves (e.g., leaving the area where respirators are necessary or changing the sorbent cartridge or canister). When warning properties must be relied on as part of a respiratory protection program, the employer should accurately, validly, and reliably screen each prospective wearer for the ability to detect the warning properties of the hazardous substance(s) at exposure levels that are less than the exposure limits for the substance(s). Warning properties should be regarded with caution and with recognition of their unreliability.

- **Service Life Information**

  For essentially all gases and vapors, no adequate service life information is available to respirator wearers or to those responsible for respiratory protection programs. When this information is not available, respirators with air-purifying sorbent elements should be used with caution and with recognition of the wide variability of service lives under differing use conditions. Employers should possess valid and reliable estimates of service lives for all sorbent elements used in the respiratory protection program. Service life test data should be representative of all conditions of intended use that can be reasonably anticipated. Factors known to affect the service lives of sorbent elements include, but are not limited to, the make and model of sorbent element, airborne concentrations of contaminant(s), and relative humidity through each sorbent element. When appropriate service life data is available, any reliance on the data should be undertaken with caution and with recognition of the limitations and uncertainties of the information.

- **Determination of Protection Factor Levels Required for Adequate Protection**

  Workers are never exposed to a single unvarying concentration of a contaminant. In a given work area, individual exposures may vary widely between workers, during a workshift, and between days. The range of potential exposures should be appropriately determined for all workers and for all circumstances that can be reasonably anticipated. The highest anticipated exposure for each respirator wearer should be used to compute the protection factor required for each wearer. Required protection factors should be used with caution and with recognition of their uncertainties.

II. RESPIRATOR DECISION LOGIC

This decision logic contains a series of questions regarding situations which may require the use of respirators. (See Respirator Decision Logic Sequence, page 8.) In answering these questions, the user of this decision logic is assisted in identifying specific classes of respirators, applicable restrictions, and the appropriate respirator selection table to use. When using one of the tables to identify a suitable class of respirators, the user must keep in mind the restrictions identified in the question section of this decision logic.

This decision logic identifies the criteria necessary to determine the classes of respirators that will provide the minimum acceptable degree of protection for a chemical at a given concentration. Classes of respirators offering greater protection can usually be used in place of the minimum acceptable class of respirators. Respirator classes are consistent with respirator certification groupings as specified in 30 CFR 11.

The recommendations in this decision logic are based primarily on the physical, chemical, and toxicologic properties of the contaminant and on the limitations of each class of respirators, including filtration efficiency, air supply capability, and face seal characteristics and leakage. Thus this decision logic is limited to identifying classes of acceptable respirators, rather than individual respirators.

After various classes of respirators are identified as being suitable for a given situation, an evaluation is made of other factors of the particular work environment so that the best respirator within the recommended classes can be chosen. In some situations, the selection of a respirator classified as providing a higher level of protection may be advisable.

To assist the user, this decision logic contains ten subparagraphs following the Respirator Decision Logic Sequence that describe respirator limitations, use of applicable exposure limits, warning properties, protection factors, oxygen limitations, and medical evaluation of suitability to wear respirators. Additional supporting information is contained in Appendices A through E. To properly use this decision logic, the user should carefully read the subparagraphs.

The assigned protection factors (APF's) used in this decision logic were based on quantitative fit factor data developed by Los Alamos National Laboratories (LANL) under contract to NIOSH and on field evaluation data gathered by NIOSH and others. Specific references and summaries of the data used to generate certain protection factors can be found in Subparagraph 8, page 28. Fit factors determined for the individual wearer of a respirator by quantitative fit testing or by any other method used to determine fit should not be substituted for the APF given for each class of respirators. However, the fit factor determined through quantitative fit testing must be greater than the APF; otherwise, the respirator cannot be used by the worker.

A. Criteria for Selecting Respirators

To use this decision logic, the user must first assemble the necessary toxicologic, safety, and other relevant information for each contaminant, including the following:

- General use conditions, including determination of contaminant(s);
- Physical, chemical, and toxicologic properties of the contaminant(s);
- Odor threshold data;
- NIOSH recommended exposure limit (REL) or when no REL exists, OSHA permissible exposure limit (PEL) or other applicable exposure limit;
- Immediately dangerous to life or health (IDLH) concentration;
- Eye irritation potential; and
- Any service life information available (for cartridges and canisters).

Obtaining complete information on all criteria needed to use this decision logic may be difficult. When conflicting or inadequate data are found, experts should be consulted before decisions are made that could affect the proper use of this decision logic. In addition, the adequacy of the respirator selected is dependent on the validity of the exposure limit used. While the decision logic can be used with any exposure limit, NIOSH recommends that an REL be used when one exists for a given contaminant. For a more detailed discussion on the use of exposure limits, especially when selecting respirators for protection against carcinogens, see Subparagraph 2, page 21.

The information obtained on general use conditions for respirators should include a description of the actual job task, including the duration and frequency, location, physical demands, and industrial processes, as well as the comfort of the respirators. Some general use conditions may preclude the use of specific types of respirators in certain circumstances because the individual must be medically and psychologically suitable to wear a given respirator for a given task, particularly if the respirator is a self-contained breathing apparatus (SCBA).

Information obtained on the service life of the cartridge/canister under conditions of intended use should be evaluated regardless of the odor warning properties of the chemicals. These evaluations should be based on all gas(es) and vapor(s) present at the temperature and relative humidity extremes (high and low) in the workplace. NIOSH recommends that when the employer or a representative of the employer conducts the tests, the challenge concentrations of the gases and vapors should be at least 10 times the maximum use concentration of the respirator. The service life value obtained from these tests should be used to determine how long a cartridge/canister could provide protection under actual use conditions. This information can be used to set up cartridge replacement schedules and should be used in conjunction with sensory warning properties. Workers should be trained to exit the contaminated area whenever they detect the odor of the contaminant. (See Subparagraph 6, page 26, for a discussion on service life testing for chemicals with poor warning properties.)

B. Restrictions and Requirements for All Respirator Usage

The following requirements and restrictions must be considered to ensure that the respirator selected will provide adequate protection under the conditions of intended use:

1. A complete respiratory protection program should be instituted which includes regular worker training; maintenance, inspection, cleaning, and evaluation of the respirator; use of the respirator in accordance with the manufacturer's instructions; fit testing; and environmental monitoring. Whenever possible, quantitative evaluation of the protection factor in the workplace should be performed to confirm the actual degree of protection provided by the respirator to each worker. Minimum respiratory protection requirements for all contaminants can be found in the OSHA Safety and Health Standards, 29 CFR 1910.134, and in separate sections for specific contaminants (e.g., 1910.1001 for asbestos, 1910.1025 for lead, etc.).

2. Qualitative or quantitative fit tests should be provided as appropriate to ensure that the respirator fits the individual. Periodic evaluation of the effectiveness of each respirator during use in the workplace should be conducted to ensure that each wearer is being provided with adequate respiratory protection. When quantitative fit testing (QNFT) is used, the fit factor screening level should be chosen with caution and with the recognition of the uncertainty of its effectiveness since no studies have demonstrated what fit factor values provide adequate accept/reject criteria for quantitative fit screening.

3. Negative pressure respirators should not be used when facial scars or deformities interfere with the face seal.

4. No respirator (including positive pressure respirators) should be used when facial hair interferes with the face seal.

5. The respirators should be properly maintained, correctly used, and conscientiously worn.

6. The usage limitations of air-purifying elements, particularly gas and vapor cartridges, should not be exceeded.

7. The respirators must be approved by the Mine Safety and Health Administration and the National Institute for Occupational Safety and Health (MSHA/NIOSH).

8. Workers should be instructed to leave the contaminated area immediately upon suspicion of respirator failure and then to determine the problem.

9. Workers are not exposed to a single unvarying concentration of a hazardous substance, rather individual exposures may vary throughout a workshift and between days. The highest anticipated concentration should therefore be used to compute the required protection factor for each respirator wearer.

10. Respirator wearers should be aware of the variability in human responses to the warning properties of hazardous substances. When warning properties must be relied on as part of a respiratory protection program, the employer should screen each prospective wearer for the ability to detect the warning properties of the hazardous substance(s) at exposure concentrations that are less than the REL for each given substance. (See Subparagraph 6, page 26, and Appendix C, page 48, for additional information.)

11. The assigned protection factors (APF's) that appear in this decision logic are based for the most part on laboratory studies. However, a few APF's have been validated and revised as necessary after consideration of data obtained from studies of workplace protection factors (WPF's). As more WPF testing of respirators is undertaken by NIOSH and others, the APF values may be further revised. For the present, the APF's should be regarded as approximate if they are not based on WPF's.

C. Respirator Decision Logic Sequence

After all criteria have been identified and evaluated and after the requirements and restrictions of the respiratory protection program have been met, the following sequence of questions can be used to identify the class of respirators that should provide adequate respiratory protection:

1. Is the respirator intended for use during fire fighting?

   a. If yes, only a self-contained breathing apparatus (SCBA) with a full facepiece operated in pressure demand or other positive pressure mode is recommended.

   b. If no, proceed to Step 2.

2. Is the respirator intended for use in an oxygen-deficient atmosphere, i.e., less than 19.5% oxygen at sea level? (Refer to Subparagraph 1, page 21, for a discussion of oxygen deficiency.)

   a. If yes, any type of SCBA or supplied-air respirator (SAR) with an auxiliary SCBA is recommended. Auxiliary SCBA must be of sufficient duration to permit escape to safety if the air supply is interrupted. If additional contaminants are present, proceed to Step 3.

b. If no, proceed to Step 3.

3. Is the respirator intended for use during emergency situations?

a. If yes, two types of respirators are recommended: a SCBA with a full facepiece operated in pressure demand or other positive pressure mode or an SAR with a full facepiece operated in pressure demand or other positive pressure mode in combination with an auxiliary SCBA operated in pressure demand or other positive pressure mode. Auxiliary SCBA must be of sufficient duration to permit escape to safety if the air supply is interrupted.

b. If no, proceed to Step 4.

4. Is the contaminant regulated by the Department of Labor as a potential occupational carcinogen or identified by NIOSH as a potential human carcinogen in the workplace, and is the contaminant detectable in the atmosphere?

a. If yes, two types of respirators are recommended: a SCBA with a full facepiece operated in pressure demand or other positive pressure mode or an SAR with a full facepiece operated in pressure demand or other positive pressure mode in combination with an auxiliary SCBA operated in pressure demand or other positive pressure mode. Auxiliary SCBA must be of sufficient duration to permit escape to safety if the air supply is interrupted.

b. If no, proceed to Step 5.

5. Is the exposure concentration of the contaminant, as determined by acceptable industrial hygiene methods, less than the NIOSH REL or other applicable exposure limit? (Whenever a worker is given a respirator to use on a voluntary basis when ambient levels are below applicable limits, OSHA requires the implementation of a complete respiratory protection program, which includes medical evaluation, training, fit testing, periodic environmental monitoring, and all other requirements in 29 CFR 1910.134.)

a. If yes, a respirator would not be required except for an escape situation. Proceed to Step 7.

b. If no, proceed to Step 6.

6. Are conditions such that a worker who is required to wear a respirator can escape from the work area and not suffer loss of life or immediate or delayed irreversible health effects if the respirator fails, i.e., are the conditions <u>not</u> immediately dangerous to life or health (IDLH)? (Refer to Subparagraph 3, page 22, for additional information on IDLH's.)

a. If yes, conditions are not considered to be IDLH. Proceed to Step 7.

b. If no, conditions are considered to be IDLH. Two types of respirators are recommended: a SCBA with a full facepiece operated in pressure demand or other positive pressure mode or an SAR with a full facepiece operated in pressure demand or other positive pressure mode in combination with an auxiliary SCBA operated in pressure demand or other positive pressure mode. The auxiliary SCBA must be of sufficient duration to permit escape to safety if the air supply is interrupted.

7. Is the contaminant an eye irritant, or can the contaminant cause eye damage at the exposure concentration? (Refer to Subparagraph 4, page 23, for a discussion of eye irritation and damage.)

a. If yes, a respirator equipped with a full facepiece, helmet, or hood is recommended. Proceed to Step 8.

b. If no, an orinasal respirator may still be an option, depending on the exposure concentration. Proceed to Step 8.

8. Divide the 8-hour time-weighted average (TWA) exposure concentration for the contaminant (or maximum exposure concentration for a contaminant with a ceiling limit) determined in Step 5 by the NIOSH REL or other applicable exposure limit to determine the minimum protection factor required. For escape respirators, determine the potential for generation of a hazardous condition caused by an accident or equipment failure. If a potentially hazardous condition could occur or a minimum protection factor has been calculated, proceed to Step 9.

9. If the physical state of the contaminant is a particulate (solid or liquid) during periods of respirator use, proceed to Step 10; if it is a gas or vapor, proceed to Step 11; if it is a combination of gas or vapor and particulate, proceed to Step 12.

10. Particulate Respirators

10.1. Is the particulate respirator intended only for escape purposes?

a. If yes, refer to Subparagraph 5, page 24, for a discussion and selection of "escape only" respirators.

b. If no, the particulate respirator is intended for use during normal work activities. Proceed to Step 10.2.

10.2. A filter medium that will provide protection against exposure to the particulate in question is recommended. (Refer to Subparagraph 9, page 29, for a discussion on limitations of approvals for filter media.) Proceed to Step 10.3.

10.3. Respirators that have not been previously eliminated from Table 1 and that have APF's equal to or greater than the minimum protection factor determined in Step 8 are recommended. (Refer to Subparagraph 8, page 28, and Appendix D, page 50, for a discussion of protection factors, and to Subparagraph 9, page 29, for a discussion on limitations of filter approvals.) Maximum airborne concentrations for each level of respiratory protection can be calculated by multiplying the NIOSH REL or other applicable exposure limit by the APF for that class of respirators. Workers wearing respirators should meet the medical guidelines discussed in Subparagraph 10, page 30.

11. Gas/Vapor Respirators

11.1. Is the gas/vapor respirator intended for "escape only" purposes?

a. If yes, refer to Subparagraph 5, page 24, for a discussion on selection of "escape only" respirators.

b. If no, the gas/vapor respirator is intended for use during normal work activities. Proceed to Step 11.2.

11.2. Are the warning properties for the gas/vapor contaminant adequate at or below the NIOSH REL or other applicable exposure limit? (Refer to Subparagraph 6, page 26, and Appendix C, page 48, for additional information on requirements for adequate warning properties.)

a. If yes, proceed to Step 11.3.

b. If no, an air-purifying respirator equipped with an effective end-of-service-life indicator (ESLI), a supplied-air respirator, or a self-contained breathing apparatus is recommended. (Refer to Appendix A, page 43, for additional information on approval of air-purifying respirators with ESLI's.) Proceed to Step 11.4.

11.3. An air-purifying chemical cartridge/canister respirator is recommended that has a sorbent suitable for the chemical properties of the anticipated gas/vapor contaminant(s) and for the anticipated exposure levels. (Refer to Subparagraph 7, page 27, for the recommended maximum use concentrations of air-purifying chemical cartridge/canister respirators.) Proceed to Step 11.4.

11.4. Respirators that have not been previously eliminated from Table 2 and that have APF's equal to or greater than the minimum protection factor determined in Step 8 are recommended. (Refer to Subparagraph 8, page 28, and Appendix D, page 50, for a discussion of protection factors.) Maximum airborne concentrations for each class of respiratory protection can be calculated by multiplying the NIOSH REL or other applicable exposure limit by the APF for that class of respirators. The calculated maximum use concentration limits should not exceed the limitations noted in Subparagraph 7, page 27. Workers wearing respirators should meet the medical guidelines discussed in Subparagraph 10, page 30.

12. Combination Particulate and Gas/Vapor Respirators

12.1. Is the combination respirator intended for "escape only" purposes?

a. If yes, refer to Subparagraph 5, page 24, for a discussion and selection of "escape only" respirators.

b. If no, the combination respirator is intended for use during normal work activities. Proceed to Step 12.2.

12.2. Does the gas/vapor contaminant have adequate warning properties at or below the NIOSH REL or other applicable exposure limit? (Refer to Subparagraph 6, page 26, and Appendix C, page 48, for additional information on requirements for adequate warning properties.)

a. If yes, proceed to Step 12.3.

b. If no, either an air-purifying respirator equipped with an effective ESLI (Appendix A, page 43), a supplied-air respirator, or a self-contained respirator is recommended. Proceed to Step 12.4.

12.3. An air-purifying chemical cartridge/canister is recommended that has a particulate prefilter suitable for the specific type(s) of gas/vapor and particulate contaminant(s) and for the exposure concentrations. (Refer to Subparagraphs 7, page 27, and Subparagraph 9, page 29, for recommended maximum use concentrations and filter limitations.) Proceed to Step 12.4.

12.4. Respirators that have not been previously eliminated from Table 3 and that have APF's equal to or greater than the minimum protection factor determined in Step 8 are recommended. (Refer to Subparagraph 8, page 28, and Appendix D, page 50, for a discussion of protection factors and Subparagraph 9, page 29, for a discussion on limitations of filter approvals.) Maximum airborne concentrations for each level of respiratory protection can be calculated by multiplying the NIOSH REL or other applicable exposure limit by the APF for that class of respirators. The calculated maximum use concentration limits should not exceed the limitations noted in Subparagraph 7, page 27. Workers wearing respirators should meet the medical guidelines discussed in Subparagraph 10, page 30.

Table 1.--Assigned protection factor classifications of respirators for protection against particulate exposures[1]

Assigned protection factor	Type of respirator
5	Single-use (see definition in Glossary) or quarter mask[2] respirator
10	Any air-purifying half-mask respirator including disposable[3] (see definition in Glossary) equipped with any type of particulate filter except single use[2,4]
	Any air-purifying full facepiece respirator equipped with any type of particulate filter[5]
	Any supplied-air respirator equipped with a half-mask and operated in a demand (negative pressure) mode[2]
25	Any powered air-purifying respirator equipped with a hood or helmet and any type of particulate filter[4]
	Any supplied-air respirator equipped with a hood or helmet and operated in a continuous flow mode[4]
50	Any air-purifying full facepiece respirator equipped with a high efficiency filter[2]
	Any powered air-purifying respirator equipped with a tight-fitting facepiece and a high efficiency filter[4]
	Any supplied-air respirator equipped with a full facepiece and operated in a demand (negative pressure) mode[2]
	Any supplied-air respirator equipped with a tight-fitting facepiece and operated in a continuous flow mode[4]

1 Only high efficiency filters are permitted for protection against particulates having exposure limits less than 0.05 mg/m^3.

2 The assigned protection factors (APF's) were determined by Los Alamos National Laboratories (LANL) by conducting quantitative fit testing on a panel of human volunteers [6].

3 An APF factor of 10 can be assigned to disposable particulate respirators if they have been properly fitted using a quantitative fit test.

4 APF's were based on workplace protection factor (WPF) data or laboratory data more recently reported than the LANL data [7-11, 14-17].

5 The APF was based on consideration of efficiency of dust, fume, and/or mist filters.

Table 1.--Assigned protection factor classifications of respirators for protection against particulate exposures[1]--Continued

Assigned protection factor	Type of respirator
50 cont.	Any self-contained respirator equipped with a full facepiece and operated in a demand (negative pressure) mode[2]
1,000	Any supplied-air respirator equipped with a half-mask and operated in a pressure demand or other positive pressure mode[2]
2,000	Any supplied-air respirator equipped with a full facepiece and operated in a pressure demand or other positive pressure mode[2]
10,000	Any self-contained respirator equipped with a full facepiece and operated in a pressure demand or other positive pressure mode[2]
	Any supplied-air respirator equipped with a full facepiece operated in a pressure demand or other positive pressure mode in combination with an auxiliary self-contained breathing apparatus operated in a pressure demand or other positive pressure mode[2]

1 Only high efficiency filters are permitted for protection against particulates having exposure limits less than 0.05 mg/m^3.

2 The assigned protection factors (APF's) were determined by Los Alamos National Laboratories (LANL) by conducting quantitative fit testing on a panel of human volunteers [6].

3 An APF of 10 can be assigned to disposable particulate respirators if they have been properly fitted using a quantitative fit test.

4 The APF's were based on workplace protection factor (WPF) data or laboratory data more recently reported than the LANL data [7-11, 14-17].

5 The APF was based on consideration of efficiency of dust, fume, and/or mist filters.

Table 2.--Assigned protection factor classifications of respirators for protection against gas/vapor exposures

Assigned protection factor[1]	Type of respirator
10	Any air-purifying half mask respirator (including disposable) equipped with appropriate gas/vapor cartridges[2]
	Any supplied-air respirator equipped with a half mask and operated in a demand (negative pressure) mode[2]
25	Any powered air-purifying respirator with a loose-fitting hood or helmet[3]
	Any supplied-air respirator equipped with a hood or helmet and operated in a continuous flow mode[3]
50	Any air-purifying full facepiece respirator equipped with appropriate gas/vapor cartridges or gas mask (canister respirator)[2]
	Any powered air-purifying respirator equipped with a tight-fitting facepiece and appropriate gas/vapor cartridges or canisters[3]
	Any supplied-air respirator equipped with a full facepiece and operated in a demand (negative pressure) mode[2]
	Any supplied-air respirator equipped with a tight-fitting facepiece operated in a continuous flow mode[3]
	Any self-contained respirator equipped with a full facepiece and operated in a demand (negative pressure) mode[2]
1,000	Any supplied-air respirator equipped with a half-mask and operated in a pressure demand or other positive pressure mode[2]

1 The assigned protection factor (APF) for a given class of air-purifying respirators may be further reduced by considering the maximum use concentrations for each type of gas and vapor air-purifying element.

2 The APF's were determined by Los Alamos National Laboratories (LANL) by conducting quantitative fit testing on a panel of human volunteers [6].

3 The APF's were based on workplace protection factor (WPF) data or laboratory data more recently reported than the LANL data [7-11, 14-17].

Table 2.--Assigned protection factor classifications of respirators for protection against gas/vapor exposures--Continued

Assigned protection factor[1]	Type of respirator
2,000	Any supplied-air respirator equipped with a full facepiece and operated in a pressure demand or other positive pressure mode[2]
10,000	Any self-contained respirator equipped with a full facepiece and operated in a pressure demand or other positive pressure mode[2]
	Any supplied-air respirator equipped with a full facepiece operated in a pressure demand or other positive pressure mode in combination with an auxiliary self-contained breathing apparatus operated in a pressure demand or other positive pressure mode[2]

1 The assigned protection factor (APF) for a given class of air-purifying respirators may be further reduced by considering the maximum use concentrations for each type of gas and vapor air-purifying element.

2 The APF's were determined by Los Alamos National Laboratories (LANL) by conducting quantitative fit testing on a panel of human volunteers [6].

3 The APF's were based on workplace protection factor (WPF) data or laboratory data more recently reported than the LANL data [7-11, 14-17].

Table 3.--Assigned protection factor classifications of respirators for protection against combination gas/vapor and particulate exposures[1]

Assigned protection factor[2]	Type of respirator
10	Any air-purifying half-mask respirator equipped with appropriate gas/vapor cartridges in combination with any type of particulate filter[3]
	Any full facepiece respirator with appropriate gas/vapor cartridges in combination with a dust or mist or fume; dust and mist; or dust, mist, and fume filter[4]
	Any supplied-air respirator equipped with a half-mask and operated in a demand (negative pressure) mode[3]
25	Any powered air-purifying respirator equipped with a loose-fitting hood or helmet[5]
	Any supplied-air respirator equipped with a hood or helmet and operated in a continuous flow mode[5]
50	Any air-purifying full facepiece respirator equipped with appropriate gas/vapor cartridges in combination with a high efficiency filter or an appropriate canister incorporating a high efficiency filter[3]
	Any powered air-purifying respirator with a tight-fitting facepiece equipped with appropriate gas/vapor cartridges in combination with a high efficiency filter or an appropriate canister incorporating a high efficiency filter[5]
	Any supplied-air respirator equipped with a full facepiece and operated in a demand (negative pressure) mode[3]

1 Only high efficiency filters are permitted for protection against particulates having exposure limits less than 0.05 mg/m^3.

2 The assigned protection factor (APF) for a given class of air-purifying respirators may be further reduced by considering the maximum use concentrations for each type of gas and vapor air-purifying element.

3 The APF's were determined by Los Alamos National Laboratories (LANL) by conducting quantitative fit testing on a panel of human volunteers [6].

4 The APF was based on consideration of efficiency of dust, fume, and/or mist filters.

5 The APF's were based on workplace protection factor (WPF) data or laboratory data more recently reported than the LANL data [7-11, 14-17].

Table 3.--Assigned protection factor classifications of respirators for protection against combination gas/vapor and particulate exposures[1]--Continued

Assigned protection factor[2]	Type of respirator
50 cont.	Any supplied-air respirator equipped with a tight-fitting facepiece and operated in a continuous flow mode[5]
	Any self-contained respirator equipped with a full facepiece and operated in a demand (negative pressure) mode[3]
1,000	Any supplied-air respirator equipped with a half-mask and operated in a pressure demand or other positive pressure mode[3]
2,000	Any supplied-air respirator equipped with a full facepiece and operated in a pressure demand or other positive pressure mode[3]
10,000	Any self-contained respirator equipped with a full facepiece and operated in a pressure demand or other positive pressure mode[3]
	Any supplied-air respirator equipped with a full facepiece operated in a pressure demand or other positive pressure mode in combination with an auxiliary self-contained breathing apparatus operated in a pressure demand or other positive pressure mode[3]

1 Only high efficiency filters are permitted for protection against particulates having exposure limits less than 0.05 mg/m^3.
2 The assigned protection factor (APF) for a given class of air-purifying respirators may be further reduced by considering the maximum use concentrations for each type of gas and vapor air-purifying element.
3 The APF's were determined by Los Alamos National Laboratories (LANL) by conducting quantitative fit testing on a panel of human volunteers [6].
4 The APF was based on consideration of efficiency of dust, fume, and/or mist filters.
5 The APF's were based on workplace protection factor (WPF) data or laboratory data more recently reported than the LANL data [7-11, 14-17].

The Respirator Decision Logic Sequence is presented in Figure 1 in the form of a flow chart. This flow chart can be used to identify suitable classes of respirators for adequate protection against specific environmental conditions. Refer to the corresponding narrative section for additional information pertaining to a specific part of the flow chart.

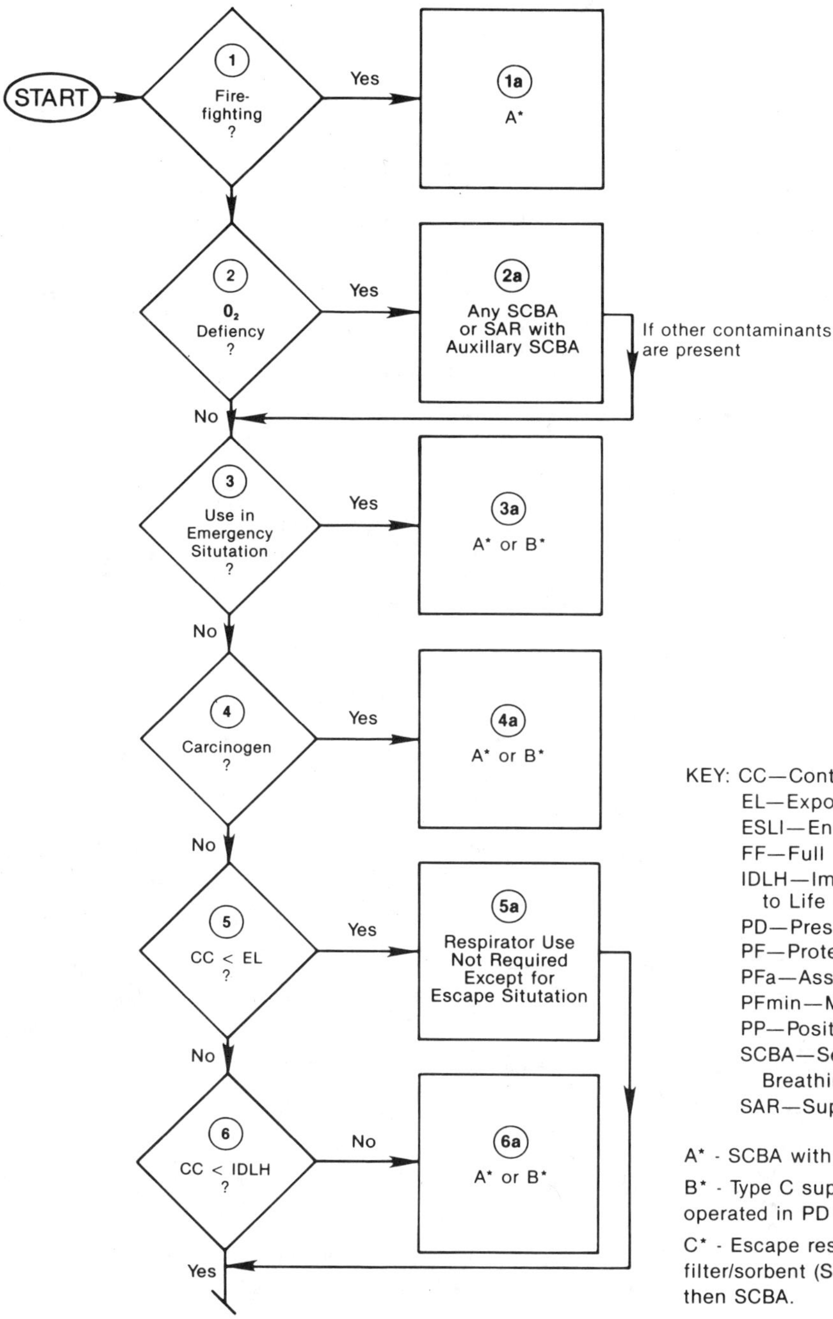

KEY: CC—Contaminant Concentration
EL—Exposure Limit
ESLI—End of Service Life Indicator
FF—Full Facepiece
IDLH—Immediately Dangerous to Life or Health
PD—Pressure Demand
PF—Protection Factor
PFa—Assigned PF
PFmin—Minimum PF
PP—Positive Pressure
SCBA—Self-Contained Breathing Apparatus
SAR—Supplied-Air Respirator

A* - SCBA with FF operated in PD or PP mode.

B* - Type C supplied-air respirator (airline) operated in PD or PP mode with auxiliary SCBA.

C* - Escape respirator or gas mask with appropriate filter/sorbent (Subparagraph 5); if 0_2 deficient, then SCBA.

Figure 1. — Flow Chart of Respirator Decision Logic Sequence

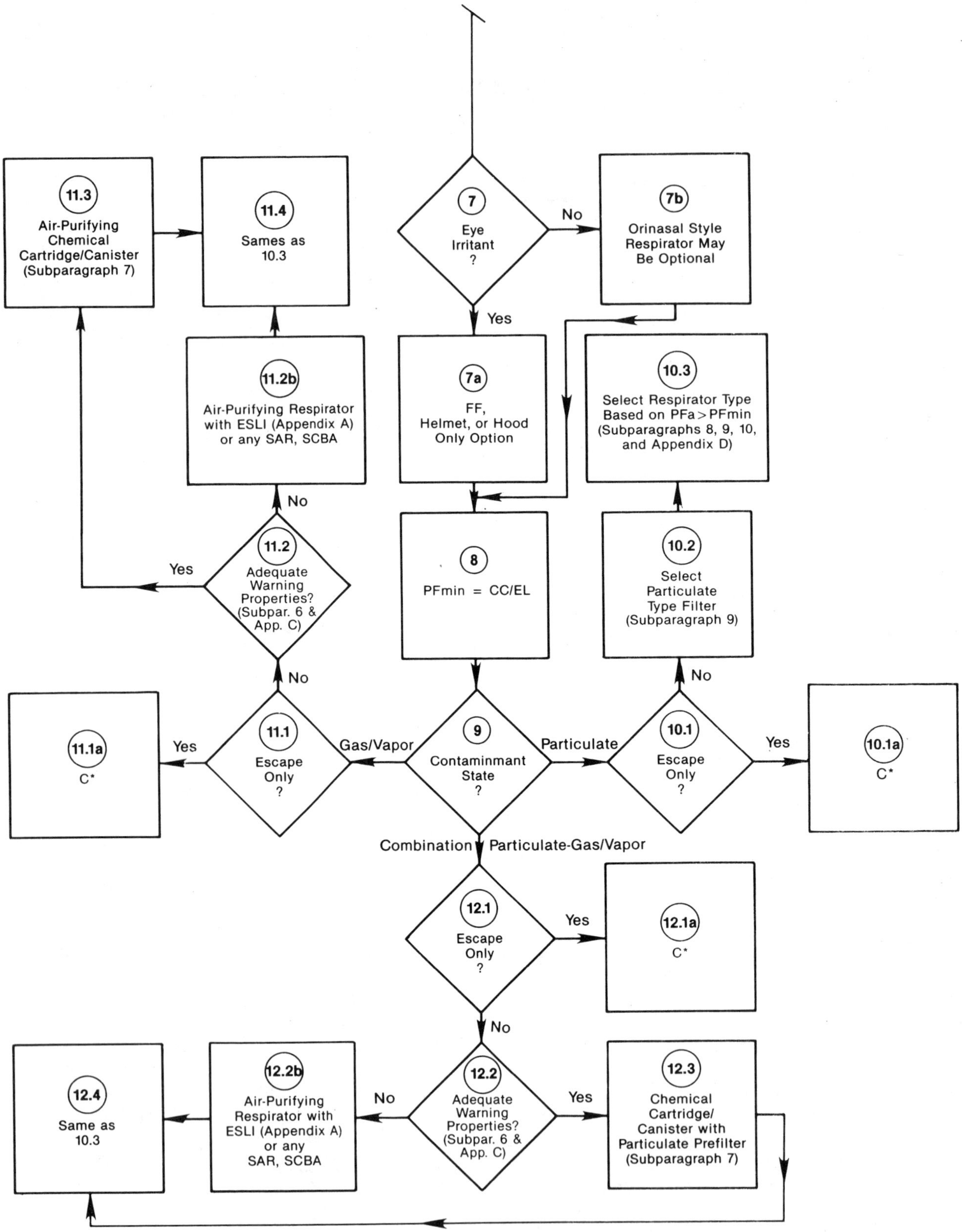

Figure 1. — Flow Chart of Respirator Decision Logic Sequence — Continued

D. Subparagraphs

The following subparagraphs provide additional information to assist the reader in using the Respirator Decision Logic Sequence:

Subparagraph 1: Oxygen-Deficient Atmosphere

The National Institute for Occupational Safety and Health (NIOSH) defines an oxygen-deficient atmosphere as any atmosphere containing oxygen at a concentration below 19.5% at sea level [1]. NIOSH certification of air-line or air-purifying respirators is limited to those respirators used in atmospheres containing at least 19.5% oxygen, except for those air-line respirators equipped with auxiliary self-contained breathing apparatus (SCBA).

The minimum requirement of 19.5% oxygen at sea level provides an adequate amount of oxygen for most work assignments and includes a safety factor. The safety factor is needed because oxygen-deficient atmospheres offer little warning of the danger, and the continuous measurement of an oxygen-deficient atmosphere is difficult.

At oxygen concentrations below 16% at sea level, decreased mental effectiveness, visual acuity, and muscular coordination occur. At oxygen concentrations below 10%, loss of consciousness may occur, and below 6% oxygen, death will result. Often only mild subjective changes are noted by individuals exposed to low concentrations of oxygen, and collapse can occur without warning [2,3,4].

Since oxygen-deficient atmospheres are life-threatening, only the most reliable respirators are recommended; the most reliable respirators are the self-contained breathing apparatus or the supplied-air respirators with auxiliary self-contained units. Because a high protection factor is not necessary to ensure an adequate supply of oxygen even in an atmosphere containing no oxygen, any certified self-contained unit is adequate. All aspects of a respiratory protection program must be instituted for these recommendations to be valid.

Subparagraph 2: Exposure Limits

The majority of the OSHA PEL's were adopted from the American Conference of Governmental Industrial Hygienists (ACGIH) TLVs® published in 1968. The difficulty in changing PEL's through promulgation of standards when new toxicologic information is identified has caused many standards to become outdated. The effectiveness of this decision logic is limited to the adequacy of the selected exposure limits in protecting the health of workers. Exposure limits based on a thorough evaluation of more recent or extensive data should be given priority.

For all chemicals that cause irritation or systemic effects but do not cause carcinogenic effects, it is currently believed that a threshold exposure concentration exists such that virtually all persons in the working population (with the possible exception of hypersensitive individuals) would experience no adverse health effects.

For many carcinogenic substances, most available data provide no evidence for the existence of a threshold exposure concentration below which the substance would be safe. As with noncarcinogenic substances, there appears to be a dose-response relationship for carcinogenic substances. If no threshold exists for a carcinogen, then there is no safe exposure concentration; however, lower exposures would be associated with lower risks.

For some carcinogens, NIOSH attempts to identify the lowest REL on the basis of the quantitative detection limit for the method used to monitor exposures. For other carcinogens, NIOSH does not identify a precise exposure limit but recommends instead that the employer control worker exposures to the lowest feasible limit.

Regardless of the selected exposure limit for a carcinogen, the best engineering controls and work practices should be instituted. Respirators should not be used as a substitute for proper control measures. When respiratory protection is required to achieve the lowest exposure concentration, then only the most effective respirators should be used. Two types of respirators are recommended: a full facepiece SCBA operated in a pressure-demand or other positive pressure mode or a full facepiece supplied-air respirator (SAR) operated in a pressure-demand or other positive pressure mode in combination with a SCBA operated in a pressure demand or other positive pressure mode. The practicality of each situation must be assessed to determine the most technically feasible protection for the worker.

Other variables such as the specific situation, worker, or job may influence the selection of the appropriate exposure limit for a given contaminant. For example, the effects of some hazardous substances may be increased due to exposure to other contaminants present in the workplace or the general environment or to medications or personal habits of the worker. Such factors, which would affect the toxicity of a contaminant, would not have been considered in the determination of the specific exposure limit. Also, some substances are absorbed by direct contact with the skin and mucous membranes, thus potentially increasing the total exposure.

Subparagraph 3: Immediately Dangerous to Life or Health (IDLH)

An IDLH exposure condition is defined in this decision logic as one that poses a threat of exposure to airborne contaminants when that exposure is likely to cause death or immediate or delayed permanent adverse health effects or prevent escape from such an environment. The purpose of establishing an IDLH exposure level is to ensure that the worker can escape from a given contaminated environment in the event of failure of the respiratory protection equipment. The IDLH is considered a maximum level above which only a highly reliable breathing apparatus providing maximum worker protection is permitted. Any appropriate approved respirator may be used to its maximum use concentration up to the IDLH concentration.

In establishing the IDLH concentration, the following conditions must be assured:

a. The ability to escape without loss of life or immediate or delayed irreversible health effects. (Thirty minutes is considered the maximum time for escape so as to provide some margin of safety in calculating the IDLH.)

b. The prevention of severe eye or respiratory irritation or other reactions that would hinder escape.

Sources of information for determining whether the exposure limit for a contaminant represents an IDLH condition are as follows:

a. Specific IDLH guidelines provided in the literature such as the American Industrial Hygiene Association (AIHA) Hygienic Guides and the NIOSH Pocket Guide for Hazardous Chemical Substances (previous editions were published jointly by NIOSH and OSHA), and/or

b. Human exposure and effects data, and/or

c. Animal exposure and effects data, and/or

d. Where such data specific to the contaminant are lacking, toxicologic data from analogous substances and chronic animal exposure data may be considered.

Subparagraph 4: Eye Irritation

Eye protection in the form of respirators with full facepieces, helmets, or hoods is required for routine exposures to airborne contaminants that cause any irritation to the mucous membranes of the conjunctivae or the cornea or cause any reflex tearing. Eye protection is required for contaminants that cause minor subjective effects as well as for those that cause any damage, including disintegration and sloughing of conjunctival or corneal epithelium, edema, or ulceration. NIOSH is not aware of any standards for gas-tight goggles that would permit NIOSH to recommend such goggles as providing adequate eye protection.

For escape, some eye irritation is permissible if the severity of irritation does not inhibit the escape and if no irreversible scarring or ulceration of the eyes or conjunctivae is likely.

When data on threshold levels for eye irritation are insufficient, quarter- or half-mask respirators can be used, provided that the worker experiences no eye discomfort and no pathologic eye effects develop. Workers should be told that if any eye discomfort is experienced, they will be provided with respirators that have full facepieces, helmets, or hoods and that provide protection equivalent to the quarter- or half-mask respirators.

Subparagraph 5: Escape Apparatus

Escape devices have a single function: to allow a person working in a normally safe environment sufficient time to escape from suddenly occurring respiratory hazards.

Escape devices can be separated into two categories: air-purifying respirators and self-contained breathing apparatus. Air-purifying respirators remove contaminants from the air by sorbent and/or filter media, but because they do not provide air, these respirators cannot be used in an oxygen-deficient atmosphere. Air-purifying escape respirators include the escape gas mask (canister) respirator, the gas mask (canister) respirator, and the filter self-rescuer. The escape gas mask consists of a half-mask or a mouthpiece respirator. The mouthpiece respirator can be used for short periods of time to escape from low concentrations of organic vapor or acid gas. The escape gas mask, which utilizes a half-mask, filters contaminants from the air. These respirators may also be used to escape from low concentrations of organic vapor or acid gas. Escape gas mask respirators equipped with full facepieces can also be used for escape from IDLH conditions but not from oxygen-deficient atmospheres. No air-purifying device is suitable for escape from a potentially oxygen-deficient atmosphere. The filter self-rescue unit is the mouthpiece device, which is designed to protect specifically against less than 1% carbon monoxide.

A self-contained breathing apparatus (SCBA) provides air to the user for escape from oxygen-deficient environments. Escape SCBA devices are commonly used with full facepieces or hoods and, depending on the supply of air, are usually rated as 3- to 60-minute units. Self-contained self-rescuer (SCSR) devices have been approved by MSHA/NIOSH for escape from mines, but these devices may also have application in other similar environments. SCSR's are mouthpiece respirators that provide a source of oxygen-enriched air for up to 60 minutes. All SCBA devices can be used in oxygen-deficient atmospheres.

When selecting escape apparatus, careful consideration must be given to potential eye irritation. This consideration is important for determining whether a gas mask or SCBA equipped with a full facepiece should be selected rather than a device equipped with a half-mask or mouthpiece.

The majority of gas masks or escape gas masks can be used in situations involving gas(es), vapor(s), or particulates. For escape from particulate-contaminated environments, an air-purifying element must be selected that will provide protection against the given type of particulate. The information in Table 4 should be used to select the appropriate escape apparatus.

Table 4.--Selection options for escape respirators

Escape conditions	Type of respirator
Short distance to exit, no obstacles (no oxygen deficiency)	Any escape gas mask[1] (canister respirator) or gas mask[2] (canister respirator)
	Any escape self-contained breathing apparatus having a suitable service life[3]
	Any acceptable device for entry into emergency situations
Long distance to exit or obstacles along the way (no oxygen deficiency)	Any gas mask[2]
	Any escape self-contained breathing apparatus having a suitable service life[3]
	Any self-contained self-rescuer having a suitable service life
Potential oxygen deficiency	Any escape self-contained breathing apparatus having a suitable service life[3]
	Any self-contained self-rescuer having a suitable service life

1 An escape gas mask is a respirator designed for use during escape only from immediately dangerous to life or health (IDLH) or non-IDLH atmospheres. It may consist of a half mask facepiece or mouthpiece, appropriate air-purifying element for the contaminant, and associated connections. Maximum use concentrations for these types of respirators are designated by the manufacturer.

2 A gas mask consists of a full facepiece and either chin-style or front- or back-mounted canisters with associated connections. Maximum use concentrations for canister air-purifying elements are listed in Table 5.

3 Escape self-contained breathing apparatus can have rated service lives of 3 to 60 minutes. All acceptable devices for entry into emergency situations can also be used.

Subparagraph 6: Potential Warning Properties for Use With Cartridge/Canister Air-Purifying Respirators

For the purpose of this decision logic, warning properties are defined according to odor, taste, eye irritation, or respiratory irritation. Adequate warning properties imply that the gas or vapor of interest has a persistent odor or irritant effect at concentrations at or below the OSHA PEL or NIOSH REL. Recognition of an odor depends on a person's sensory ability to detect it. Since the range of odor recognition thresholds within a population is very large, odor recognition should not be relied on as the only means for determining that a cartridge or canister is no longer effectively removing a contaminant from the air. A more detailed discussion of variability of odor detection within a population is provided in Appendix C.

NIOSH recommends that the employer ensure that each worker who is required to wear an air-purifying cartridge or canister respirator is capable of recognizing the odor of the substance of concern at a concentration at or below the applicable exposure limit. Such a determination will necessitate that an odor screening test be conducted on each individual for each substance of concern in the particular workplace.

It is recognized that existing screening tests are subjective in nature and not sufficiently sensitive and that conducting screening tests for a group of workers exposed to several substances may be impractical. Therefore, NIOSH knows of no compelling reason not to develop quantitative service life test data to supplement or replace odor screening test results if it can be demonstrated that such a procedure will afford the wearer a level of protection at least equivalent to that indicated by odor screening. Even when service life test data are used, the employer and the respirator wearer should not ignore the usefulness of sensory detection properties (for those who can detect the contaminant's presence) to serve as a warning that the cartridge/canister has failed or that the integrity of the respirator face seal has been compromised.

It is important to realize that 30 CFR 11 [specifically, 30 CFR 11.90(b) (note 4) for gas masks (canister respirators) and 30 CFR 11.150 (note 7) for chemical cartridge respirators], which provides for approval of air-purifying (organic vapor) devices, prohibits their approval for use against organic vapors with poor warning properties unless there is an OSHA standard which permits their use. A more detailed discussion appears in Appendix C.

A recent policy decision by NIOSH allows the use of respirators with effective end-of-service-life indicators for protection against contaminants with poor warning properties, provided that certain conditions are met. These conditions are described in that policy statement, which is reproduced in Appendix A.

Subparagraph 7: Limitations of Respirators for Gases and Vapors

Air-purifying respirators cannot be used in IDLH atmospheres or in atmospheres containing less then 19.5% oxygen by volume. Gas masks (canister respirators) may be used for escape if the atmosphere is not oxygen-deficient.

If, after the APF is multiplied by the REL or other applicable exposure limit (APF X REL), the product exceeds the IDLH value, then the IDLH value shall be the maximum use concentration. (See Tables 1, 2, and 3.) In addition, there are maximum use concentrations associated with all gas and vapor air-purifying elements. (See Table 5.)

Air-purifying devices should not be allowed for either entry into or escape from hazardous environments when supporting evidence exists to demonstrate that unreasonably short service life would occur at the maximum use concentration.

Where there is reason to suspect that a sorbent has a high heat of reaction with a substance, use of that sorbent is not recommended. For such a substance, only non-oxidizable sorbents should be allowed.

Air-purifying respirators cannot be used for protection against gases and vapors with poor warning properties unless the respirator is approved with an effective ESLI. (See Appendix A.)

Although limited in number, there are specific air-purifying respirators that are approved by MSHA/NIOSH for protection against gases and vapors when respirators approved for a given class of contaminants (e.g., organic vapors) cannot be used due to sorbent deficiencies.

Subparagraph 8: Assigned Protection Factors (APF's)

APF's (sometimes referred to in the literature as respirator protection factors), which appear in the 1975 and 1978 versions of the OSHA/NIOSH Respirator Decision Logic, in the 1980 American National Standards Institute (ANSI) standards for respiratory protection, and in all OSHA health standards, are based on quantitative fit testing (QNFT) of respirators [6]. (See definition of fit factors in Appendix D.) No data have been reported in the literature to demonstrate that the results of QNFT are sufficiently indicative of the protection that a given respirator provides in the workplace. Recent studies by NIOSH [7-9] and others [10-12] have suggested that fit factors do not correlate with the workplace protection factors provided by powered air-purifying respirators (PAPR's) and negative pressure half-mask respirators. (See definition of workplace protection factors in Appendix D.)

Table 5.--NIOSH recommended maximum use concentrations (expressed in ppm) for gas and vapor air-purifying elements

Type of gas or vapor	Cartridge(s)	Chin-style canister	Front- or back-mounted canister
	Classification of gas and vapor air-purifying elements		
Organic vapors	1,000*	5,000†	20,000†
Acid gases			
Sulfur dioxide (SO_2)	50	100	100
Chlorine (Cl_2)	10	25	25
Hydrochloric (HCl)	50	100	100
Ammonia (NH_3)	300	500	500
Methyl amine (CH_3NH_2)	100	--	--
Carbon monoxide (CO)	NA	NA	1,500

* Maximum use concentration will be 1,000 ppm or the immediately dangerous to life or health (IDLH) value for the specific organic vapor, whichever is lower.

† Maximum use concentration for "entry into" will be limited to the value listed or to the IDLH value for the specific organic vapor, whichever is lower.

APF's that are still based on the fit factors determined by Los Alamos National Laboratories (LANL) can be used for those classes of respirators for which no WPF data or simulated workplace protection factor (SWPF) data are available. However, as WPF data are developed, these APF's will be revised, as have the current APF's for powered air-purifying respirators (PAPR's) [7-9,11,14-16]. It should be noted that a number of studies [17-20] on the workplace performance of respirators have appeared in the literature. However, the results of these studies are of little value for establishing APF's because their protocols did not require proper fit or correct use and conscientious wearing of the respirator while in-facepiece sampling was done. A notable exception is the study by Revoir (1974) [21].

When WPF data existed, NIOSH utilized the point estimate equation proposed by Myers et al. [13] to help establish the APF's recommended in this decision logic. The point estimate equation is as follows:

$$\text{protection factor (PF)} = \mu g/Sg^{Zp}$$

where μg = the geometric mean of the measured WPF

Sg = the geometric standard deviation of the measured WPF

Zp = the value corresponding to the selected proportion (p) on the log-normal probability distribution

When WPF data existed, NIOSH selected a confidence limit of p=0.95. Thus for a given set of data and given class of respirators, NIOSH would expect that 95% of the WPF's would exceed the calculated point estimate value.

Despite the fact that some of the PF's have a statistical basis, they are still only estimates of an approximate level of protection. It must not be assumed that the numerical values of the APF's presented in this decision logic represent the absolute minimum level of protection that would be achieved for all workers in all jobs against all respiratory hazards. The industrial hygienist or other professional responsible for providing respiratory protection or evaluating respiratory protection programs is therefore encouraged to evaluate as accurately as possible the actual protection being provided by the respirator.

Subparagraph 9: Particulate Filter Respirators

MSHA/NIOSH particulate respirators are certified according to seven basic categories. These categories consist of the following types of exposures:

- Dusts: Airborne exposure limit not less than 0.05 mg/m^3 or 2 mppcf (see Appendix B);

- Fumes: Airborne exposure limit not less than 0.05 mg/m^3 or 2 mppcf;

- Mists: Airborne exposure limit not less than 0.05 mg/m^3 or 2 mppcf (see Appendix B);

- Dusts, Fumes, and Mists: Airborne exposure limit less than 0.05 mg/m^3 or 2 mppcf and radionuclides;

- Radon Daughters;

- Asbestos-Containing Dusts and Mists (see Appendix B); and

- Single-Use Dust and Mist Respirators (see Appendix B).

Subparagraph 10: Suggested Medical Evaluation and Criteria for Respirator Use

The following NIOSH recommendations allow latitude for the physician in determining a medical evaluation for a specific situation. More specific guidelines may become available as knowledge increases regarding human stresses from the complex interactions of worker health status, respirator usage, and job tasks. While some of the following recommendations should be part of any medical evaluation of workers who wear respirators, others are identified as being applicable for specific situations.

a. A Physician Should Make the Determination of Fitness to Wear a Respirator by Considering the Worker's Health, the Type of Respirator, and the Conditions of Respirator Use.

The recommendation above satisfies OSHA regulations and leaves the final decision of an individual's fitness to wear a respirator to the person who is best qualified to evaluate the multiple clinical and other variables. Much of the clinical and other data could be gathered by other personnel. It should be emphasized that the clinical examination alone is only one part of the fitness determination and that collaboration with foremen, industrial hygienists, and others may often be needed to better assess the work conditions and other factors that affect an individual's fitness to wear a respirator.

b. A Medical History and At Least a Limited Physical Examination are Recommended.

The medical history and physical examination should emphasize the evaluation of the cardiopulmonary system and should elicit any history of respirator use. The history is an important tool in medical diagnosis and can be used to detect most problems that might require further evaluation. Objectives of the physical examination should be to confirm the clinical impression based on the history and to detect important medical conditions (such as hypertension) that may be essentially asymptomatic.

c. While Chest X-Ray and/or Spirometry May Be Medically Indicated in Some Fitness Determinations, These Should Not Be Routinely Performed.

In most cases, the hazardous situations requiring the wearing of respirators will also mandate periodic chest X-ray and/or spirometry for exposed workers. When such information is available, it should be used in the determination of fitness to wear respirators. (See Recommendation h, page 33.)

Routine chest X-rays and spirometry are not recommended solely as data for determining if a respirator should be worn. In most cases, with an essentially normal clinical examination (history and physical) these data are unlikely to influence the respirator fitness determination; additionally, the X-ray would be an unnecessary source of radiation exposure to the worker. Chest X-rays in general do not accurately reflect a person's cardiopulmonary physiologic status, and limited studies suggest that mild to moderate impairment detected by spirometry would not preclude the wearing of respirators in most cases. Thus it is recommended that chest X-ray and/or spirometry be done only when clinically indicated. (See Appendix E, page 52, for further discussion on the pulmonary effects of wearing respirators.)

d. The Recommended Periodicity of Medical Fitness Determinations Varies According to Several Factors but Could Be as Infrequent as Every 5 Years.

Federal or other applicable regulations shall be followed regarding the frequency of respirator fitness determinations. The guidelines for most work conditions for which respirators are required are shown in Table 6. These guidelines are similar to those recommended by ANSI, which recommends annual determinations after age 45 [22]. The more frequent examinations with advancing age relate to the increased prevalence of most diseases in older people. More frequent examinations are recommended for individuals performing strenuous work involving the use of SCBA. These guidelines are based on clinical judgment and, like the other recommendations in this section, should be adjusted as clinically indicated.

e. The Respirator Wearer Should Be Observed During a Trial Period to Evaluate Potential Physiological Problems

In addition to considering the physical effects of wearing respirators, the physician should determine if wearing a given respirator would cause extreme anxiety or claustrophobic reaction in the individual. This could be done during training, while the worker is wearing the respirator and is engaged in some exercise that approximates the actual work situation.

Present regulations state that a worker should be provided the opportunity to wear the respirator "in normal air for a long familiarity period..." [23]. This trial period should also be used to evaluate the ability and tolerance of the worker to wear the respirator [24]. This trial period need not be associated with respirator fit testing and should not compromise the effectiveness of the vital fit testing procedure.

Table 6.--Suggested frequency of medical fitness determinations*

	Worker age (years)		
	<35	35 - 45	>45
Most work conditions requiring respirators	Every 5 yrs	Every 2 yrs	1-2 yrs
Strenuous work conditions with SCBA†	Every 3 yrs	Every 18 mos	Annually

* Interim testing would be needed if changes in health status occur.
† SCBA = self-contained breathing apparatus

f. Examining Physicians Should Realize that the Main Stress of Heavy Exercise While Using a Respirator Is Usually on the Cardiovascular System and that Heavy Respirators (e.g., Self-Contained Atmosphere Supplying) Can Substantially Increase this Stress. Accordingly, Physicians May Want To Consider Exercise Stress Tests with Electrocardiographic Monitoring When Heavy Respirators Are Used, When Cardiovascular Risk Factors Are Present, or When Extremely Stressful Conditions Are Expected.

Some respirators may weigh up to 35 pounds and may increase workloads by 20 percent. Although a lower activity level could compensate for this added stress [25], a lower activity level might not always be possible. Physicians should also be aware of other added stresses, such as heavy protective clothing and intense ambient heat, which would increase the worker's cardiac demand. As an extreme example, firefighters who use SCBA inside burning buildings may work at maximal exercise levels under life-threatening conditions. In such cases, the detection of occult cardiac disease, which might manifest itself during heavy stress, may be important. Some authors have either recommended stress testing [26] or at least its consideration in the fitness determination [22]. Kilbom [26] has recommended stress testing at 5-year intervals for firefighters below age 40 who use SCBA and at 2-year intervals for those aged 40-50. He further suggested that firemen over age 50 not be allowed to wear SCBA.

Exercise stress testing has not been recommended for medical screening for coronary artery disease in the general population [27,28]. It has an estimated sensitivity and specificity of 78% and 69%, respectively, when the disease is defined by coronary angiography [27,29]. In a recent 6-year prospective study, stress testing to determine the potential for heart attack indicated a positive predictive value of 27% when the prevalence of disease was 3 1/2% [30,31]. While stress testing has limited effectiveness in medical screening, it could serve to detect those individuals who may not be able to complete the heavy exercise required in some jobs.

A definitive recommendation regarding exercise stress testing cannot be made at this time. Further research may determine whether this is a useful tool in selected circumstances.

g. An Important Concept Is that "General Work Limitations and Restrictions Identified for Other Work Activities Also Shall Apply for Respirator Use" [22].

In many cases, if a worker is able to do an assigned job without an increased risk to health while not wearing a respirator, the worker will in most situations not be at increased risk when performing the same job while wearing a respirator.

h. Because of the Variability in the Types of Respirators, Work Conditions, and Workers' Health Status, Many Employers May Wish to Designate Categories of Fitness To Wear Respirators, Thereby Excluding Some Workers from Strenuous Work Situations Involving the Wearing of Respirators.

Depending on the various circumstances, there could be several permissible categories of respirator usage. One possible scheme would consist of three overall categories: full respirator use, no respirator use, and limited respirator use including "escape only" respirators. The latter category excludes heavy respirators and strenuous work conditions. Before identifying the conditions that would be used to classify workers into various categories, it is critical that the physician be aware that these conditions have not been validated and are presented only for consideration. The physician should modify the use of these conditions based on actual experience, further research, and individual worker sensitivities. The physician may wish to consider the following conditions in selecting or permitting the use of respirators:

- History of spontaneous pneumothorax;

- Claustrophobia/anxiety reaction;

- Use of contact lens (for some respirators);

- Moderate or severe pulmonary disease;

- Angina pectoris, significant arrhythmias, recent myocardial infarction;

- Symptomatic or uncontrolled hypertension; and

- Age.

It seems unlikely that wearing a respirator would play any significant role in causing lung damage such as pneumothorax. However, without good evidence that wearing a respirator would not cause such lung damage, it may be prudent to prohibit the individual with a history of spontaneous pneumothorax from wearing a respirator.

Moderate lung disease is defined by the Intermountain Thoracic Society [32] as being a forced expiratory volume in one second (FEV_1) divided by the forced vital capacity (FVC) (i.e., FEV_1/FVC) of 0.45 to 0.60 or an FVC of 51 to 65% of the predicted FVC value. Similar arbitrary limits could be set for age and hypertension. It would seem more reasonable, however, to combine several risk factors into an overall estimate of fitness to wear respirators under certain conditions. Here the judgment and clinical experience of the physician are needed. Even many impaired workers would be able to work safely while wearing respirators if they could control their own work pace, including having sufficient time to rest.

Conclusion

Individual judgment is needed in determining the factors affecting an individual's fitness to wear a respirator. While many of the preceding guidelines are based on limited evidence, they should provide a useful starting point for a respirator fitness screening program. Further research is needed to validate these recommendations and others currently in use. Of particular interest would be laboratory studies involving physiologically impaired individuals and field studies conducted under actual day-to-day work conditions.

REFERENCES

1. Code of Federal Regulations, Title 30, Part 11, revised July 1, 1986.

2. Guyton AC. Textbook of medical physiology, 3rd ed, Philadelphia: W.B. Saunders Co., 1966, p. 578.

3. Clayton GD, Clayton FE, ed. Patty's industrial hygiene and toxicology, 3rd ed, Vol 1, New York: John Wiley & Sons, 1978.

4. A guide to industrial respiratory protection. Cincinnati: U.S. Department of Health, Education, and Welfare, Public Health Service, Centers for Disease Control, National Institute for Occupational Safety and Health, 1976; HEW (NIOSH) publication no. 76-189.

5. Goodman LS, Gilman A. The pharmacological basis of therapeutics. 3rd ed, New York: The Macmillan Co, 1968, p. 897.

6. Hyatt EC. Respirator protection factors. New Mexico: Los Alamos scientific laboratory of the University of California, informal report no. LA-6084-MS, 1976.

7. Myers WR, Peach MJ III, Allender J. Workplace protection factor measurements on powered air-purifying respirators at a secondary lead smelter--test protocol. Am Ind Hyg Assoc J 1984;45(4):236-41.

8. Myers WR, Peach MJ III, Cutright K, Iskander W. Workplace protection factor measurements on powered air-purifying respirators at a secondary lead smelter--results and discussion. Am Ind Hyg Assoc J 1984;45(10):681-88.

9. Myers WR, Peach MJ III. Performance measurements on a powered air-purifying respirator made during actual field use in a silica bagging operation. Ann Occup Hyg 1983;27(3):251-59.

10. Dixon SW, Nelson TJ. Workplace protection factors for negative pressure half-mask facepiece respirators. J Int Soc Respir Prot 1984;2(4):347-61.

11. Dixon SW, Nelson TJ, Wright JE. Program protection factor study on the 3M W316 Airhat™. Presented at the American Industrial Hygiene Conference, May 22, 1984, Michigan. Detroit: E.I. du Pont de Nemours & Co.

12. Hinton JJ. Reliability of quantitative fit protection factors in assessing face-to-facepiece seals. [Unpublished thesis]. Houston, TX: University of Texas, Health Science Center, 1980.

13. Myers WR, Lenhart SW, Campbell D, Provost G. [Letter]. Am Ind Hyg Assoc J 1983;44(3):B25-26.

14. Myers WR, Peach MJ III, Cutright K, Iskander W. Field test of powered air-purifying respirators at a battery manufacturing facility. J Int Soc Respir Prot 1984;4(1):62-89.

15. Lenhart SW, Campbell DL. Assigned protection factors for two respirator types based upon workplace performance testing. Ann Occup Hyg 1984;28(2):173-82.

16. Linauskas SH, Kalos F. Study of efficiency and current use of respiratory protective devices. [Report prepared for the Atomic Energy Control Board. Ottawa, Canada]. Atomic Energy of Canada Limited, 1984.

17. Bentley RA, Bostock GJ, Longson DJ, Roff MW. Determination of the quantitative fit factors of various types of respiratory protective equipment. J Int Soc Respir Prot 1984;2(4):313-37.

18. Moore DE, Smith TJ. Measurement of protection factors of chemical cartridge, half-mask respirators under working conditions in a copper smelter. Am Ind Hyg Assoc J 1976;37(8):453-58.

19. Toney CR, Barnhart WL. Performance evaluation of respiratory protective equipment used in paint spraying operations, NIOSH Technical Information, HEW publication no. (NIOSH) 76-177, 1976.

20. Smith TJ, Ferrell WC, Varner MO, Putnam RD. Inhalation exposure of cadmium workers: effects of respirator usage. Am Ind Hyg Assoc J 1980;41:624-28.

21. Revoir WH. Respirators for protection against cotton dust. Am Ind Hyg Assoc J 1974;35(8):503-10.

22. American National Standards Institute, Inc. American national standard for respirator protection-respirator use-physical qualifications for personnel, ANSI Z88.6-1984. New York: ANSI, Inc., 1984, pp. 7-15.

23. Code of Federal Regulations, Title 29, Part 1910, Section 134(e)(5), revised July 1, 1986.

24. Harber P. Medical evaluation for respirator use. J Occup Med 1984;26(7):496-502.

25. Manning JE, Griggs TR. Heart rates in fire fighters using light and heavy breathing equipment: similar near-maximal exertion in response to multiple work load conditions. J Occup Med 1983;25(3):215-18.

26. Kilbom A. Physical work capacity of firemen. Scand J Work Environ Health 1980;6:48-57.

27. Weiner DA, Ryan TJ, McCabe CH, et al. Exercise stress testing: correlations among history of angina, ST-segment response and prevalence

of coronary-artery disease in the coronary artery surgery study (CASS). N Engl J Med 1979;301(5):230-35.

28. Epstein SE. Limitations of electrocardiographic exercise testing [Editorial]. N Engl J Med 1979;301(5):264-65.

29. Nicklin D, Balaban DJ. Exercise EKG in asymptomatic normotensive subjects [Letter to the editor]. N Engl J Med 1984;310(13):852.

30. Giagnoni E, Secchi MB, Wu SC, et al. Prognostic value of exercise EKG testing in asymptomatic normotensive subjects. N Engl J Med 1983;309(18):1085-89.

31. Folli G. Exercise EKG in asymptomatic normotensives subjects [Reply to letter to the editor]. N Engl J Med 1984;310(13):852-53.

32. Kanner RE, Morris AH, ed. Clinical pulmonary function testing: a manual of uniform laboratory procedures for the intermountain area. 1st ed, Salt Lake City, Utah: Intermountain Thoracic Society, 1975.

33. Amoore JE, Hautala E. Odor as an aid to chemical safety: odor thresholds compared with threshold limit values and volatilities for 214 industrial chemicals in air and water dilution. J Appl Toxicol 1983;3(6):272-90.

34. Williams FT. Photometric measurement of respirator quantitative fit test protection factors and their interpretation, use and meaning, Dynatech Frontier Technical Note, 108-0008, 1978.

35. Halperin WE, Ratcliffe JM, Frazier TM, Becker SP, Schulte PA. Medical screening in the workplace: proposed principles. J Occup Med 1986;28(8):547-52.

36. Raven PB, Dodson AT, Davis TO. The physiological consequences of wearing industrial respirators: a review. Am Ind Hyg Assoc J 1979;40(6):517-34.

37. James RH. Breathing resistance and dead space in respiratory protective devices. U.S. Department of Health, Education, and Welfare, National Institute for Occupational Safety and Health, Cincinnati, Ohio, October 1976.

38. Gee JBL, Burton G, Vassallo C, Gregg J. Effects of external airway obstruction on work capacity and pulmonary gas exchange. Am Rev Respir Dis 1968;98:1003-12.

39. Hodous TK, Petsonk L, Boyles C, Hankinson J, Amandus H. Effects of added resistance to breathing during exercise in obstructive lung disease. Am Rev Respir Dis 1983;128:943-48.

40. Raven PB, Jackson AW, Page K, et al. The physiological responses of mild pulmonary impaired subjects while using a "demand" respirator during rest and work. Am Ind Hyg Assoc J 1981;42(4):247-57.

41. Hodous TK, Boyles C, Hankinson J. Effects of industrial respirator wear during exercise in subjects with restrictive lung disease. Am Ind Hyg Assoc J 1986;47:176-80.

42. Altose MD, McCauley WC, Kelsen SG, Cherniack NS. Effects of hypercapnia and inspiratory flow-resistive loading on respiratory activity in chronic airways obstruction. J Clin Invest 1977;59:500-07.

43. Bentley RA, Griffin OG, Love RG, Muir DCF, Sweetland KF. Acceptable levels for breathing resistance of respiratory apparatus. Arch Environ Health 1973;27:273-80.

44. Love RG, Muir DCF, Sweetland KF, Bentley RA, Griffin OG. Acceptable levels for the breathing resistance of respiratory apparatus: results for men over the age of 45. Br J Ind Med 1977;34:126-29.

45. Deno NS, Kamon E, Kiser DM. Physiological responses to resistance breathing during short and prolonged exercise. Am Ind Hyg Assoc J 1981;42(8):616-23.

46. Raven PB, Davis TO, Shafer CL, Linnebur AC. Maximal stress test performance while wearing a self-contained breathing apparatus. J Occup Med 1977;19(12):802-06.

47. Craig FN, Blevins WV, Cummings G. Exhausting work limited by external resistance and inhalation of carbon dioxide. J Appl Physiol 1970;29(6):847-51.

48. Stemler FW, Craig FN. Effects of respiratory equipment on endurance in hard work. J Appl Physiol 1977;42:28-32.

49. Myhre LG, Holden RD, Baumgardner FW, Tucker D. Physiological limits of firefighters. Air Force School of Aerospace Medicine, Brooks AFB, TX, ESL-TR-79-06, 1979.

50. James R, Dukes-Dobos F, Smith R. Effects of respirators under heat/work conditions. Am Ind Hyg Assoc J 1984;45(6):399-404.

51. Hermansen L, Vokac Z, Lereim P. Respiratory and circulatory response to added air flow resistance during exercise. Ergonomics 1972;15(1):15-24.

52. Meyer E, Gurtner HP, Scherrer M. Physiological appraisal of a new respirator with positive pressure. Pneumonology 1975;153:61-72.

53. Dahlback GO, Balldin UI. Physiological effects of pressure demand masks during heavy exercise. Am Ind Hyg Assoc J 1984;45(3):177-181.

54. Arborelius M, Dahlback GO, Data P-G. Cardiac output and gas exchange during heavy exercise with a positive pressure respiratory protective apparatus. Scand J Work Environ Health 1983;9:471-477.

55. Bjurstedt H, Rosenhamer G, Lindborg B, Hesser CM. Respiratory and circulatory responses to sustained positive-pressure breathing and exercise in man. Acta Physiol Scand 1979;105:204-14.

56. Black LF, Hyatt RE. Maximal respiratory pressures: normal values and relationship to age and sex. Am Rev Respir Dis 1969;99:696-702.

57. Bates DV, Macklem PT, Christie RV. Respiratory function in disease: an introduction to the integrated study of the lung, 2nd ed, Philadelphia: W.B. Saunders Co., 1971, p. 43.

58. Raven PB, Bradley O, Rohm-Young D, McClure FL, Skaggs B. Physiological response to "pressure-demand" respirator wear. Am Ind Hyg Assoc J 1982;43(10):773-81.

59. Harber P, Tamimie RJ, Bhattacharya A, Barber M. Physiologic effects of respirator dead space and resistance loading. J Occup Med 1982;24(9):681-84.

60. Petsonk EL, Hancock J, Boyles C. Physiologic effects of a self-contained self-rescuer. Am Ind Hyg Assoc J 1983;44(5):368-73.

61. Morgan WP. Psychological problems associated with the wearing of industrial respirators: a review. Am Ind Hyg Assoc J 1983;44(9):671-76.

62. Morgan WP. Psychological problems associated with the wear of industrial respirators. J Int Soc Respir Prot 1983;1:67-108.

63. Ronk R, White MK. Hydrogen sulfide and the probabilities of "inhalation" through a tympanic membrane defect. J Occup Med 1985;27(5):337-40.

64. Cantekin EI, Bluestone CD, Saez CA, Bern SA. Airflow through the eustachian tube. Ann Otol 1979;88:603-612.

65. daRoza RA, Weaver C. Is it safe to wear contact lenses with a full-facepiece respirator? Lawrence Livermore National Laboratory manuscript UCRL-53653, 1985, pp. 1-3.

IV. GLOSSARY

The following definitions of terms are provided to assist in the understanding and application of this decision logic.

ASSIGNED PROTECTION FACTOR (APF): See **PROTECTION FACTOR**.

BREAKTHROUGH: The penetration of challenge material(s) through a gas or a vapor air-purifying element. The quantity or extent of breakthrough during service life testing is often referred to as the percentage of the input concentration.

DISPOSABLE RESPIRATORS: A respirator that is discarded after the end of its recommended period of use, after excessive resistance or physical damage, or when odor breakthrough or other warning indicators render the respirator unsuitable for further use.

DUST: A solid, mechanically produced particle with a size ranging from submicroscopic to macroscopic.

EMERGENCY RESPIRATOR USE SITUATION: A situation that requires the use of respirators due to the unplanned generation of a hazardous atmosphere (often of unknown composition) caused by an accident, mechanical failure, or other means and that requires evacuation of personnel or immediate entry for rescue or corrective action.

ESCAPE GAS MASK: A gas mask that consists of a half-mask facepiece or mouthpiece, a canister, and associated connections and that is designed for use during escape only from hazardous atmospheres (see Subparagraph 5).

ESCAPE ONLY RESPIRATOR: Respiratory devices that are designed for use only during escape from hazardous atmospheres.

FILTERING FACEPIECE: A particulate respirator with a filter as an integral part of the facepiece or with the entire facepiece composed of the filtering medium. (See **SINGLE-USE DUST or DUST and MIST RESPIRATORS** and **DISPOSABLE RESPIRATORS**.)

FIT FACTOR: A quantitative measure of the fit of a specific respirator facepiece to a particular individual. (For further discussion of fit factors, refer to Appendix D.)

FUME: A solid condensation particulate, usually of a vaporized metal.

GAS: An aeriform fluid that is in a gaseous state at standard temperature and pressure.

IMMEDIATELY DANGEROUS TO LIFE OR HEALTH (IDLH): Acute respiratory exposure that poses an immediate threat of loss of life, immediate or delayed irreversible adverse effects on health, or acute eye exposure that would prevent escape from a hazardous atmosphere.

MIST: A liquid condensation particle.

ORINASAL RESPIRATOR: A respirator that covers the nose and mouth and that generally consists of a quarter- or half-facepiece.

PLANNED or UNPLANNED ENTRY into an IDLH ENVIRONMENT, AN ENVIRONMENT OF UNKNOWN CONCENTRATION of HAZARDOUS CONTAMINANT, or an ENVIRONMENT of UNKNOWN COMPOSITION: A situation in which respiratory devices are recommended to provide adequate protection to workers entering an area where the contaminant concentration is above the IDLH or is unknown.

POTENTIAL OCCUPATIONAL CARCINOGEN: Any substance, or combination or mixture of substances, which causes an increased incidence of benign and/or malignant neoplasms, or a substantial decrease in the latency period between exposure and onset of neoplasms in humans or in one or more experimental mammalian species as the result of any oral, respiratory, or dermal exposure, or any other exposure which results in the induction of tumors at a site other than the site of administration. This definition also includes any substance that is metabolized into one or more potential occupational carcinogens by mammals (29 CFR 1990.103, OSHA Cancer Policy).

PROTECTION FACTORS (See Appendix D):

ASSIGNED PROTECTION FACTOR (APF): The minimum anticipated protection provided by a properly functioning respirator or class of respirators to a given percentage of properly fitted and trained users.

SIMULATED WORKPLACE PROTECTION FACTOR (SWPF): A surrogate measure of the workplace protection provided by a respirator.

WORKPLACE PROTECTION FACTOR (WPF): A measure of the protection provided in the workplace by a properly functioning respirator when correctly worn and used.

RECOMMENDED EXPOSURE LIMIT (REL): An 8- or 10-hour time-weighted average (TWA) or ceiling (C) exposure concentration recommended by NIOSH that is based on an evaluation of the health effects data.

SERVICE LIFE: The length of time required for an air-purifying element to reach a specific effluent concentration. Service life is determined by the type of substance being removed, the concentration of the substance, the ambient temperature, the specific element being tested (cartridge or canister), the flow rate resistance, and the selected breakthrough value. The service life for a self-contained breathing apparatus (SCBA) is the period of time, as determined by the NIOSH certification tests, in which adequate breathing gas is supplied.

SINGLE-USE DUST or DUST AND MIST RESPIRATORS: Respirators approved for use against dusts or mists that may cause pneumoconiosis and fibrosis.

VAPOR: The gaseous state of a substance that is solid or liquid at temperatures and pressures normally encountered.

V. APPENDICES

APPENDIX A. NIOSH POLICY STATEMENT ON APPROVAL OF AIR-PURIFYING RESPIRATORS WITH END-OF-SERVICE-LIFE INDICATORS

Department of Health and Human Services
Public Health Service
Centers for Disease Control
National Institute for Occupational Safety and Health

NIOSH/MSHA TESTING AND CERTIFICATION OF AIR-PURIFYING RESPIRATORS WITH END-OF-SERVICE-LIFE INDICATORS

Agency: National Institute for Occupational Safety and Health (NIOSH)

Action: Notice of Acceptance of Applications for Approval of Air-Purifying Respirators with End-of-Service-Life Indicators

Summary: 30 CFR 11; Sec. 11.150 states that NIOSH and MSHA may, after a review of the effects on wearers' health and safety, approve respirators for gases and vapors not specifically listed in that section. The current regulations also permit the use of "window indicators" for gas masks to warn the wearer when the canister will no longer remove a contaminant [11.102-5(c)(2)]. Although indicators are not mentioned in Subpart L, Chemical Cartridge Respirators, there is nothing in the regulations which explicitly prohibits their use. A NIOSH policy to allow end-of-service-life indicators (ESLI's) on air-purifying respirators for gases and vapors with adequate warning properties has already been established (Letter to All Respirator Manufacturers from Dr. Elliott Harris, June 18, 1975).

Use of ESLI's on chemical cartridge respirators for use against gases and vapors with poor warning properties could also be approved, because 30 CFR 11; Sec. 11.150; footnote 7 states:

> "Not for use against gases or vapors with poor warning properties (except where MSHA or Occupational Safety and Health Administration standards may permit such use for a specific gas or vapor)...." Thus, air-purifying respirators with ESLI's could be approved for substances such as acrylonitrile, because the OSHA acrylonitrile standard permits the use of chemical cartridge respirators.

Under the present regulations, NIOSH can also require "any additional requirements deemed necessary to establish the quality, effectiveness, and safety of any respirator used as protection against hazardous atmospheres" [30 CFR 11; Sec. 11.63 (c)]. NIOSH must notify the applicants in writing of these additional requirements [30 CFR 11; Sec. 11.63 (d)].

The purpose of this notification is to inform respirator manufacturers and users of the NIOSH requirements for approving air-purifying respirators with either effective passive or active ESLI's for use against gases and vapors with adequate warning properties or for use against gases and vapors with inadequate warning properties whenever there is a regulatory standard already permitting the use of air-purifying respirators.

For additional information, contact: Chief, Certification Branch, 944 Chestnut Ridge Road, Morgantown, WV 26505, (304) 291-4331.

Supplemental Information

Because human senses are not foolproof in detecting gases and vapors and because many gases and vapors found in the workplace do not have adequate warning properties, NIOSH has been investigating alternate means of detection for respirator wearers. In 1976, NIOSH adopted its current policy which allows acceptance of applications for certification of air-purifying respirators, provided that the respirators are equipped with active ESLI's for use against gases and vapors with poor warning properties and are not specifically listed in 30 CFR 11.

An active ESLI is defined as an indicator that invokes an automatic and spontaneous warning signal (e.g., flashing lights, ringing bells, etc.). An active indicator does not require monitoring by the wearer although a passive indicator (normally color change indicator) does.

During the past several years, NIOSH has received notices of concern from respirator manufacturers, regulatory agencies, and general industry regarding the Institute's policy of accepting only active ESLI's for certification. At the October 1983 Mine Health Research Advisory Council (MHRAC) meeting, NIOSH presented a document briefing on "Consideration of Use of End-of-Service-Life Indicators in Respiratory Protective Devices," and requested that MHRAC provide recommendations to the Institute with regard to the appropriateness of the use of both active and passive ESLI's. MHRAC asked their Respirator Subcommittee to review the issue.

The Respirator Subcommittee held a public meeting in Washington, D.C., on December 19, 1983, to solicit comments from interested parties. The Subcommittee reviewed the comments and then reported back to the full committee at the February 2, 1984, MHRAC meeting. Based on the public comments, the Subcommittee also suggested a few additions or modifications be made to the NIOSH proposed evaluation criteria. NIOSH incorporated the recommendations. MHRAC also recommended that active and passive ESLI's are appropriate for use with respiratory protective devices provided that criteria are established for their certification and use to ensure that the user is not exposed to increased risk as a consequence of relying upon such ESLI's.

In order for NIOSH to determine the potential effects of ESLI's on user safety and health, NIOSH recommends that all applications for approval of gas and vapor respirators with ESLI's contain the following information:

CRITERIA FOR CERTIFICATION OF END-OF-SERVICE-LIFE INDICATORS

An applicant for certification of an ESLI for use against substances with poor warning properties must provide NIOSH with the following information:

1. Data demonstrating that the ESLI is a reliable indicator of sorbent depletion ($\leq$ 90% of service life). These shall include a flow-temperature study at low and high temperatures, humidities, and contaminant concentrations which are representative of actual workplace conditions where a given respirator will be used. A minimum of two contaminant levels must be utilized: the exposure limit (PEL, REL, TLV®, etc.) and the exposure limit multiplied by the assigned protection factor for the respirator type.

2. Data on desorption of any impregnating agents used in the indicator, including a flow-temperature study at low and high temperatures and humidities which are representative of actual workplace conditions where a given respirator will be used. Data shall be sufficient to demonstrate safe levels of desorbed agents.

3. Data on the effects of industrial interferences which are commonly found in workplaces where a given respirator will be used. Data should be sufficient to show which interferences could impair the effectiveness of the indicator and the degree of impairment, and which substances will not affect the indicator.

4. Data on any reaction products produced in the reaction between the sorbent and the contaminant gases and vapors, including the concentrations and toxicities of such products.

5. Data which predict the storage life of the indicator. (Simulated aging tests will be acceptable).

In addition to the foregoing, all passive ESLI's shall meet the following criteria:

1. A passive ESLI shall be placed on the respirator so that the ESLI is visible to the wearer.

2. If the passive indicator utilizes color change, the change shall be such that it is detectable to people with physical impairments such as color blindness.

3. If the passive indicator utilizes color change, reference colors for the initial color of the indicator and the final (end point) color of the indicator shall be placed adjacent to the indicator.

All ESLI's shall meet the following criteria:

1. The ESLI shall not interfere with the effectiveness of the face seal.

2. The ESLI shall not change the weight distribution of the respirator to the detriment of the facepiece fit.

3. The ESLI shall not interfere with required lines of sight.

4. Any ESLI that is permanently installed in the respirator facepiece shall be capable of withstanding cleaning and a drop from a height of 6 feet. Replaceable ESLI must be capable of being easily removed and shall also be capable of withstanding a drop from a height of 6 feet.

5. A respirator with an ESLI shall still meet all other applicable requirements set forth in 30 CFR 11.

6. If the ESLI uses any electrical components, they shall conform to the provisions of the National Electrical Code and be "intrinsically safe." Where permissibility is required, the respirator shall meet the requirements for permissibility and intrinsic safety set forth in 30 CFR 18, Subpart D. Also, the electrical system shall include an automatic warning mechanism that indicates a loss of power.

7. Effects of industrial substances interferences which are commonly found where a given respirator will be used and which hinder ESLI performance, shall be identified. Substances which are commonly found where the respirator is to be used must be investigated. Data sufficient to indicate whether the performance of the respirator would be affected must be submitted to NIOSH. The user shall be made aware of use conditions that could cause false positive and negative ESLI responses.

8. The ESLI shall not create any hazard to the wearer's health or safety.

9. Consideration shall be given to the potential impact of common human physical impairments on the effectiveness of the ESLI.

APPENDIX B. NIOSH POLICY STATEMENT ON USE OF SINGLE-USE AND DUST AND MIST RESPIRATORS FOR PROTECTION AGAINST ASBESTOS

June 21, 1984, OSHA Public Hearings

Under Title 30, Code of Federal Regulations, Part 11 (30 CFR 11), NIOSH is required to test and certify respirators within the categories specified therein when such devices are submitted to NIOSH by applicants. Currently, 30 CFR 11, Subpart K defines a number of dust, fume, and mist respirators which may be used for protection against certain hazardous particulate atmospheres. Among the respirators defined in Subpart K are single-use dust respirators designed as respiratory protection against pneumoconiosis-producing and fibrosis-producing dusts, or dusts and mists. Subpart K lists asbestos as one of the dusts against which the single-use dust respirator is designed to protect [Subpart K, Sec. 11.130(H)]. Although at the time of the promulgation of Subpart K, it may have been assumed appropriate to list asbestos as a fibrosis-producing particulate against which the single-use disposable respirator could be reasonably expected to provide adequate protection, NIOSH is no longer confident that such an assumption is reasonable because asbestos is also a potent carcinogen.

The current requirements as (specified in 30 CFR 11) for approval of a single-use dust respirator or dust and mist respirator do not include any tests with fibrous challenge aerosol. NIOSH is currently in the process of doing a comprehensive revision of 30 CFR 11 and intends to address the issue of appropriate respiratory protection for use against asbestos, and to require that any respirator for which such approval is sought be proven to provide effective protection against asbestos. NIOSH may change the regulations included in 30 CFR 11 only in accordance with procedures set forth in the Administrative Procedures Act. In the interim, NIOSH will continue to consider applications for approval of single-use and replaceable dust/mist respirators for use against asbestos only because of the legal requirement in the current approval regulations. However, NIOSH does not recommend the use of such respirators where exposures to asbestos may occur because such a recommendation would not be prudent based on the occupational health risk.

This policy position is contained in "The Statement of the National Institute for Occupational Safety and Health--The Public Hearings on Occupational Exposure to Asbestos."

APPENDIX C. ODOR WARNING: BACKGROUND INFORMATION

It is important to realize that 30 CFR 11 prohibits the use of MSHA/NIOSH approved air-purifying (organic vapor) respirators for protection against organic vapors with poor warning properties unless there is an OSHA standard that permits such use. Specifically, 30 CFR 11, Section 11.90(b), footnote 4 gives the standards for gas masks (canister devices), while 30 CFR 11, Section 11.150, footnote 7 gives the standards for chemical cartridge respirators. Thus the "organic vapor respirator" shall be approved only for organic vapors with adequate warning properties. In addition, the requirement for adequate warning properties also applies to all MSHA/NIOSH-approved air-purifying respirators for protection against organic gases and vapors.

A recent policy decision by NIOSH allows the use of respirators for protection against contaminants with poor warning properties, provided that certain conditions are met. These conditions are outlined in the policy statement in Appendix A. MSHA/NIOSH approval may be granted for a respirator designed for use against gases and vapors with poor warning properties if the respirator incorporates an effective end-of-service-life indicator (ESLI).

However, unless the respirator incorporates an ESLI, wearers of air-purifying chemical cartridge/canister respirators must rely on adequate warning properties to alert them to the breakthrough of the sorbent in the cartridge or canister. Amoore and Hautala [33] have noted:

> The ability of members of the population to detect a given odor is strongly influenced by the innate variability of different persons' olfactory powers, their prior experience with that odor, and by the degree of attention they accord to the matter.

Amoore and Hautala [33] found that on the average, 95% of a population will have a personal odor threshold that lies within the range from about one-sixteenth to sixteen times the reported mean "odor threshold" for a substance. That is, about 2.5% of a population will be able to detect a substance's odor at concentrations less than one-sixteenth of the "odor threshold" for a substance. Correspondingly, about 2.5% of the individuals will need to be exposed to concentrations exceeding by a factor of 16 the "odor threshold" in order to perceive the odor. Thus for many substances the width of distribution of personal odor threshold is over two orders of magnitude of concentration. The "odor thresholds" reported in the literature generally are the median values for wide population distributions. Also, 50% of prospective respirator wearers can detect a substance's odor only at levels that must exceed the reported "odor threshold," and about 15% cannot detect the odor at levels that exceed the "odor threshold" by fourfold [33].

OSHA incorporated into the lead standard a new isoamyl acetate qualitative fit test protocol, developed by Du Pont, which requires odor threshold screening [29 CFR 1910.1025, Appendix D (I)(A)]. Du Pont realized that a qualitative fit test depending on odor recognition would be ineffective if every individual were not first screened for the ability to detect the odor of isoamyl acetate at some minimum concentration. This is also true for detection of the odor of the gas or vapor used to alert the wearer of sorbent element (cartridge or canister) breakthrough. Thus NIOSH recommends screening tests for workers who wear air-purifying gas or vapor respirators to determine their ability to detect the odor below the exposure limit for that gas or vapor.

APPENDIX D. PROTECTION FACTOR: BACKGROUND INFORMATION

The U.S. Bureau of Mines referred to the term "Decontamination Factor" in their Approval Schedule 21B, first issued in 1965, and defined it to be "the ratio of the concentration of dust, fume, or mist present in the ambient atmosphere to the concentration of dust, fume, or mist within the facepiece while the respirator is being worn." The decontamination factor is now referred to as the respirator protection factor. The original definition and application given in schedule 21B has been somewhat generalized over the years.

The protection factor of a respirator is an expression of performance based on the ratio of two measured variables, C_I and C_O. The variable C_I is defined only as the measured concentration of a contaminant inside the respirator facepiece cavity, and C_O is defined only as the measured contaminant concentration outside the respirator facepiece. The relationship between these two variables can be expressed not only as the protection factor (C_O/C_I) but also as the penetration (C_I/C_O) or efficiency $[(C_O-C_I)/C_O]$.

The protection factor can be related to the penetration (p) and efficiency (E) as follows:

$$PF = C_O/C_I = 1/p = 1/(1-E)$$

A further implicit condition on the PF function is that $C_I \leq C_O$; therefore, the PF will always be greater than unity.

Protection factor assessments are made almost exclusively on man/respirator systems, while penetration and efficiency assessments are made only on component parts of the respirator system. It is important to recognize that on a man/respirator system, the measured variable C_I becomes a complicated function of many individual sources of penetration (e.g., air-purifying element penetration, exhalation valve penetration, face seal penetration, and other inboard penetration) and those environmental conditions that would effect penetration. To deal with the multiple methods for determining and applying protection factors, a number of definitions have been proposed [13]. These definitions, described below in greater detail than in the Glossary, are as follows:

ASSIGNED PROTECTION FACTOR (APF): A special application of the general protection factor concept, APF is defined as a measure of the minimum anticipated workplace level of respiratory protection that would be provided by a properly functioning respirator or class of respirators to a percentage of properly fitted and trained users. The maximum specified use concentration for a respirator is generally determined by multiplying the exposure limit for the contaminant by the protection factor assigned to a specific class of respirators [13].

SIMULATED WORKPLACE PROTECTION FACTOR (SWPF): A surrogate measure of the workplace protection factor (WPF) of a respirator, SWPF differs from the WPF only in that it is measured in a laboratory simulation of a workplace setting rather than in the actual workplace. The definitions and restrictions of C_O and C_I are as described for the WPF. For laboratory protection factor testing to reliably estimate WPF's, a relationship must be demonstrated between the two tests. No such relationship has been identified in the literature. Until such a relationship can be shown to exist, the laboratory protection factor is of questionable use in determining or predicting the WPF [13].

WORKPLACE PROTECTION FACTOR (WPF): A measure of the actual protection provided in the workplace under the conditions of that workplace by a properly functioning respirator when correctly worn and used, WPF is defined as the ratio of the estimated contaminant concentration outside the respirator facepiece (C_O) to the contaminant concentration inside the respirator facepiece (C_I). The sampling restrictions placed on C_O and C_I are that both C_O and C_1 should be TWA samples taken simultaneously while the respirator is being properly worn and used during normal work activities. In practice, the WPF would be determined by measuring the concentration inside and outside the facepiece during the activities of a normal workday [13].

FIT FACTOR: A special application of the protection factor ratio that represents a quantitative measure of the fit of a particular respirator facepiece to a particular individual, the fit factor is defined under the conditions of quantitative fit testing as the aerosol concentration in the test chamber (C_O) divided by the penetration that occurs through the respirator face seal interface (C_I) [34]. For C_I to reflect only face seal leakage, high efficiency filters [greater than 99.97% efficient against 0.3 μm aerodynamic mass median diameter (AMMD) dioctylphthalate aerosol] are installed on the respirator. It is assumed that either no leakage or only a negligible amount of leakage into the facepiece occurs through the exhalation valve or any source other than the face seal. The fit factor is measured on a complete respirator worn by a test subject who follows a regimen of slow head movements, deep breathing, and talking; a polydispersed oil mist or sodium chloride aerosol is used that has an AMMD of approximately 0.6 $\pm$ 0.1 μm (with a geometric standard deviation of approximately 2 to 2.4).

APPENDIX E. MEDICAL ASPECTS OF WEARING RESPIRATORS: BACKGROUND INFORMATION

In recommending medical evaluation criteria for respirator use, one should apply rigorous decision-making principles [35], using knowledge of screening test sensitivity, predictive value, etc. Unfortunately, many gaps in knowledge in this area exist. The problem is complicated by the large variety of respirators, their conditions of use, and individual differences in the physiologic and psychologic responses to them. For these reasons, the preceding guidelines (see Subparagraph 10) are to be considered as informed suggestions rather than established NIOSH policy recommendations. The following information is intended primarily to assist the physician in developing medical evaluation criteria for respirator use.

Health Effects of Wearing Respirators

Brief descriptions of the health effects associated with wearing respirators are summarized below. Interested readers are referred to recent reviews for more detailed analyses of the data [36,37].

Pulmonary: In general, the added inspiratory and expiratory resistances and dead space of most respirators cause an increased tidal volume and decreased respiratory rate and ventilation (including a small decrease in alveolar ventilation). These respirator effects have usually been small both among healthy individuals and, in limited studies, among individuals with impaired lung function [38-42]. This generalization is applicable to most respirators meeting Federal regulations when resistances (particularly expiratory resistance) are low [1,43,44]. While most studies report minimal physiologic effects during submaximal exercise, the resistances commonly lead to reduced endurance and reduced maximal exercise performance [45-49]. The dead space of a respirator (reflecting the amount of expired air that must be rebreathed before fresh air is obtained) tends to cause increased ventilation. At least one study has shown substantially increased ventilation with a full-face respirator, a type which can have a large effective dead space [50]. However, the net effect of a respirator's added resistances and dead space is usually a small decrease in ventilation [39,45,46-48,51].

The potential for adverse effects, particularly decreased cardiac output, from the positive pressure feature of some respirators has been reported [52]. However, several recent studies suggest that this is not a practical concern, at least not in healthy individuals [53-55].

Theoretically, the increased fluctuations in thoracic pressure while breathing with a respirator might constitute an increased risk to subjects with a history of spontaneous pneumothorax. Few data are available in this area. While an individual is using a negative pressure respirator with relatively high resistance during very heavy exercise, the usual maximal peak negative oral pressure during inhalation is about 15-17 cm of water [53]. Similarly, the usual maximal peak positive oral pressure during exhalation is about 15-17 cm of water, which might occur with a respirator in a positive pressure mode, again during very heavy exercise [53]. By comparison, maximal positive pressures, such as those during a vigorous cough, can generate 200 cm of water pressure [56]. The normal maximal negative pleural pressure at full inspiration is -40 cm of water [57], and normal subjects can generate -80 to -160 cm of negative water pressure [56]. Thus while vigorous exercise with a respirator does alter pleural pressures, the risk of barotrauma would seem to be substantially less than that of the cough maneuver.

In some asthmatics, an asthmatic attack may be exacerbated or induced by a variety of factors including exercise, cold air, and stress, all of which may be associated with wearing a respirator. While most asthmatics who are able to control their condition should not have problems with respirators, a physician's judgment and a field trial may be needed in selected cases.

Cardiac: The added work of breathing from respirators is small and could not be detected in several studies [38,39]. A typical respirator might double the work of breathing from 3 to 6% of the oxygen consumption, but this is probably not of clinical significance [38]. In concordance with this view is the finding of several studies that at the same workloads heart rate does not change with the wearing of a respirator [39,54,58-60].

In contrast, the added cardiac stress due to the weight of a heavy respirator may be considerable. A self-contained breathing apparatus (SCBA), particularly one that uses compressed air cylinders, may weigh up to 35 pounds. Heavier respirators have been shown to reduce maximum external workloads by 20% and similarly increase heart rate at a given submaximal workload [46]. In addition, it should be appreciated that many uses of SCBA (e.g., for firefighting and hazardous waste site work) also necessitate the wearing of 10-25 pounds of protective clothing.

Raven et al. [40,58] found significantly higher systolic and/or diastolic blood pressures during exercise for persons wearing respirators (although increases were minimal, i.e., $\leq$10 mmHg systolic, 0-2 mmHg diastolic). Arborelius et al. [54] did not find significant differences for persons wearing respirators during exercise.

Body Temperature: Proper regulation of body temperature is primarily of concern with the closed circuit, self-contained breathing apparatus that produces oxygen via an exothermic chemical reaction. Inspired air within these respirators may reach 120°F (49°C), thus depriving the wearer of a minor cooling mechanism and causing discomfort. Obviously this can be more of a problem with heavy exercise and when ambient conditions and/or protective clothing further reduce the body's ability to lose heat. The increase in heart rate due to increasing temperature represents an additional cardiac stress.

Closed-circuit breathing units of any type have the potential for heat stress since warm expired gases (after exothermic carbon dioxide removal with or without oxygen addition) are rebreathed. Respirators with large dead space also have this potential problem, again because of partial rebreathing of warmed expired air [50].

Diminished Senses: Respirators may reduce visual fields, decrease voice clarity and loudness, and decrease hearing. Besides the potential for reduced productivity, these effects may result in reduced industrial safety. These factors may also contribute to a general feeling of stress [61].

Psychologic: This important topic is discussed in recent reviews by Morgan [61,62]. There is little doubt that virtually everyone suffers some discomfort when wearing a respirator. The large variability and the subjective nature of the psycho-physiologic aspects of wearing a respirator, however, make studies and specific recommendations difficult. Fit testing obviously serves an important additional function in providing a trial to determine if the wearer can psychologically tolerate the respirator. General experience indicates that the great majority of workers can tolerate respirators and that experience aids in this tolerance [62]. However, some individuals are likely to remain psychologically unfit for wearing respirators.

Local Irritation: Allergic skin reactions may occur occasionally from wearing a respirator, and skin occlusion may cause irritation or exacerbation of preexisting conditions such as pseudofolliculitis barbae. Facial discomfort from the pressure of the mask may occur, particularly when the fit is unsatisfactory.

In addition to the health effects associated with wearing respirators (described above) specific groups of respirator wearers may be affected by the following factors:

Perforated Tympanic Membrane: While inhalation of toxic materials through a perforated tympanic membrane (ear drum) is possible, recent evidence indicates that the airflow would be minimal and rarely if ever of clinical importance [63,64]. In highly toxic or unknown atmospheres, use of positive pressure respirators should ensure adequate protection [63].

Contact Lens: Contact lenses are generally not recommended for use with respirators, although little documented evidence exists to support this viewpoint [65]. Several possible reasons for this recommendation are noted below:

a. Corneal irritation or abrasion might occur with the exposure. This would, of course, be a problem primarily with quarter- and half-face masks, especially with particulate exposures. However, exposures could occur with full-face respirators due to leaks or inadvisable removal of the respirator for any reason. While corneal irritation or abrasion might also occur without contact lenses, their presence is known to substantially increase this risk.

b. The loss or misplacement of a contact lens by an individual wearing a respirator might prompt the wearer to remove the respirator, thereby resulting in exposure to the hazard as well as to the potential problems noted in "a." above.

c. The constant airflow of some respirators, such as powered air-purifying respirators (PAPR) or continuous flow air-line respirators, might irritate a contact lens wearer.

APPENDIX F

BREATHING AIR SYSTEMS FOR USE WITH
PRESSURE-DEMAND SUPPLIED AIR RESPIRATORS
IN ASBESTOS ABATEMENT

Breathing Air Systems for Use with Pressure-Demand Supplied Air Respirators in Asbestos Abatement

a Technical Report

by

Clifton M. McClure

Consumer Fuels, Inc.
7250 Governors Drive West
Huntsville, Alabama 35805

for

U.S. Department of Health and Human Services
Public Health Service
Centers for Disease Control
National Institute for Occupational Safety and Health
Division of Safety Research

ACKNOWLEDGEMENTS

The author is indebted to the following individuals who provided invaluable suggestions during the development of this Appendix:

William L. Bowers
Daboco, Inc.
3319 E. 10 Mile Rd.
Warren, MI 48091

Dorothy Rushton
Deltech Engineering, Inc.
Century Park, Box 667
New Castle, Delaware 19720

Table of Contents

Figures and Tables

List of Tables

Appendix F. Breathing Air Systems for Use with Pressure-Demand Supplied Air Respirators in Asbestos Abatement

I. INTRODUCTION

The National Institute for Occupational Safety and Health (NIOSH) and the Environmental Protection Agency (EPA) recommend that either self-contained breathing apparatus (SCBA) or combination pressure-demand supplied air respirators (SAR) with escape SCBA be used to protect workers from detectable airborne concentrations of asbestos. Since SCBA are often impractical for abatement due to their size and weight, the combined SAR/SCBA will probably offer the best protection for workers on abatement jobs. Only those respirators tested and certified by NIOSH (U.S. Department of Health and Human Services) and the Mine Safety and Health Administration (MSHA, U.S. Department of Labor) and therefore which bear the NIOSH/MSHA approval label (See Appendix B) are recommended.

As the term "supplied air" indicates, these respirators receive breathable air from an external source through a system that typically consists of compression, purification, storage, and distribution components. The subject of this Appendix is the system which produces breathable air and supplies it to the recommended respirators. The intent is to (1) acquaint employers with the characteristics of available types of breathing air systems (Part II), (2) emphasize the caution required in the use of such systems (Part III), and (3) examine the cost benefits of supplied air versus air-purifying respirator systems (Part IV). The names and addresses of suppliers of equipment used in and with breathing air systems are provided in the final section (Part V).

II. BREATHING AIR SYSTEMS

A. Performance Requirements

A breathing air system must accomplish the following:

(1) provide a continuous sufficient supply of Grade D breathing air

(2) provide adequate reserve or escape time

(3) provide breathing air temperature control

(4) provide a continuous monitor and alarm against carbon monoxide (CO) in the breathing airstream.

(1) Continuous Sufficient Supply of Grade D Breathing Air

A **continuous sufficient supply** of breathing air means that both the air pressure and air volume requirements necessary for respirator operation are supplied directly to each respirator. **Grade D breathing air** is air that meets certain criteria established by the Compressed Gas Association, Inc., and is required to be used in air supplied respirators (see Table 1). Producing and supplying a continuous sufficient supply of Grade D breathing air is accomplished by the combined effect of compression, purification, and delivery processes.

(a) Compression

Any person interested in specification of, purchasing, or operation of any breathing air system for use with pressure-demand supplied air respirators in asbestos removal should know the basics of air compression.

Theoretical Compression Process. For a moment, let us consider the compression process apart from compressors. Forget low or high pressure or any other type of mechanical compressor. Consider only a parcel of air, A, as in Figure 1. Parcel A has a spherical diameter of about 4.0 inches, and the air is at room or ambient conditions; its pressure is about 14.7 pounds per square inch atmospheric (psia), its temperature is about 70°F.

This air parcel, as do all air parcels, carries water vapor and contaminants. In atmospheric air, water vapor is not usually considered a contaminant. In compressed air for breathing purposes, however, water vapor should be considered as a major contaminant. In order to produce breathable air, water vapor must be properly processed out of the compressed air. Water in compressed air is itself a contaminant and it traps and carries other contaminants.

If this air parcel were suddenly compressed to 100 psi over and above it's ambient pressure of 14.7 psia, its absolute pressure would become 114.7 psia. The volume of the parcel of air is reduced by compression to about ⅛ of its original volume, or about one-half inch in spherical diameter.

Even with no outside heat added, because of compression the temperature of the compressed air parcel would jump to about 350°F. The water vapor and contaminants would also be compressed. Compressing air reduces its ability to hold water vapor. However, increasing the temperature increases the ability to hold water vapor. Because of these two opposite effects, the water vapor would not condense immediately upon compression, but most certainly would condense as the air temperature decreases. In a compressor, the compression itself increases contamination levels in the air. These increased contamination levels must be controlled so that they do not become a human hazard.

If the parcel of air were to be compressed to 1/300 of its initial volume, the 4-inch diameter spherical air parcel would be reduced to only 0.01 inches diameter. The air temperature in this high compression parcel would be very hot, 1500° to 2500°F. The water vapor and contaminants would also be equally highly compressed.

If either compressed air parcel in the above examples were held for a time at its higher pressure, the heat would eventually transfer out. Even in its compressed state, the initial high air temperature would decrease back toward the ambient temperature of 70°F. Once compressed air has cooled back to ambient temperature, a large amount of the water will have condensed. Condensed water can be mechanically collected and simply drained out of the air parcel. Even after all the condensation is removed, the air parcel is still saturated with the remaining water vapor. (Being saturated simply means that any further reduction in temperature of the air parcel below 70°F will also result in additional water condensation.)

After the air temperature has cooled back to 70°F, if we were then to expand the air back to its original spherical diameter of 4.0 inches, the air temperature would drop dramatically. Such a re-expansion of the air parcel would, in effect, dry the air enabling it to carry more moisture again.

There are several important things to remember about theoretical compression of air:

- Air temperature always rises with compression. The more compression, the greater the temperature rise. Even at low pressures, there are substantial temperature elevations.

- In theoretical compression, this temperature rise does not come from mechanical heating effects due to the action of pistons, vanes, compressor drive motors, etc., but only from compression.

- Compression always heats air, but the compression process can be designed to provide cooling effects in the air. This cooling is available only if sufficient heat exchanger design and time is available to remove the heat of compression from the air before delivery of the air to the workers.

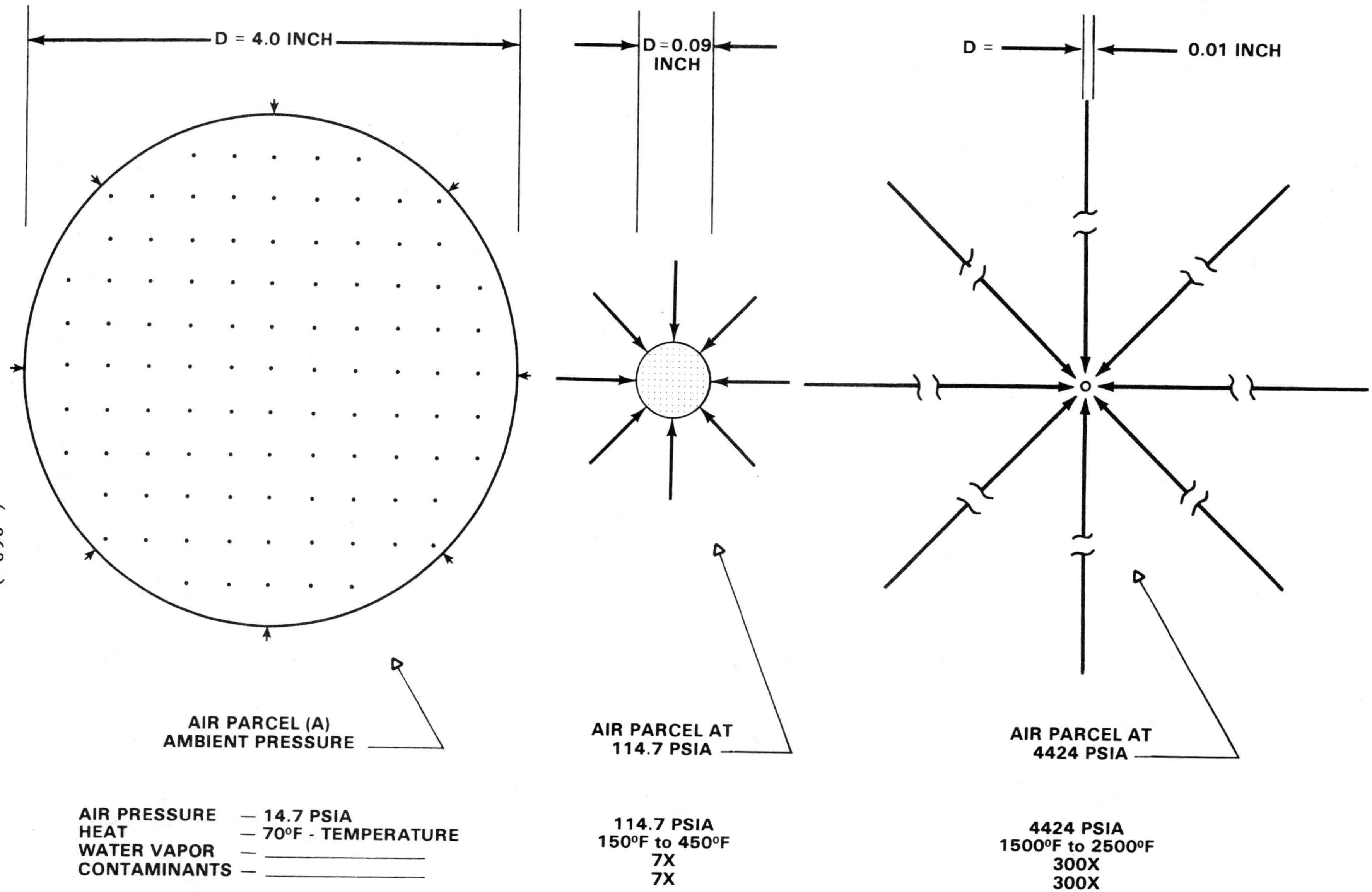

Figure F1. Theoretical Air Compression

Table 1. Characteristics of Grade D and Better Breathing Air

Limiting Characteristics	GRADES D	E	F	G	H	I
% O_2 (v/v) Balance predominately N² (Note 1)	atm. 19.5-23.5	atm. 19.5-23.5	atm. 19.5-23.5	atm. 19.5-23.5	atm. 19.5-23.5	atm. 19.5-23.5
Water	note 2	note 2	note 2	note 2	note 2	1 -10.4°F
Hydrocarbons (condensed) in Mg/m³ of gas at NTP (Note 3)	5	5				
CO	20	10	5	5	5	1
Odor	*	*	*	*	*	*
CO_2	1000	500	500	500	0.5	
Gaseous Hydrocarbons (as methane)			25	15	10	0.5
Nitrogen Dioxide				2.5	0.5	0.1
Nitrous Oxide						0.1
Sulfur Dioxide				2.5	1	0.1
Halogenated Solvents				10	1	0.1
Acetylene						0.05

*Adapted from Compressed Gas Association, Inc., Air Specification G-7.1

[Note 1: The term "atm" (atmospheric) denotes the normal oxygen content of atmospheric air numbers indicate oxygen limits for synthesized air.

Note 2: The water content of compressed air required for a particular grade can vary from saturated to dry depending upon the intended use. If a specific water limit is required, it should be specified as a limiting dewpoint (expressed in temperature °F at one atmosphere absolute pressure) or concentration in ppm (v/v).

Note 3: No limits are given for condensed hydrocarbons beyond Grade E since gaseous hydrocarbon limits could not be met if condensed hydrocarbons were present.]

- The water vapor is also compressed, and if high temperatures are lowered, will easily condense.
- Water vapor in compressed air is a major contaminant. Condensed water in compressed air is itself a contaminant and it traps and carries other contaminants.
- Concentrations of contaminants are increased and may become hazardous unless removed.

Practical Compression. Real compression requires a mechanical compressor of some type. Additional heat from the drive motor and frictional heat will be added in the real compression process. In addition, the compressor will add wear particles such as metal, carbon, etc. The compressor may also add lubricant oil as either liquid oil or oil vapor. If the compressor operates at excessive temperatures, it may actually form deadly carbon monoxide (CO) within the machine, although such CO formation is rare.

A compressor may be suited for only the tasks or types of jobs for which it was originally designed and built. For instance, a compressor built to power other industrial air machines may not need heat, water, and oil removal. In fact, some compressors actually have "oilers" in the output air to increase the oil being carried in the air. A compressor whose basic design was unsuitable could easily overpower the finest air purifier assembly. Operating with such an unsuitable machine would require more frequent filter and canister replacement than normal to maintain the required air quality. The cost of maintaining the air purifier in such a case would be prohibitive. The cost of redesigning and re-building such a compressor could be more than buying a compressor of a different design.

The real effect of water as a contaminant can be understood with an example: Consider a low pressure breathing air system with a normal piston or screw-type compressor and an air purifier assembly, such as depicted in Figure 1. This actual machine is pumping 100 standard cubic feet per minute (SCFM) of air on a day when the ambient temperature is 70°F and the relative humidity is 75%. This machine will take in about 16.5 gallons of water in vapor form every 24 hours. If the machine is properly designed for breathing air applications, it will have an aftercooler to cool the air and to condense most of this water. This breathing air compressor will also have water removal traps to drain the condensate out of the machine. If the air is being cooled in the compressor aftercooler back to near ambient temperature, then about 11.5 gallons of liquid water will condense. This condensing water has many of the other contaminants entrained. This contaminated liquid water can be mechanically removed from the aftercooler drain trap. This leaves about 5.0 gallons of water as water vapor still moving with the compressor output air. Most of this 5.0 gallons of water vapor will be removed along with any other contaminants by the air purifier assembly that is downstream of the compressor.

Proper design of the compressor with sufficient intercooling, aftercooling, and proper water removal traps can mechanically remove about 65% to 90% of all water and contaminants. Since mechanical removal methods are more or less permanent removal methods, the overall compressor design is important for final breathing air quality. The final polishing of the air quality to obtain Grade D or better will be accomplished by stages in the air purifier assembly.

(b) Purification

Ordinary compressed air cannot be used to supply breathing air to work crews working in hazardous atmospheres. Ambient breathing air, when pumped through an ordinary compressor, is not fit for human respiration. Even if the compressed air is filtered to remove dust and other particulates, it still contains the contaminants in ordinary atmospheric air, plus the localized contaminants near the compressor intake, plus any contaminants and wear particles added during compression. The compressor may add oil vapor, hydrocarbons, even carbon monoxide.

The compressor intake is especially vulnerable to all types of carbon monoxide sources. Sources of CO, such as transient vehicles and other mobile internal combustion engines, are especially hard to control on the typical asbestos abatement job.

Various contaminants are potentially present in air from ordinary compression. Where present, these contaminants are concentrated by the compression process. For these reasons, breathing apparatus will NOT provide protection unless the breathing air is purified.

Purification of air is a very precise technology which has developed over many years. Purification is considerably more than filtration. Filtration is simply capture and removal of particulates by a filter. Filtration is almost always included in the overall purification process, although it is a small part of the overall purifying process.

Adsorption. Purifiers are based primarily on the design and use of ADSORPTION. Adsorption of vapor and chemical contaminants is done by proper design and use of the class of materials known as adsorbers. The common adsorbers used in design of air purifier assemblies may include:

molecular sieves

silica gel

activated alumina (Al_2O_3)

activated charcoal

Adsorbers are porous type materials with large quantities of interconnected, submicroscopic internal voids, pores, or capillaries. This internal porous structure gives these adsorber materials very large surface areas in contact with the gases to which the adsorber is exposed. Adsorbers also have the property of being physiochemically "active" or can be "activated." This means that these adsorbers can hold onto, or adsorb onto their active surfaces, various physiologically active contaminants. The adsorbant thereby effectively removes the contaminants from the airstream and leaves the air pure and uncontaminated. These adsorbers are not all equally effective with all contaminants.

Water is an active contaminant for most adsorbers. Water is also processed in large quantities by air compression. Ninety percent of the water and entrained contaminants can regularly be removed by proper compression, cooling, and water traps, all of which are designed into the breathing air compressor section. Much of the remaining water must still be removed in order to allow adsorption of other vapor contaminants.

For the adsorber design to be effective, the appropriate types, quantities, and sequence of adsorber materials must be selected.

Pressure Level and Adsorbers. The effectiveness of all adsorbers increases with increasing pressure. As the pressure of the air increases, the density of the air increases. More dense air exposed to any adsorber material simply means that more of the air is pushed into more intimate contact within the adsorber. Therefore, as air pressure increases, less adsorber is needed to do the same job.

Table 2 shows the typical operating pressure range and the relative density increase for both typical types of breathing air systems for use in asbestos removal work.

Table 2. Typical Pressure and Relative Adsorber Effectiveness

Type of Breathing Air System	Typical Pressure Range	Relative Air Density (and Adsorber Effectiveness)
Low Pressure	100-200 psi	6x to 12x
High Pressure	2000-4000 psi	150x to 300x

Adsorbers must be periodically replaced. Adsorber cartridges can be equipped with a color change reaction that will show the progress of adsorber use. Such cartridges can be changed based on coloration changes through a visual canister. Adsorption canisters may also be changed on a simple operational time basis.

The Carbon Monoxide Catalyst. The action of this catalyst, which is used to eliminate carbon monoxide, is unique. On the catalyst surface, carbon monoxide, in the low concentration ranges of 10 ppm to 600 ppm, is brought into contact with oxygen in the air. These conditions cause the chemical reaction $2CO + O_2 = 2\ CO_2$. The end result is that dangerous CO is changed to CO_2, which is not harmful in these low concentrations. Theoretically, catalysts last forever, but in practice they permanently adsorb trace chemicals and become "inactive." Most manufacturers recommend yearly replacement of their catalyst-type filters.

Even very small amounts of water vapor contamination on the catalytic adsorber "poison" the catalyst and reduce its activity. For such a catalyst to operate for a reasonable period of time, the air entering the catalyst must be very dry, below 5% relative humidity.

The most effective way to dry air to these conditions is to use drying adsorbents before the air reaches the catalyst. If a drying adsorber of the throwaway type were considered for use in a low pressure purifier assembly, enormous quantities of this disposable adsorber material would be required for each 8-hour shift. In order to avoid having to use such quantities of water adsorber material in the low pressure purifiers, a different design solution has been used.

The Regenerative Water Adsorber Dryer. The heatless air regenerated dryer has evolved as the simplest and most rugged method to continously regenerate the required adsorber material. It consists of airline plumbing, two central air dryer towers, and a tower switching system. In action, this system has one tower drying the process airstream while the other tower is "off-cycle." From 10% to 20% of the dry air output of the "on-cycle" tower (depending on system operating pressure) is split off and sent back down in reverse through the "off-cycle" tower. This regeneration air removes the water previously adsorbed in the "off-cycle" tower and is vented to the atmosphere. In this way the off-cycle adsorber material is renewed or regenerated. Every few minutes on a regular basis, the cycle switches, alternating between the two towers.

A typical adsorber design for 100 SCFM process air flow, which has 50 pounds of activated alumina in each tower, can be expected to run regeneratively for several years before this activated alumina stops being regenerated. Replacement of 100 pounds of activated alumina only one time every 5 to 7 years is inexpensive. In comparison, a single column of activated alumina in a throwaway canister design would need about 100 pounds of new activated alumina every 8 hours.

If the activated alumina regenerated dryer were the first step in the purifying process just following the breathing air compressor, it would "see" significant amounts of oil and oil vapor as well as water vapor. The regenerative dryer is based on the alternate adsorption and desorption of water from the adsorber. In these cycling towers oil will not desorb. The regenerative dryer will operate only a few days if no oil adsorption media is placed in front of the regenerative drying section. An oil adsorption prefilter must precede the dryer towers.

The Oil Adsorption Prefilter. The active media in the oil adsorption prefilter is chosen for its ability to selectively retain oil and oil vapor. It can be formulated with a color change reaction and placed into a visual canister for visual determination of the filter media remaining. The oil vapor adsorption prefilter may quickly be saturated if "slugs" of oil and water come from the compressor. Removal of liquid "slugs" just prior to the oil prefilter is accomplished by the coalescing filter and drain trap.

The Coalescing Filter and Drain Trap. Compressors used for breathing air need great attention paid to removal of heat, which causes condensed liquids to be formed. These breathing air machines also provide special liquid removal devices called "liquid traps." Liquids are retained in the traps and can be drained from them.

Heat exchangers and drain traps do not remove vapors. Water vapor and oil vapor move through liquid traps. Also, microscopic drops of both liquid water and liquid oil (aerosols) act similar to vapor and move through ordinary liquid traps. The coalescing element is designed to cause these aerosols to impact on a myriad of mechanical elements within the coalescing filter. This action makes big drops out of the aerosols so they can be removed.

Summary of Important Points About Adsorption Purification:

- Purification of air requires adsorption as well as filtration.
- Purification and adsorber design is a highly developed science. Proper design of adsorber must include:
  - proper choice of adsorber material
  - sufficient quantities of adsorber
  - proper sequencing of the correct adsorbers.
- All adsorbers must be changed periodically.
- Systems with higher working pressures will require less adsorber material to do the same job.
- A low pressure adsorber should include a regenerative dryer or enormous quantities of adsorber material will need to be replaced every eight (8) hours.

Grade D breathing air is specified by OSHA 29 CFR 1910.134(d)(1) as that listed by the Compressed Gas Association Specification G-7.1. Table 1 shows the criteria for Grade D and better breathing air. Most established American manufacturers of both high and low pressure breathing air purifying systems design and test their systems to produce Grade D or better breathing air.

(c) Distribution

Breathing air must be delivered to the respirators in a continuous and sufficient supply, which means that both air pressure and air volume requirements must be maintained through the purification and delivery processes. Required air pressure can be ensured:

- by measuring and controlling the air pressure within the air delivery system at the entrance to the respirator hoses

(Air pressure is adjusted to the required pressure specified by the manufacturer for each respirator.)

- by maintaining the required pressure under all flow conditions when all the respirators are being used.

Two factors which affect the respirator pressure during air flow are (1) the inside diameters of hoses and their connectors, and (2) the overall length of air supply hose. Respirator hose-line pressures must typically be maintained in the 65-100 pounds per square inch gauge (psig) range. The Occupational Safety and Health Administration (OSHA) and NIOSH regulations prohibit the actual hose length from the respirator manifold to exceed 300 feet in length.

In order to add low pressure supply hose beyond 300 feet, the respirator input pressure should be maintained at the required and specified value for the respirators being used. Extra large diameter supply hose from the compressor to the respirator hose manifold may allow some length increases beyond the 300 feet. The simplest method to add some extra length to the low pressure supply line is to provide a compressor with output pressure higher than the pressure required by the respirators, and to provide a regulator at the respirator manifold. This regulator functions to reduce, control, and maintain the correct respirator pressure at the inlet to the respirator hoses. An accurate pressure gauge should be located at the inlet to the respirator hoses. For increases in hose length to be acceptable, this respirator inlet pressure gauge must read the correct and required value specified for the respirators being used when under maximum flow conditions (i.e., with all available respirators in use).

An easy test of the low pressure distribution system can be conducted by:

(1) laying out the required length of air transfer hoses

(2) connecting all respirator manifolds

(3) attaching the maximum number of respirator hoses and respirators to be used (up to 300 feet if needed)

(4) pressurizing the system

(5) with all respirators in use, then check the pressure at the respirator manifolds.

Should the pressure at the manifolds be less than the specified respirator pressure, increasing the pressure may be accomplished by using extra-large diameter supply hoses, or increasing compressor pressure combined with use of a control regulator at the respirator manifolds. If one of these methods will allow the required respirator pressure to be maintained, the extra length is acceptable for use. If the required respirator pressure cannot be maintained, the hose lengths must be shortened until the specified respirator hose pressure can be maintained.

Remember: providing a continuous and sufficient supply of breathing air is accomplished by maintaining the correct and specified respirator inlet air pressure under all airflow conditions.

(2) Adequate Reserve Air or Escape Time

Providing for adequate reserve air or escape time is a necessary and required function of the breathing air system. The OSHA Safety and Health Manual 29 CFR 1910.134 (d)(2)(ii) states, "A receiver of sufficient capacity to enable the respirator wearer to escape from a contaminated atmosphere in event of compressor failure and alarms to indicate compressor failure shall be installed in the system."

This poses the question of how much reserve time, and therefore how much stored air, is necessary. If a work crew were told an escape test was going to be conducted at a specified time, such a test might show that only 10 to 20 minutes were required. The escape time required under actual workplace conditions could be considerably longer. Complex airline routing and even tangling, work on scaffolding or in restricted access areas, and the requirement for the entire work crew to take showers can all lengthen escape time. For a crew size of ten workers, actual egress times have been measured at 30 to 50 minutes and more. Therefore, for most asbestos jobs a reserve time specification of 50 minutes to one hour is needed. Certain special asbestos jobs with more complicated egress conditions may need escape time of more than one hour.

Prepumped air or air stored in a pressure container is used as the method to obtain the required escape time. However, it should be noted here that low pressure systems, with pressures up to 200 psi, are not capable of storing any appreciable escape time in any practical tank volume size. However, high pressure air storage in the 2000 psi to 4000 psi range is easily capable of meeting the required escape time and more. When high pressure tanks are used to provide one hour and more escape time, the overall tank size, weight and cost are within practical limits.

The requirement to use high pressure (2000 to 4000 psi) as the only practical reserve air storage method does not adversely affect specification, choice, or the use of low pressure breathing air systems. The cost for providing a high-pressure standby reserve system with Grade D air on a low pressure breathing air system is minimal. The high pressure breathing air tanks for this standby air reserve do not need to be purchased; rental is the normal arrangement for suppliers of such high pressure tanks. High pressure tanks are routinely available from many sources nationwide. The rental cost for such tanks is usually minimal. Suppliers can be found by search of the Yellow Pages of a local telephone book under the heading, "Gas - Industrial and Medical." Since this high pressure standby reserve should be used only for the occasional emergency compressor stoppage, the actual cost of the air used from such a standby reserve system on a jobsite should also be minimal.

Cost considerations for the in-line reserve or escape air on a high pressure breathing air system are even lower. The in-line air storage bank provides more than sufficient escape time.

(3) Temperature Control of the Breathing Air

Asbestos removal during warm weather can create extremely hot working environments for abatement workers. Typically, the heating, ventilation, and air conditioning is shut down, and the building is then sealed off with plastic sheeting on all wall, overhead, and floor surfaces. This increases the retention of heat in the workplace. Then, water sprays are introduced into this hot workplace in order to minimize the airborne fibers. Such sprays create high humidities that reduce or eliminate the normal external body heat removal method of sweat evaporation. It is not at all unusual to see workplace ambient temperatures of 120° to 130°F with relative humidities in the 90% - 100% range.

The worker has other additional adverse personal circumstances. The asbestos worker is clothed with disposable garments which are very hot to wear. Although these garments are light in weight, they are made of material which is of low permeability. Such garments restrict local body air movement and, therefore, the transfer of heat from the body.

Asbestos removal work is hard physical labor. In many instances, this labor is performed from precarious or dangerous work positions, such as high up on movable scaffolding, or in the crawl space above lightweight ceiling grids where temporary flooring is placed.

It is in this hot and difficult workplace that the respiratory protective system must be used. If a low quality supplied air system is introduced, it typically may bring hot, humid, foul-smelling air, or even air that is dangerous to breathe. In such a case, it is no wonder that the worker may dislike the respiratory protective device and remove it whenever possible.

However, a supplied air system which delivers cooled, high quality breathing air, can provide the worker with relief against body heat buildup in such hot environments. Under these circumstances the respirator may even become equipment preferred by the worker.

Where hot environmental conditions exist, the asbestos worker should be provided with some type of personal cooling. The available choices of personal cooling depend on which type of breathing air system is being used. Hot air is produced in the compression process of all three basic types of breathing air systems--low pressure, high pressure, and prepumped high pressure tank systems. The already hot general working conditions of the asbestos workplace make it intolerable to deliver hot breathing air to the worker. Unless some temperature control is placed within the breathing air system to reduce and control the compressed air temperature and remove all condensables before the air is admitted to the air purifier, the air quality will also be unreliable. Reduction of temperature and removal of condensate before the air enters the purifier system are vital to ensure air quality, even if expensive and otherwise adequate purification systems are used.

Three methods of personal cooling that are in breathing air systems are the aftercooler (air-cooled or water-cooled), the Vortex tube, and adiabatic cooling.

The Aftercooler. Hot compressed air exiting a compressor may be cooled by using an aftercooler or heat exchanger. These heat exchangers may transfer the heat either to the ambient air (air-cooled) or to locally available cold water (water-cooled). Figure 2 shows the correct location of such aftercoolers within the overall breathing air processing system. For the downstream air purifier assembly to function properly and give good control to process high quality breathing air, excess heat, condensates, water, and oil must be removed. This is accomplished by first removing heat, and then removing the condensed water and oil. These are two vital sequential steps that must be taken before air is admitted to any purifier assembly or supplied to any worker.

The efficiency of the air-cooled aftercooler will be affected by the ambient air temperature. Because of this fact, the air-cooled aftercooler will not function as efficiently on the hottest days, when worker cooling is most needed. Therefore, the best type of aftercooler choice to ensure that worker cooling is available when needed may be the water-cooled aftercooler.

The Vortex Tube. The Vortex Tube (for cooling or heating) is another available method of worker temperature control (See Figure 3). The Vortex Tube is a very simple device. It is a tube of approximately ½ to 1 inch diameter and perhaps 6 to 12 inches in length. The Vortex tube is simple, lightweight, and inexpensive. Air is admitted into the side of the tube and split into two separate airstreams, each exiting at opposite ends of the tube. One airstream is hot, the other is cold. Either of these two airstreams may be directed into the worker's disposable suit or hood to provide external temperature control to the worker.

The only disadvantage of the Vortex tube is that it uses a comparatively high volume of air, approximately 15 to 20 cfm per worker. Compared to the air used by a pressure-demand type respirator, each vortex tube will use as much air as would be needed to supply 4 or 5 pressure-demand respirators. Therefore, the use of vortex worker cooling will increase the size and cost of both the compressor and the breathing air purifier.

Adiabatic Cooling. Adiabatic cooling is available when sufficient cooling capacity has been designed into each of the multistage compression steps found internally in the high pressure compressor. Provided that the high pressure compressor cooling design is adequate, cool or ambient temperature air will be produced at the high pressure compressor outlet. This air is carried into the in-line air reserve tanks and then into the asbestos work area via high pressure lines to an air control panel. The air pressure regulator on this panel reduces the high pressure air from pressures of 1000 to 4000 psig down to the required respirator line pressure (typically in the 65 to 100 psig range). The air temperature also drops dramatically with this air expansion at the control panel and the resulting cold air is directed into the respirator lines at the panel.

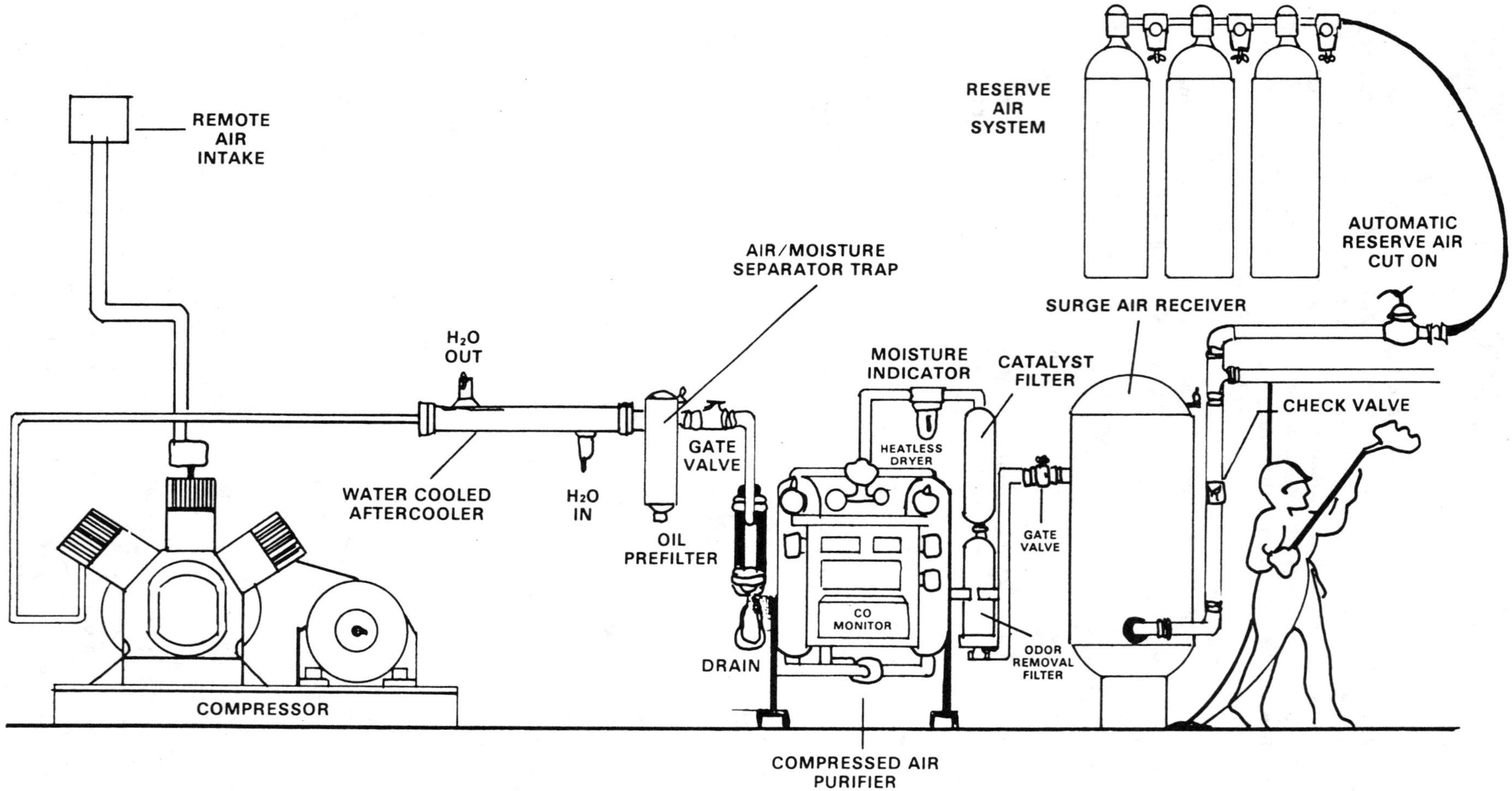

Figure F2. Typical Installation of Low Pressure Breathing Air System

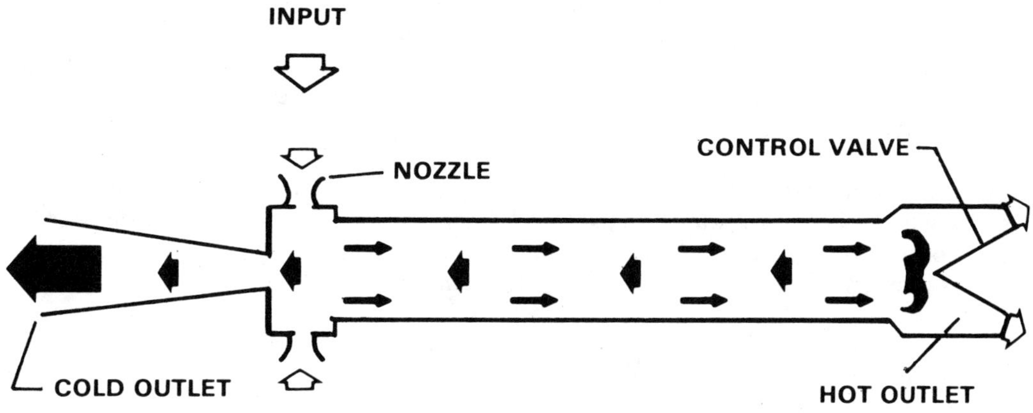

SCHEMATIC DRAWING OF A VORTEX TUBE

WHAT IS A VORTEX TUBE?

The Vortex tube is a device capable of converting an ordinary supply of compressed air into two streams, one hot and one cold. The proportions of hot and cold flow and their temperatures can be varied over a wide range. All of this is accomplished without moving parts using only compressed air as a source of power.

The temperature differences in the hot and cold outputs can be striking. With a 100 psig compressed air source, the Vortex tube can be adjusted to cool the air as much as 100° below inlet air temperature.

HOW DOES IT WORK?

The compressed air first enters nozzles which inject it at sonic speed circumferentially into the vortex generation chamber. Spinning as fast as one million revolutions per minute, the vortex moves through the tube toward the hot outlet. Air near the surface of the tube becomes hot and some of it leaves through the control valve at the hot end. The control valve imposes enough pressure on the vortex to force some of the air to the center and back through the tube to the cold end. This air becomes very cold in the process and leaves the tube through the cold outlet.

Figure F3. The Vortex Tube, Its Construction and Performance

Adiabatic cooling is very simple, lightweight, and reliable provided the compressor has been initially designed to be adequate for such cooling.

In the typical asbestos worksite, cold breathing air will aid in cooling the asbestos worker. Normal external body cooling methods have been reduced due to the previously described working conditions, while body core cooling effects of breathing cool air have not been changed. Cooling methods using cool or cold breathing air can also be used incidentally to provide cool air externally to the worker. This can be accomplished simply by directing the cool exhaust from the respirator exhalation valve down inside the asbestos worker's disposable garment. Workers generally are observed to accomplish this added cooling without special instruction or added personal equipment. With a high pressure breathing air system, a single user of a pressure-demand full facepiece type respirator (with built-in adiabatic cooling) may use a total of only 4 standard cubic feet per minute (SCFM).

When asbestos abatement is accomplished in extremely cold environments, there may be a need to provide heat to the breathing air. Heat exchangers with a warm water heat source can be used to heat and control the breathing air being delivered to the respirator hoses. Supplemental heating or cooling may be used with any type breathing air system.

(4) Continuous Carbon Monoxide (CO) Monitor and Alarm

Providing a continous CO monitor and alarm is a requirement of law and of common sense. Carbon monoxide monitors and alarms are available from many sources. A list of sources is included in Part V of this Appendix. The CO monitor should be purchased as a part of the overall breathing air system or breathing air purifier assembly. Proper choice of CO monitor and correct installation in the system are aided by the system manufacturer. Since CO monitor and alarm systems can malfunction, employers may find it prudent to install two such systems to ensure continued protection in case of failure.

Manufacturers of carbon monoxide monitors have available two basic types of sensors. One sensor type is specific or sensitive only to carbon monoxide. This sensor will ignore all other trace chemicals and alarm only in the presence of CO. The monitors based on a CO-specific sensor are usually more expensive. The other type of sensor also will alarm in the presence of carbon monoxide, but it is a non-specific sensor and may also give alarms in the presence of trace chemicals when carbon monoxide is not actually present. Non-specific systems are usually less expensive.

Some manufacturers tend to recommend the non-specific type sensor for inclusion in the asbestos removal air system. Non-specific sensors may give more alarms. The reasoning behind recommending the non-specific type is that other potentially harmful chemicals are being detected when this system gives such an alarm. For instance, off-gassing of certain synthetic compressor lubricants not recommended for use as lubricants in breathing air compressors may cause such non-CO alarms. The breathing air system would be protected against an "unfamiliar" rental compressor in which such adverse synthetic lubricants had been used by the action of such alarms.

On the other hand, the occurrence of numerous alarms will disrupt the asbestos worksite and could significantly increase the cost of removal or make job completion difficult. Such excessive alarms also create a "cry wolf" attitude in the workforce, leading to a disregard for the alarm. Disregard for the CO alarm is a very dangerous practice and MUST be avoided. Therefore, the CO monitor must be kept in calibration and all alarms equally respected. Immediate air quality samples may be taken during the alarm to verify the absense or presence of CO. Should numerous alarms be experienced, the possible sources for other chemicals being detected by the alarm should be found and eliminated.

If CO alarms continue after efforts at finding a local fix, contact the CO monitor manufacturer for aid. In this case, consider with the manufacturer or supplier of the carbon monoxide monitor either (1) obtaining a new CO monitor of the same type, to eliminate the possibility of a mechanically or electrically malfunctioning alarm, or (2) obtaining a CO monitor and alarm from a different manufacturer.

IF A LOW PRESSURE BREATHING AIR SYSTEM IS BEING USED WHEN THE ALARM SOUNDS:

When the alarm sounds, the breathing air system should immediately be switched to the high pressure standby air reserve system. Depending on the capacity of the reserve system, the workers should exit the toxic removal zone. Typically, one 220 standard cubic foot tank will provide one man equipped with a 4.0 SCFM pressure-demand respirator with fifty-five minutes of escape time.

The outside supervisors should check and make certain all workers are exiting. All respirators should be accounted for and verified as no longer in use.

With sufficent high pressure reserve or when using a high pressure breathing air system with sufficient in-line reserve capacity, CO alarms and unexpected compressor shutdown can often be handled without disruptions in the asbestos removal work.

Remember, air being processed in a low pressure air system is almost immediately being delivered to and breathed by the workers. Therefore, when using the low pressure system, there is an immediate need for switchover to the high-pressure reserve air when the CO alarm sounds. If only the minimum high pressure reserve is available, the workers should exit the area. If additional reserve air capacity is available, the workers should exit when the reserve supply approaches the minimum acceptable amount.

When using a high pressure breathing air system with an in-line high pressure air storage bank, the compressed air from the compressor is delayed and diluted by the action of the in-line storage bank before being delivered to the workers. When the CO alarm sounds in a high pressure breathing air system, the stored air at the moment of the alarm has previously been processed through the CO monitor, and is already guaranteed to be Grade D quality. The air in the in-line air bank therefore remains available for the workers' continued use.

IF A HIGH PRESSURE BREATHING AIR SYSTEM IS BEING USED WHEN THE ALARM SOUNDS:

Immediately stop the air flow from the compressor into the in-line reserve air bank by shutting the output air valve. **[Note: If so arranged, this step may be automatically accomplished through relays in the CO monitor.]**

Immediately provide a gas sample test for CO in the supply output from the air bank to the workers. (See discussion of the gas detection method which follows).

If the sample test shows no carbon monoxide in the air from the air bank going to the workers, then the workers may continue to work. They may work as long as no further air from the compressor is being admitted into the air bank, and provided more air time is stored in the bank than the required one hour reserve time. When and if the one hour reserve level is reached, the workers should be removed.

A study of formation of carbon monoxide in breathing air compressors was done by Lawrence Livermore Laboratory in 1978*. Two separate conclusions from this study which are of particular signifiance for breathing air systems used in asbestos removal are as follows:

- "Exhaust gases from combustion engines are the major threat to the quality of compressed air." (p. 6)

---

*Formation of Carbon Monoxide in Air Compressors, Lawrence Livermore Laboratory, T.M. Distler, July 26, 1978, 94550 Contract No. W-7405-Eng-48

- "The preceding observations [of the study] indicate that a high temperature shut-off or alarm, as one of the options specified by OSHA, does not significantly protect against CO contamination of compressed air. In the event of local overheating in a compressor, the effectiveness of a temperature sensor would depend on its placement near the hot spot. The oil reservoir, because of its much lower temperature, is unreliable as an indicator of overheating. Therefore, a high-temperature alarm or shut-off device should not be considered as a substitute for CO monitoring." (p. 7)

Gas Detector Tubes. As previously noted, when a CO alarm sounds in a high pressure system, a gas sample test for CO in the supply output from the air back to workers should be done immediately. Whether a low pressure or a high pressure breathing air system is in use, after all workers have exited, and all respirators have been accounted for, air testing should be conducted to determine if CO was present or not.

Although direct reading CO monitors are available, a less expensive and simple to use on-site air analysis method can be used to provide a positive backup analysis method in case a CO alarm is activated. This method uses preset chemical color change analysis. The analysis chemicals are precharged and sealed into small glass tubes. Different tubes are available for many different gases. A small case contains several sets of tubes and the constant volume sampling pump. Other tubes useful on an asbestos jobsite include those which indicate oxygen and carbon dioxide. These tubes are simple to use. The ends are broken off a tube and the tube is inserted into the pump. Operating the hand pump draws a measured volume of air sample through the tube. The results are read directly on a scale on the tube.

Practice samples taken on two known CO sources can be used to verify the detection of CO using detector tubes. Cigarette smoke can be used as a common type of low-level carbon monoxide sample test. Exhaust from an idling, non-catalytic-equipped automobile, truck, or other engine is a second example, this time of high CO content. Taking these two known CO-content samples on a CO tube will educate the crew as to what the abnormal CO reading actually looks like on the tube. The usual CO sample results on a high quality breathing air is zero CO.

Periodic gas tube sampling results should be permanently logged. This provides an additional record of the air quality on the job site.

B. Types of Breathing Air Systems

There are three (3) general types of breathing air systems potentially available for use in asbestos removal. These general types are categorized according to the pressure levels at which they are designed to operate:

(1) the low pressure system

(2) the high pressure system

(3) high pressure pre-pumped tanks

(1) The Low Pressure System

The typical low pressure system is shown in Figure 2. This system consists of:

(a) a low pressure compressor

(b) an aftercooler assembly with water removal traps

(c) an air purifier assembly

(d) a standby high pressure air reserve assembly

(e) a surge-tank or in-line air volume tank

(f) a distribution hose and distribution manifold with connections for respirator hose lines.

(a) A Low Pressure Breathing Air Compressor

The low pressure breathing air compressor produces pressures between 100 and 200 psi. It has sufficient flow capacity to provide the flow needed for the respirators being used. The compressor should also be equipped with sufficient interstage and aftercooling capacity to reduce the air temperature to within 10°F of the ambient air temperature. The low pressure compressor should be equipped with suitable moisture removal traps to be able to remove 60% to 85% of the water/oil condensed within the machine. Water removal may be either automatic and continuous or manual and periodic.

(b) An Aftercooler Assembly with Water Removal Traps

The aftercooler assembly is used immediately following the low pressure breathing air compressor. The aftercooler and its water trap may be incorporated physically in the compressor. The purpose of the aftercooler assembly is to guarantee that the air temperature is reduced to within 10°F of ambient air temperature. Such a reduction in temperature forces condensation of water/oil in the airstream. The cyclone-type water separator or water trap is also a part of the aftercooler. This separator or water trap is used to allow removal of the water/oil mixtures condensed by the action of the aftercooler in the airstream.

Aftercoolers may either be ambient air-cooled or water-cooled. Ambient air aftercoolers will not function as well on the hottest days, when the most worker cooling is needed. Water-cooled aftercoolers may work best on the low pressure system.

(c) An Air Purifier Assembly

The purpose of this purifier network (see Figure 4) is to polish the air to at least the required Grade D air quality.

The air inlet is on the upper left of the diagram. The air path is actually downward into the prefilter, and the first active element encountered by the air is an added water coalescing element in the down tubes and bottom of this prefilter. Water is mechanically collected on this coalescing section of the prefilter and drains downward into the water removal trap. Water can be drained automatically or through a manual valve added to the bottom of this trap.

[IMPORTANT NOTE: ALL CONDENSED WATER AND OIL MUST BE DRAINED AND REMOVED FROM THE AIR ADMITTED INTO THIS PREFILTER. If proper reduction of air temperature and proper removal of condensate is not accomplished at the entrance to the prefilter, the breathing air purifier may not function as well as expected and may require more filter replacements.]

The air continues moving upward through the prefilter and into the oil removal section of the prefilter. At the lowest visual level in the prefilter there is a red color-match band. Oil vapors are adsorbed by the filter media, beginning just above the red band. Oil adsorption causes a red color change in the originally white filter material above the red color-match band. As additional air quantities are passed through the prefilter, this color change will progress upward inside the prefilter material as the filter material adsorbs the oil from the airstream. When the color change approaches the top of the prefilter material, the prefilter should be changed. The above description is typical of the visual or color-change method of notice of need for filter change, which is used by several manufacturers in many types of adsorption filters.

[IMPORTANT NOTE: Some low pressure compressors that may be available for local rental may be built and set up to power industrial machines. Industrial machines such as air tools, jack-hammers, roadwork earth drills, and other such machines have very different

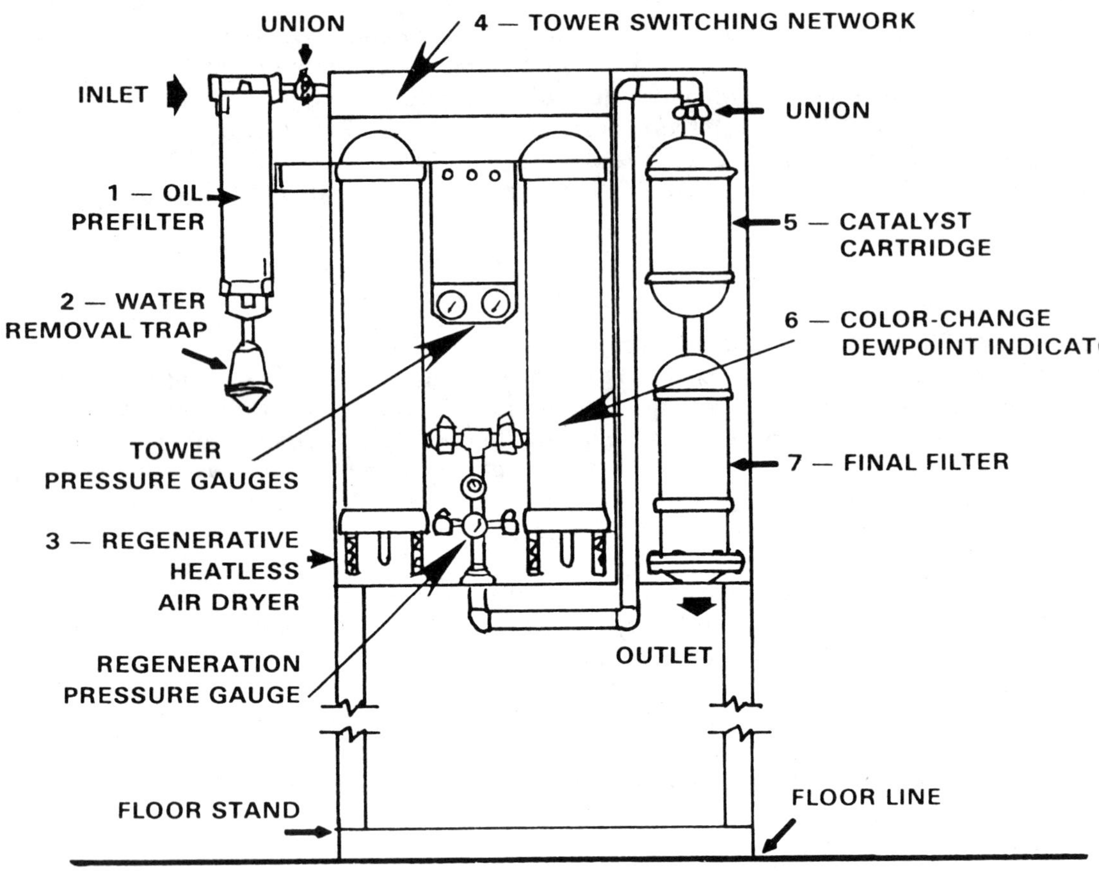

1. Oil Prefilter — removes oil mist, particulates, and entrained water. Color-change replacement notice

2. Water Removal Draintrap — removes condensed water-oil mixtures

3. Dual Regenerative Heatless Air Drying Towers — reduce water vapor content; action is to regenerate its own adsorber material

4. Tower Switching Network — acts with plumbing to provide timed dryer tower switching to effect regeneration

5. Catalyst Cartridge — removes CO by catalytic conversion to CO_2

6. Color Change Dewpoint Indicator — Color change visually shows the performance of the drying towers

7. Final Filter - effects odor removal

Figure F4. Typical Low Pressure Breathing Air Purifier Assembly

requirements from a compressor required to produce breathing air. Industrial machines may require a high oil content in the airstream. Industrial oiling requirements may be designed to be met directly in the compressor output or may be met by the addition of airline oilers. In such cases where a high oil content is found in the air, the solution is to either remove airline oilers downstream of the compressor outlet, or change to a different and suitable compressor that has low oil output.]

Air processed through the active prefilter passes into the dual dryer tower assembly, into the air-switching plumbing circuit assembly. This air-switching circuit simply directs the air into the heatless air dryer assembly. There are two of these drying towers. Each tower is alternately either on-line, drying the air, or off-line being regenerated.

The regeneration of the off-duty tower is accomplished by taking a percentage of the dry air from the output of the on-duty drying tower and running it in a reverse direction through the off-duty tower. The dewpoint of the drying air and also the amount of air to be diverted to drying the off-cycle tower is determined by the setting of the regeneration pressure gauge.

The breathing air purifier shown in Figure 4 has visual moisture indicators in each drying tower. These indicators change color in the presence of moisture. Observation of these color-change indicators allows the operator to observe the functioning of the drying operation. During operation the on-cycle tower will begin to absorb water. After approximately 2½ minutes the system will switch, the now dry off-cycle tower will become the functioning tower, and the on-cycle tower will go over to off-cycle as it begins to be de-adsorbed or regenerated.

Over a period of years in normal operation the ability of the towers to be regenerated decreases. Colorimetric indicators are available to indicate when the adsorber material in these towers must be replaced.

[<u>IMPORTANT NOTE:</u> The drying action of these towers depends on water adsorption and water de-adsorption. If the system is operated with a depleted prefilter, oil may be passed into the drying towers. The activated alumina in the drying towers will adsorb oil and therefore will provide a backup to the function of oil removal normally accomplished by the prefilter. However, oil adsorbed in the drying towers will not be desorbed in the towers. Therefore oil passing through a saturated prefilter will effectively ruin the water drying function of part or all of the tower and result in shorter-than-expected drying media lifetime and more frequent tower media replacement.]

Air from the dryer towers now enters the CO catalyst. This catalyst changes harmful CO to CO_2. The catalyst can process up to 400 ppm inlet CO and still keep the output air below the required 20 ppm limit.

[<u>Note</u>: A carbon monoxide continuous monitor and alarm is required on all breathing air systems used in asbestos removal work, even if a CO catalyst is also used.]

Periodic replacement of the CO catalyst is recommended by all purifier manufacturers.

Air now flows to the final adsorber canister where odors are removed by activated charcoal. This canister is usually replaced on a recommended interval basis. This final canister may also contain a particle filter which prevents adsorber particles from passing downstream.

The low pressure breathing air compressor plus the described breathing air purifier is time-proven and will deliver high quality breathing air.

(d) A Standby High Pressure Reserve System

The only effective method to store sufficient air for an industrial sized asbestos removal work crew is through the use of high pressure storage tanks. Such tanks are available for rental at low rates, and they can be delivered directly to the asbestos abatement worksite.

The standby reserve system functions by sensing both the line air pressure and the air quality provided by the compressor and breathing air system. Should the compressor fail and the line air pressure begin to drop or should CO levels exceed 20 ppm, the standby reserve sensing system detects dropping pressure or presence of CO and starts to supply pressure from the reserve air system. This pressure supply is automatic and immediate, and functions to continuously provide sufficient air to operate the respirators.

There are two operational notes that must be included in the startup and shutdown checklist for the operator of this system:

On Startup of the Low Pressure Breathing Air System:

(1) Start the low pressure breathing air compressor and verify air delivery at full pressure.

(2) Only then turn each reserve air tank on.

On Shutdown after workers have exited:

(1) Turn OFF each reserve air tank valve.

(2) Only then go through the procedures to shut down the breathing air compressor.

Operating any standby reserve air system without including the directions listed above could cause inadvertent loss of air from the reserve system. This could result in low or zero reserve air in the standby reserve air tanks when it is really needed.

(e) A Surge Tank or In-line Air Volume Tank

A surge tank provides air storage capacity so that peak flow conditions will not deplete the air supply.

(f) A Distribution Hose and Manifold with Connections for Respirator Hose Lines

Once air is processed through the low pressure air purifier it is directed into the delivery air line and is immediately available to the worker.

(2) The High Pressure System

The high pressure breathing air system (Figure 5) is composed of four major components:

(a) a high pressure compressor

(b) an air purifier assembly

(c) a high pressure air storage bank

(d) a high pressure control and distribution panel

(a) A High Pressure Compressor

The function of the high pressure compressor is the same as that in the low pressure system. The low pressure compressor utilized one or two successive compression steps or stages to compress the air up to 100 to 200 psi. The high pressure machine pumps the air to pressures of 2000 to 4000 psi utilizing from 3 to 5 successive stages of compression.

Each time the air is processed through a compression stage, its density and its pressure are increased, and its volume is decreased. The air temperature increases sharply through each

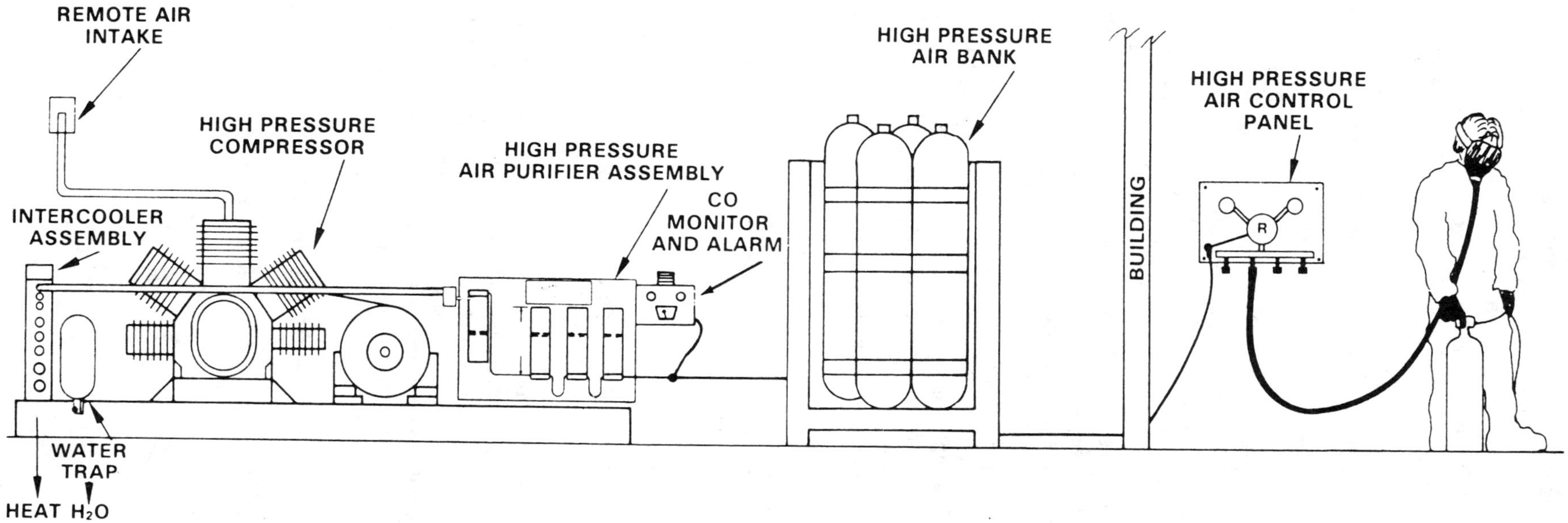

Figure F5. Typical High Pressure Breathing Air System

compression stage due to the adiabatic process. Following each stage of compression, the air is put through an intercooler that transfers considerable heat out of the air. Once the compressed air temperature is brought down, it cannot hold the moisture that it carried before that stage of compression, and the water vapor and other vapors condense. Following each intercooler stage is a cyclone-type liquid trap. The liquid trap is a vertical cylinder with a drain valve in the bottom. The air is introduced tangentially near the top of the trap, and creates a spinning vortex within the trap. The higher density condensed liquids are thrown against the cylinder walls of the trap. They drain down along the walls of the trap and can be removed from the compressor through the drain valve in the bottom. Even though water has been condensed and removed, the air is saturated. In this state, further compression or cooling will be able to remove additional water. This will be done in the following stages.

The air from the preceding compressor stage is now carried into the intake of the next compressor state. Here it is again compressed, cooled, and water is again extracted. This process of compression, cooling, and condensate removal is repeated for every succeeding state within the high pressure compressor. High pressure makes it possible to take out considerably more heat from the air than could be extracted by low pressure compression. The same is true for moisture removal within the high pressure machine. It is capable of removing much more of the water vapor that was originally being carried by the air than if the air were only compressed to a lower pressure in a single or dual state compressor.

Heat and water removal inside the compressor, by intercoolers and drain traps, is done by mechanical methods. Mechanical removal methods are more or less permanent removal methods. These methods do not require replacement adsorber cartridges nor the maintenance associated with such cartridge changes. Very high percentages of condensates are capable of being mechanically removed in high pressure processing. The result of such processing is to reduce the water vapor and other contaminants that must be removed by the following adsorber purifier.

Therefore, one of the major effects of high pressure mechnanical processing in the breathing air compressor is to reduce the required size and weight of adsorbent material needed in the follow-on high pressure purifier assembly.

(b) The Air Purifier Assembly

The high pressure purifier assembly is made up of an aftercooler, a combination coalescing filter/drain trap, and a number of successive purifier containers that hold adsorber materials.

The function of the aftercooler is similar to that of the intercoolers. Following the aftercooler, the air is put through a combination mechanical coalescing filter element/drain trap. Vapor is not removed in mechanical drain traps. There are some very tiny drops of condensed materials, called aerosols (water, oil, etc.) which act almost like vapor and also move through ordinary drain traps. In order to mechanically remove these aerosols, they are forced, in the coalescing element, to impact or squeeze together and to form big drops out of the aerosols. These coalesced liquid drops can now be drained from the air stream.

The air now moves into the adsorber section of the purifier.

Adsorber materials to be used in high pressure adsorber chambers are the same as used in low pressure designs:

molecular sieves

silica gel

activated alumina (Al_2O_3)

activated charcoal.

At this point the engineer or designer of the high pressure purifier assembly has two major advantages over designing for low pressure air purification: (1) more condensate and contaminates have already been mechanically removed within the high pressure compressor section, and (2) the density of the air is much higher. Higher density air means that any given amount of adsorber will be more effective and will process more air. Both of these facts add to a reduction in the required adsorber needed.

There is a third factor in the overall high pressure design which also allows for a reduction in the required adsorber material. One major action of the in-line high pressure storage bank is to allow a smaller compressor to be used. The high-pressure in-line air bank allows the designer to reduce compressor output, size, weight, and horsepower. Therefore overall cost of this system is reduced. Costs for the high pressure system are lower both in initial purchase and in operating costs, than if the designer were operating without the in-line high pressure air storage bank.

The combination of:

- more condensate mechanically removed by the high pressure compressor
- increased adsorber effectiveness due to higher density of air
- lower air flowrates needed because of the combination of the high pressure compressor and in-line air storage bank

make possible the use of simpler, smaller, and less costly adsorber purifiers to process the high pressure air.

As with low pressure breathing air systems, high pressure regenerative adsorber systems are available, but their high initial cost make them unattractive to the engineer/designer. They are generally not included in high pressure assemblies processing breathing air for asbestos work crews.

Following the coalescing filter trap, there are usually two (2) to four (4) successive additional disposable adsorber containers. These are usually replaced on a machine time basis, but color change or other indicators are available. Since cartridges cannot regenerate themselves it is especially important that they are changed on a regular and scheduled basis. Failure to do so could allow desiccants to reach saturation and permit contaminants to enter and contaminate the high pressure storage bank system. A typical high pressure purifier assembly, consisting of an inlet coalescing drain trap and three successive replaceable adsorber containers, is shown in Figure 6.

Continous CO Monitor and Alarm. Air passing from the high pressure purifier should be continuously monitored by an electric carbon monoxide alarm. Should any carbon monoxide be produced in the compressor or induced into the compressor air intake, it will be detected by the CO monitor. The CO alarm will visually and/or audibly warn if the CO level goes above 20 ppm. Visual warning is accomplished by meter and by a green/red system of lights. High decibel audible alarms are also available.

CO monitors can be adjusted to alarm at different levels of CO present. In order to meet the requirements of "Grade D" air, no more than 20 ppm are allowed.

(c) The High Pressure In-line Air Storage Bank

High quality air, Grade D or better, is now pumped directly into the high pressure storage bank. The function of this high pressure storage bank is to act as an air reservoir, so that:

- the peak air flow demands can be met without concern for or limitation by the maximum compressor output

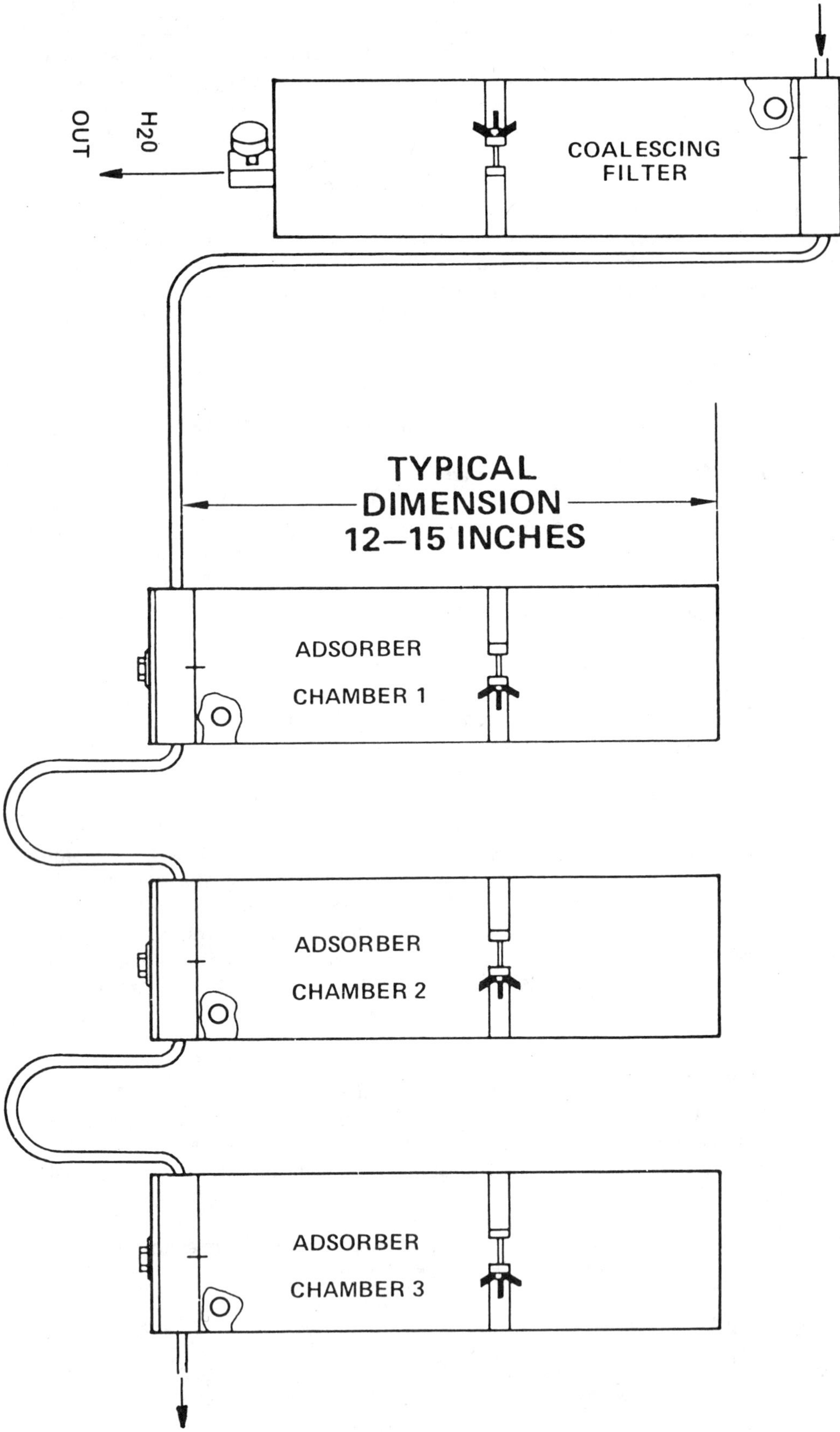

Figure F6. Typical High Pressure Purifier Assembly

- the compressor and purifier can be sized for lower flowrates than the peak flowrates required
- in emergency compressor conditions, such as power failure, compressor stoppage, etc. the work crew air supply remains uninterrupted for at least one hour
- greater capacity (typically three to six hours) than the minimum required for escape (one hour) can be used to allow routine or emergency maintenance of the system to be accomplished without interrupting the work crew.

<u>Air Reservoir for Peak Flow</u>. A compressor pumping directly to a large work crew is analogous to a water pump pumping without a water reservoir. The direct supply water pump must be sized to meet the peak flow demands. Water systems include a water storage reservoir so that the peak flows are supplied by the reservoir, while the water pump operates over longer periods of lower flow to maintain the reservoir level. This pump/storage design method is done more than just for convenience; it is done also for cost reasons. Even small community water systems would require prohibitively sized water pumps, if only direct supply from the water pump was used. Therefore the function of large storage capacities is included in all municipal water systems. We see large water tanks located strategically around cities.

<u>Air Reservoir to Lower Costs</u>. Air storage is different from storage of water. Water density is the same for all water pumps, while air density is a function of air pressure. Low pressures simply do not have enough density to store air effectively. Therefore low pressure air compressors must deliver and use the air almost immediately, since no effective storage is available. Higher pressure increases air density. Increased air density makes possible the compressor/storage combination which can more effectively accomplish the air supply to large crews. Therefore smaller, lighter weight, lower horsepower and lower cost high pressure air compressors can compress air into and maintain the high pressure reservoir. The high pressure reservoir can supply peak flowrates without being limited by lower maximum compressor flowrates.

The major reason for the use of in-line high pressure air storage is economic. The in-line high pressure air storage bank allows a lower cost of smaller high pressure compressor to provide breathing air to a large asbestos removal work crew. Without the in-line air storage bank, a larger and more costly air compressor and larger and more costly air purifier assembly would be needed to support the same crew.

Reserve air time in excess of one to one and a half hours is also available from the high pressure system. Extra time above the one hour escape time may be called the working reserve. Working reserve time, stored in a high pressure storage bank, is very valuable in that unscheduled or scheduled maintenance can be done without interupting the work crew.

<u>Air Reservoir for Emergency Conditions</u>. The working reserve allows the severity of emergency conditions to be lessened. For instance, an inadvertent compressor stoppage with a low pressure system requires an immediate switchover to the high pressure air reserve. A normally open air valve is held closed until switchover is required to provide adequate egress time. The reserve air tanks must be fully charged. It is recommended that a low pressure sensor and alarm be used to monitor the standby reserve. In the high pressure system with in-line storage and reserve, the worker does not enter the toxic zone in the first place unless he is drawing air from the reserve air bank. Both outside and inside toxic zone pressure gauges show at all times the number of hours of reserve time for any crew size. Should the power fail and the high pressure compressor stop, there is no requirement for a switch to operate in order for the "reserve air" to be brought on line.

The working reserve also decreases the severity of the other conditions which might constitute real emergency conditions in other systems. For instance, consider that the CO alarm sounds. The CO alarm has auxiliary relays which can be used in the high pressure system to protect the air previously stored in the air bank. (Likewise, such relays can switch the low pressure system over to the reserve air bank.) It does this by providing power to close the air valve on the compressor output (high pressure system) or open the air valve to the backup reserve bottles (low pressure system). At the first moment of alarm, this valve is shut. Also, for both high and low pressure systems, manual valving on the compressor output can be used to shut off flow upon CO alarm. With Grade D air stored in the air bank, there is no CO emergency for the inside workers. The outside supervisors and outside workers can deal with this alarm as a potential CO problem. The inside workers are using the previously processed air stored in the bank, which will supply them for the next several hours. The problem can be identified and the condition corrected.

(d) A High Pressure Control and Distribution Panel

Air is delivered into the toxic zone from the high pressure air bank through small high pressure lines. These lines may be flexible or solid high pressure lines and may be several hundred feet in length. This high pressure line is led into the building to a lightweight air control and air distribution panel. The panel has a high pressure guage that may be marked off in pressure units or it may be rated in time units (hours) for any size work crew. Each worker attached by respirator hose to this panel can at all times see exactly how much working reserve time (and escape time) is available.

As with the low pressure breathing air system manifold, this panel also contains a regulator and low pressure gauge. The regulator sets, controls and maintains the respirator hose-line pressure to a precise value. Momentary fluctuations in the low pressure hose lines are removed by the action of the regulator. The regulator holds the respirator hose-line pressure at a constant value, which allows for more consistent respirator performance.

Respirator low pressure hose-line lengths are still limited to not more than 300 feet.

Filling SCBA Tanks. If equipped with filling devices, high pressure SCBA tanks can be filled from any part of a high pressure system.

Worker Cooling with the High Pressure Breathing Air System. Providing worker cooling is a consistent problem in asbestos removal work. Both the high and low pressure breathing air systems have built-in worker cooling. Because of its higher working pressures, high pressure cooling is more noticeable. The air supplied to the air panel is at high pressure and is also at ambient temperature (2000 to 4000 psi and about 70° - 85°F). The air panel regulator reduces this pressure to 80 to 100 psi. When this pressure reduction takes place, the air temperature drops 25° to 40°F or more. This cold low pressure air is supplied to the respirator hose lines. These hose lines may moderate the air temperature somewhat, but the result is that very desirable cold air is available for the worker to breathe. This adiabatic method of cooling is reliable, lightweight, and requires no added heat exchanger or other worker or work area equipment. It does not increase airflow requirements, and adds no cooling air burden to the compressor designer's air supply requirements.

(3) High Pressure Pre-Pumped Tanks

Sufficient breathing air for small jobs may be supplied by using pre-pumped high pressure air. There are two different choices of supply:

- rental cylinders from commercial speciality gas suppliers (This is the same source used to provide the high pressure standby air reserve.)
- the pre-pumped in-line reserve air bank from a high pressure breathing air system.

Either of these air sources can supply a small crew of one to four workers with enough air for one to three days. Operating in this manner, no electrical, gasoline, or diesel power is required at the jobsite. The pre-pumped air has already been processed through a CO monitor; therefore, job-site monitoring is not required. Special designs of larger air storage banks are possible so that this simple method of operation can be extended for larger crews and for longer times. A single high pressure air source located either at a major job site or at home base can function effectively to support one or more additional off-site jobs.

(4) Other

The Non-Lubricated Compressor. There are certain models of industrial-crew sized compressors which use solid state lubrication, rather than liquid lubrication. These machines, if recommended by the manufacturer, can be used to pump air for human consumption. Most of these special machines are more expensive than their oil-lubricated equivalents. They generally have to be rebuilt with less running time than the oil lubricated models.

The majority of breathing air around the world is pumped from oil-lubricated machines, and purified to Grade D air using the adsorber technology described in this report. Whether high or low pressure air, whether commercial divers, sport divers, industrial plant breathing apparatus, fire and rescue crews, all use Grade D air produced from adsorption-based air purifiers.

Unless there is a very special reason, and unless the extra cost can be justified, there is no need to operate the special class of non-lubricated compressor.

The Ambient Air Pump. The ambient air pump is a low power (½ h.p. to 5 h.p.) pump. These pumps take ambient air and supply it to the respirator through the appropriate hose line. They are not intended to improve the quality of the air being pumped.

Ambient air pumps provide an output air pressure in a range from 8 psig to 30 psig. They do not provide sufficient pressure to operate any currently approved NIOSH/MSHA pressure-demand combination SAR/SCBA respirator. Therefore, ambient air pumps cannot be used with the respirator recommended by NIOSH for use in asbestos abatement operations.

(5) Use of Breathing Air Systems in Multi-story Buildings

Large and heavy breathing air system components, including the compressor, the air-purification system, and the reserve air tanks, are best located on ground or basement floor levels. The lightweight components, such as the feed air lines and air distribution manifolds or air panels, are all that is necessary to install at upper floor levels.

The respirator manufacturers' specified pressure for the respirators being used must be maintained at all times at the inlet to the respirator hose. The Occupationsl Safety and Health Administration (OSHA) and NIOSH regulations prohibit the actual hose length to exceed 300 feet in length.

The simplest method to provide the manufacturer-specified pressure on the upper floor level is to provide a ground level compressor with output pressure sufficiently higher than the pressure required by the respirator, and use a control regulator on the respirator manifold. Highest compressor output pressures will achieve satisfactory performance at the highest floor level.

III. CAUTIONS IN THE USE OF BREATHING AIR SYSTEMS

1. Gross contaminations of the inlet air to the air compressor will adversely affect purifier performance. Therefore,

CAUTION: The compressor intake should be properly located to intake ordinary uncontaminated ambient air.

2. Inlet air must not be oxygen deficient. No breathing air system will increase the oxygen content of the intake air being processed. Therefore,

   CAUTION: The compressor intake should be located to ensure that air with normal ambient air oxygen content (19.5% - 23.5%) is always available.

3. The inlet to the compressor should be located away from known or mobile (transient) sources of carbon monoxide. That is, it should be located away from and protected from the engine exhaust of any diesel or gasoline drive compressor, or away from the exhaust from automobiles, trucks, lawnmowers, and other mobile (transient) internal combustion engines. Therefore,

   CAUTION: The compressor intake should be remotely located from the compressor and all possible mobile exhausts to ensure that carbon monoxide (CO) is excluded from the intake. The intake should be remotely plumbed to a safe position at each worksite.

4. The potential for carbon monoxide poisoning through the intake of the compressor of the breathing air system is high enough so that further protection from carbon monoxide is required by OSHA regulation. Such additional CO protection should be part of any breathing air system at any asbestos removal worksite.

   The General Industry OSHA Safety and Health Standards (29 CFR 1910.134), states "If an oil lubricated compressor is used, it shall have a high-temperature or carbon monoxide alarm, or both. If only a high-temperature alarm is used, the air from the compressor shall be frequently tested for carbon monoxide to insure that it meets the specifications."

   Since the asbestos removal workplace is usually a temporary worksite, the expectation is that mobile sources of carbon monoxide may pose more hazard than in a permanent worksite. If carbon monoxide is introduced into the intake it will NOT be detected by a high temperature alarm. Therefore, due to the conditions at the asbestos removal worksite, the recommendation is made that additional protection from carbon monoxide be provided by a continuous carbon monoxide monitor with alarm. This choice of a continuous carbon monoxide monitor and alarm is the preferred choice rather than using a high temperature alarm on the compressor.

   Catalysts that under ideal conditions can cause oxidation of carbon monoxide to the less dangerous carbon dioxide (CO_2) are a feature to help protect against carbon monoxide in breathing air. However, OSHA requires the protection of a monitor and alarm against CO in the breathing air. Therefore,

   CAUTION: A continuous carbon monoxide monitor and alarm should be installed and functioning in the compressor output breathing air stream.

5. When operating a diesel or gasoline driven compressor, addition precautions should be taken to plumb both compressor intake and exhaust away from the compressor and into a safe location. Therefore,

   CAUTION: Any internal combustion engine-driven compressor should also have the exhaust line plumbed to a safe location, as well as having the intake line plumbed to a safe (separate) location.

6. An open-ended or broken pneumatic line or hose may create a hose "whipping" or moving hose hazard. Therefore all pneumatic lines, low or high pressure, should be restrained. Simple and inexpensive restraints such as sandbags are usually sufficient. Therefore,

   CAUTION: Air supply hose or lines should be restrained every 15 feet of their length. (This does not include the length of hose from the distribution manifold to the respirator.)

7. Asbestos removal worksites create the possible hazard of airborne toxic fibers. Therefore standard practices to contain these fibers must be used. The compressor is a concentrator of any airborne contaminants. The compressor intake inlet and the entire length of intake hose should be free of airborne asbestos fiber contamination. Therefore,

CAUTION: The compressor intake point and intake hose should never be operated in air contaminated with asbestos fibers. The compressor and air intake hose should be located in a clean air environment outside the asbestos work zone.

8. Compressor oil suitable for use in breathing air applications should be used. The only proper source for such oil type recommendation is the manufacturer of the breathing air compressor or breathing air system. Therefore,

CAUTION: Use only compressor oil suitable for use in breathing air applications.

and

CAUTION: The recommendation for oil suitable for use in compressors for breathing air applications should only be made by the compressor or breathing air system manufacturer.

9. The user of any breathing air system should recognize the importance of running the system at the correct design conditions. The heat, moisture and oil removal abilities designed within the compressor are important. If the high air temperatures generated by compression are not reduced, the water/oil vapors will not be condensed and therefore may pass through the water traps without being removed. This circumstance may present an overload of water/oil to any breathing air purification assembly that follows the compressor and aftercooler. Such purifier assembly overload will cause the adsorber assemblies within the purifier assembly to be replaced on a more frequent than normal schedule. Unnecessary canister replacement increases the expense of maintaining the breathing air purifier. Therefore,

CAUTION: Compressors equipped with breathing air purifier assemblies should be used. Breathing air purifier assemblies should be used as designed and not overloaded.

10. Pure oxygen gas must not be pumped by or utilized in a breathing air system for use with air supplied respirators. Only air is pumped by these systems. Pure oxygen gas is never to be used in the standby escape time or reserve air system. Only compressed air is used in the standby reserve air system. Pure oxygen is not to be supplied from any source into the respirator systems used in asbestos removal. Therefore,

CAUTION: Never use pure oxygen gas in any part of the gas supply system supplying the air supplied respirators. Respirators are supplied only with Grade D air.

11. High pressure air reserve bottles are, and all compressed air systems have, pressurized vessels. Therefore, an explosive hazard potential exists.

CAUTION: Before starting and operating a compressor and purifier system, inspect all system components for structural damage which could result in an explosion. Inspect safety relief valves carefully, and verify that they are in good working order.

IV. COST ANALYSIS: COMBINATION SUPPLIED AIR VERSUS AIR-PURIFYING RESPIRATOR SYSTEMS

This part of the Appendix presents an analysis of the comparative cost of equipping equal sized crews with combination supplied air respirator/breathing air systems versus air-purifying respirators.

Some important conclusions of this cost comparison, which follows in detail, are:

(1) A breathing air supply system used with pressure-demand, combination supplied air respirators, is considerably lower in cost than an air-purifying respirator system.

(2) The initial cost of outfitting an asbestos removal crew is lower when equipped with air-purifying respirators than the initial cost of obtaining a breathing air system and equipping the same crew with pressure demand combination supplied air respirators.

(3) The yearly cost for the asbestos removal crew equipped with air-purifying respirators is much higher than the same size crew equipped with the breathing air system and combination supplied air respirators. This higher yearly cost is the result of the recurring daily costs of the required replacement filters for the air-purifying respirators.

(4) The higher initial cost of the pressure-demand combination supplied air respirators and breathing air system over the cost of the air-purifying respirators is usually returned to the owner of the breathing air system within only 6 months to one year of operational use.

(5) Following this short time of operational use, the pressure-demand combination supplied air respirators with the breathing systems continue to save the owner the cost of the entire system approximately every 6 months to one year throughout its subsequent operational lifetime.

---

*Based on the average yearly cost of $20,509.00 of the Supplied Air System.

RESULTS COMPARATIVE INITIAL COSTS

Crew Size 15 Workers All Cases

I.	Initial cost full facepiece PAPR-HEPA	8,985.00
II.	Initial cost full facepiece negative pressure	1,425.00
III.	Initial cost breathing air system with pressure demand combination respirators	26,000.00 to 38,000.00

[NOTE: Low pressure rental breathing air compressors have not been calculated; however, they are sometimes locally available. If rental compressors were calculated, it would reduce the initial purchase cost and increase the yearly costs of the low pressure breathing air system in this comparative study. High pressure breathing air compressors are not generally available for rent.]

RESULTS COMPARATIVE YEARLY COSTS

I.	Full facepiece positive pressure air purifying powered air high efficiency particulate filtration respirator (PAPR-HEPA)	$57,030.00 to $110,168.00/yr.
II.	Full facepiece negative pressure air purifying respirator	30,617.00 to 60,617.00/yr.
III.	Breathing air system with full facepiece pressure demand combination respirators	18,709.00 to 22,309.00/yr.

Conclusion:

On a yearly cost basis, breathing air systems cost considerably less than air purifying replaceable filter respirators. The higher yearly costs of the replaceable filter air purifying respirators are due almost entirely to the recurring daily costs of replacement filter canisters.

COSTS OF FULL FACEPIECE POSITIVE PRESSURE DEMAND AIR-PURIFYING HIGH EFFICIENCY PARTICULATE FILTER TYPE RESPIRATORS (PAPR-HEPA)

Initial Purchase:

15 each PAPR-HEPA at $599.00 each	$8,985.00
Yearly cost:	
Amortize in three years	$2,995.00/yr.
Unscheduled maintenance at 10% per year	898.00/yr.
Scheduled maintenance for HEPA cartridge replacement at $14.17/day or $28.35/day based on one shift per day, 5 days per week, for 50 weeks per year or 250 days per year	53,137.00/yr. to 106,275.00/yr.
TOTAL COSTS YEARLY	**$57,030.00 to $110,168.00**

[NOTE: Inclusion of the air purifying respirator types in this comparative cost study should not be inferred as a recommendation for their suitability for use in any given asbestos removal circumstance. Breathing air systems, either low pressure (100 to 200 psi) or high pressure (2000 psi or more), used with pressure-demand full-facepiece respirators, or pressure-demand self-contained breathing apparatus provide higher levels of protection and the high reliability needed for asbestos removal.]

COSTS OF FULL FACEPIECE NEGATIVE PRESSURE AIR-PURIFYING RESPIRATORS

Initial purchase:

15 each negative pressure full facepiece respirators at $95.00	$1,425.00

Yearly cost:

Amortize in three years	$475.00/yr.
Unscheduled maintenance at 10% per year	142.00/yr.
Scheduled maintenance for daily replacement of filter canisters averaging either $8.00 or $16.00 per man per pay day for 250 days	30,000.00/yr. to 60,000.00/yr.
TOTAL COSTS YEARLY	**$30,617.00 to $60,617.00**

[NOTE: Inclusion of the air purifying respirator types in this comparative cost study should not be inferred as a recommendation for their suitability for use in any given asbestos removal circumstance. Breathing air systems, either low pressure (100 to 200 psi) or high pressure (2000 psi or more), used with pressure-demand full-facepiece respirators, or pressure-demand self-contained breathing apparatus provide higher levels of protection and the high reliablility needed for asbestos removal.]

COSTS OF BREATHING AIR SYSTEM WITH FULL FACEPIECE COMBINATION PRESSURE DEMAND RESPIRATORS

Initial purchase:	
Breathing air compressor	$8,000.00 to $12,000.00
Air purifier system	$9,000.00 to $17,000.00
15 each combination respirators complete with fittings and hoses at $600.00 each	9,000.00
Yearly costs:	
Cost of compressor operation at 21¢/1000 SCFM	$6,623.00/yr.*
Purge air costs at 21¢/1000 SCFM	$1,325.00/yr.*
Amortize breathing air system in five years	$3,400.00 to $5,800.00/yr.
Unscheduled maintenance at 10% per year	$2,598.00 to $3,798.00/yr.
Scheduled maintenance for breathing air purifying canister replacement* (see below)	$1,763.00/yr.
Amortize respirators three years	$3,000.00/yr
TOTAL COSTS YEARLY:	**$18,709.00/yr. to $$22,309.00/yr.**
*Scheduled maintenance:	
Oil purifier prefilter 6x per year at $60.00 - 80.00	$480.00/yr.
$A1_2O_3$ dryer towers 1x every 3 years at $100.00	$33.00/yr.
CO catalyst filter 1x per year at $750.00 - $1,800.00	$1,800.00/yr.
Odor removal charcoal filter 2x per year at $90.00 - 120.00	$240.00/yr.
Total scheduled maintenance per year	**$1,763.00/yr.**

*The cost figures given above represent "worst case" estimates because they are based on 24-hour day, 365-day year operations (8760 hours/yr.). Actual costs will be proportionately less depending upon actual use.

V. SUPPLIERS OF BREATHING AIR EQUIPMENT

INCLUDING SUPPLIERS OF

High and Low Pressure Breathing Air Compressors
High and Low Pressure Breathing Air Purifiers
Carbon Monoxide Monitors
Gas Detection Tubes
Heat Exchangers
Particle Filters
Vortex Tubes

American Bristol Industries
1600 West 240th Street
Harbor City, California 90710

Asbestos Control Technology
P.O. Box 183
Maple Shade, New Jersey 08052

Atlas Copco Turbonetics
20 School Road
Voorheesville, New York 12186

Bauer
1328 Azalea Garden Drive
Norfolk, Virginia 23502

E. D. Bullard Co.
2680 Bridgeway
Sausalito, California 94965

Consumer Fuels, Inc.
7250 Governors Drive West
Huntsville, Alambama 35805

Critical Services, Inc.
2828 Broad
Houston, Texas 77087

Control Resource Systems, Inc.
670 Mariner Drive
Michigan City, Indiana 46360

Ingersol Rand
11 Greenway Plaza
Houston, Texas 77046

Joy Manufacturing Company
Montgomery Industrial Park
Montgomeryville, Pennsylvania 18936

3M Company
3M Center Building 230-B
St. Paul, Minnesota 55101

Daboco, Inc.
3319 E. Ten Mile
Warren, Michigan 48091

Davey Compressor Company
11060 Kenwood Road
Cincinnati, Ohio 45242

Deltech Engineering, Inc.
Century Park, P.O. Box 667
New Castle, DE 19720

Dynamation, Inc.
3748 Plaza Drive
Ann Arbor, Michigan 48104

Dynatech Frontier, Inc.
5655 Kircher Blvd. NE
Albuquerque, New Mexico 87109

Enmet Corporation
2307 South Industrial Highway
Ann Arbor, Michigan 48104

Hankison Corporation
1000 Philadelphia Street
Cannonsburg, Pennsylvania 15317

Industrial Pump & Compressor
12014 Chain Lake Road
Snohomish, Washington 98290

Industrial Safety Products
1502 Telegraph Road
Mobile, Alambama 36611

Rix Industries
6460 Hollis Street
Emeryville, California 94608

Sullair Corporation
3700 East Michigan Blvd.
Michigan City, Indiana 46360-9990

Mine Safety Appliances Company
600 Penn Center Blvd.
Pittsburgh, Pennsylavania 15235

National Draeger
101 Technology Drive
Pittsburgh, Pennsylvania 15235

North Safety Equipment
2000 Plainfield Pike
Cranston, Rhode Island 02816

RhineAir, Inc.
8402 Magnolia Avenue
Santee, California 92071

Racal Airstream Inc.
7209A Grove Road
Frederick, Maryland 21701

Vortec Corporation
10125 Carver Road
Cincinnati, Ohio 45242

Willson Safety Products
2nd and Washington Streets
P.O. Box 622
Reading, Pennsylvania 19603

☆ U.S. GOVERNMENT PRINTING OFFICE: 1993—750-160 / 80013